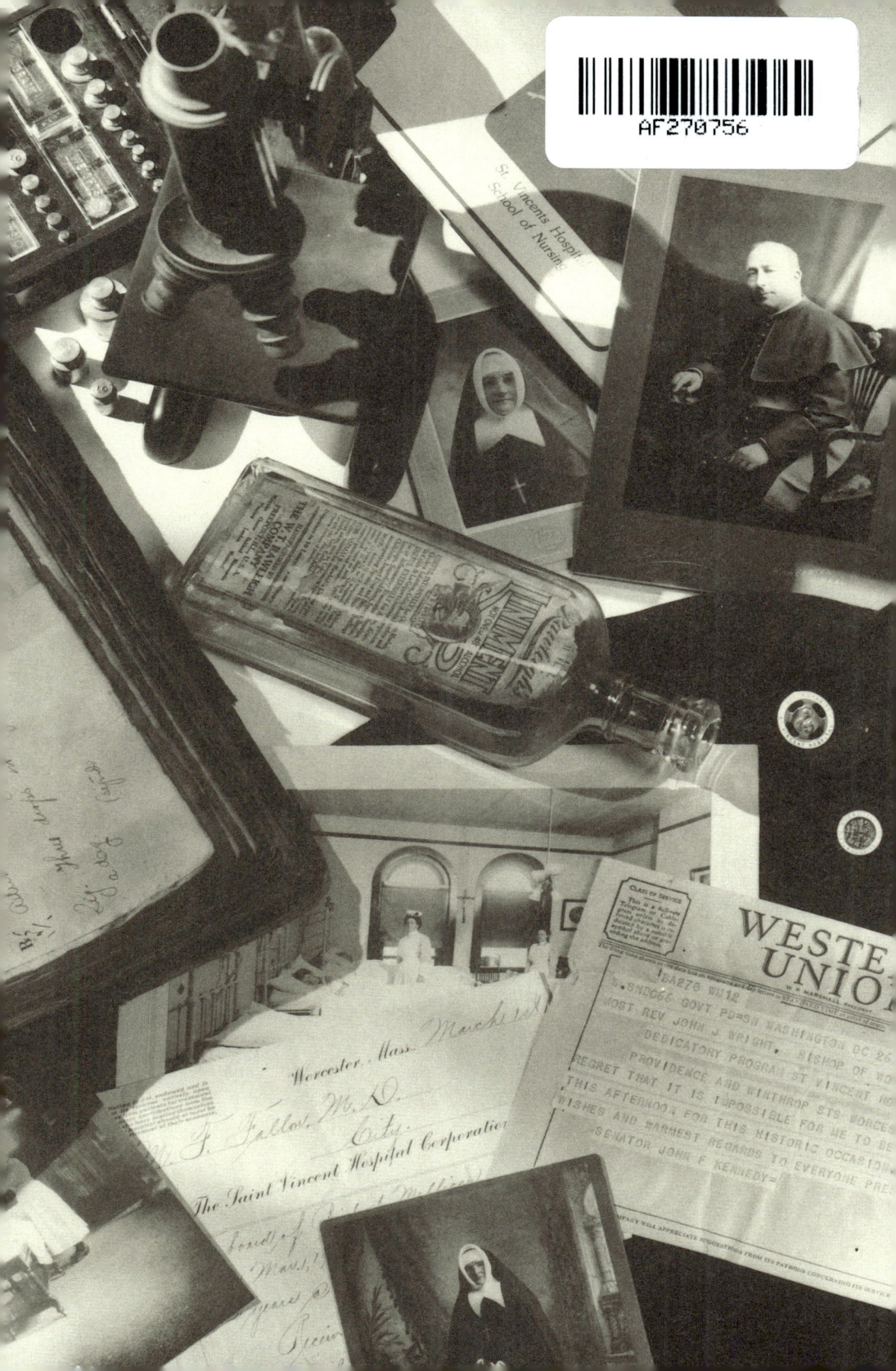

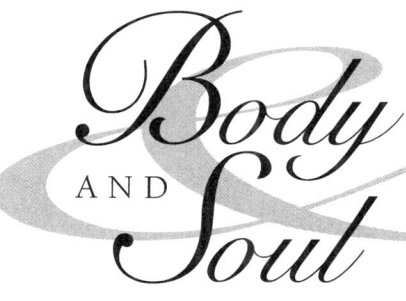

Body AND Soul

100 YEARS AT
SAINT VINCENT
HOSPITAL
1893–1993

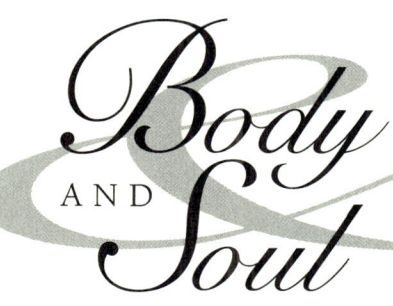

Body
AND Soul

100 YEARS AT
SAINT VINCENT
HOSPITAL
1893–1993

by

DAVID P. KOWAL

International Standard Book Number: ISBN 0-9636277-3-2

Library of Congress Catalog Card Number: 93-086119

First Edition

Published by the

Saint Vincentennial Celebration Committee

Printed in the United States of America

by Lafayette Graphics Inc.

Worcester, Massachusetts 01608   U.S.A.

Dedication

Any book which attempts to chronicle historical events can, at best, reflect only a limited perspective on the many things that happened. Body and Soul is the result of research and the selective memories of only a few of the many individuals who participated in important episodes from our past. We nevertheless hope this compilation of fact and opinion presents a true story of Saint Vincent Hospital.

This book is dedicated to everyone who participated or continues to play a vital role in our unfolding history. We hope it sparks some memories of your own.

THE SAINT VINCENTENNIAL CELEBRATION COMMITTEE

Foreword

Body and Soul commemorates and celebrates the 100th anniversary of the founding of Saint Vincent Hospital. Commissioned by the Saint Vincentennial Celebration Committee, this book offers us the opportunity to reflect upon all that Saint Vincent Hospital has given to us throughout its long history of service to the community. The title *Body and Soul* is a metaphor for the constancy of certain timeless values (SOUL) held by the special people who work within the continually changing walls of brick and mortar (BODY). This book is truly a retrospective that can be read on many levels.

On one level, *Body and Soul* explores the heritage, contributions and legacy of the "hospital on the hill." This work traces the history of Saint Vincent Hospital from its origins as a small, twelve-bed, Catholic hospital managed by the Sisters of Providence, through its long development as a unique health-care facility, and on to its current configuration as the foundation of a comprehensive health-care delivery system. This story focuses on a complex interplay of forces: medical and financial challenges, changing standards of medical practice and the increasing need for expansion and growth. Indeed, this work can be seen as much a chronicle of the evolution of medical care in this century as a chronology of one special institution in the city.

On a more fundamental level, *Body and Soul* is about the people who have played a role in the development of Saint Vincent Hospital. It's about doctors, nurses, religious and volunteers. It's about their dreams, their work, their sacrifices and their contributions to medicine. Most especially, however, it is about their care of patients. From the founding days of Saint Vincent Hospital, the Sisters of Providence provided a model of compassion, selflessness and dedication that still echoes in the corridors of the hospital today. Indeed, one of the enduring strengths of Saint Vincent Hospital has always been its patient-centered approach, the inviolability of the relationship between the patient and the health-care team. At its core, Saint Vincent Hospital has always been about people caring for people.

On a deeper level still, this book hopefully reflects the virtues and values of the people of Saint Vincent Hospital, highlighted in the Vincentennial motto "Making life better is our life's work." It's about a tangible moral code rooted in the basics: respect, accountability, participation and integrity. In this respect, the history contained in this book is valuable not only as a record so that we may learn from our collective successes and failures, but also as a mirror so that we might better understand who we are. Only then can we reflect upon the special responsibility of Saint Vincent Hospital in its unique role as a Catholic hospital, a teaching hospital and a community hospital. And only then can we really understand the mission of Saint Vincent Hospital to deliver compassionate, quality medical care to each and every patient we serve.

It is my hope that each of us can read this work with an eye toward appreciating the role that all these levels play in the rich tradition of Saint Vincent Hospital. In a time of uncertainty concerning the future directions of medical care, we have many challenges yet to be faced as a hospital community. I believe that in such times all of us may draw strength and pride from the legacy, sacrifices and vision of Saint Vincent Hospital captured in *Body and Soul*.

Denis J. FitzGerald, M.D., M.H.A.
President and Chief Executive Officer
Saint Vincent Hospital

Acknowledgements

Dr. Michael F. Fallon, the first chief of surgery at St. Vincent Hospital, observes in the hospital's 1911 annual report that "the success of the hospital depends upon brains, not upon bricks."

Indeed, while bricks mark the milestones in the progress of the hospital, it is the people themselves — the "brains" — who have been responsible for its success during its first 100 years. While this history makes note of the "bricks," it is really about the people who have dedicated themselves to St. Vincent Hospital.

Many of the people who were, or continue to be, part of St. Vincent Hospital's history contributed to Body and Soul. Many contributed their time for interviews, others contributed historical materials or helped in some other way. I wish to acknowledge Dr. Denis J. FitzGerald, Kenneth P. Heekin and Michael S. Wronski not only for editing this book, but also for their guidance, insight and understanding. Others I would like to acknowledge include the following:

Dr. Robert A. Abodeely, Dr. Lambi N. Adams, Sister Mary Adrianella, Lorraine Bachand, James Baker, Dr. Olier L. Baril, Charlene Baron, Christy W. Bell, Dr. Robert D. Blute, Sr., Sister Mary John Bosco, Dr. William A. Carey, Dr. Gerald J. Carroll, Sister Mary Clare, Mildred Collins, Jeanette Couillard, Thomas J. Cullinane, Mary Darcy, Dr. George E. Deering, Sister Mary Denise, Sister Mary Devota, Filomena DiTomaso, Sister Mary Dolorum, Frances G. Donahue, Dr. John H. Donovan Jr., Dr. John A. Duggan, Deborah Fahey, John Fallon Jr., Bishop Bernard J. Flanagan, Shirley Fornier, Sister Mary Francis, Dr. Raymond W. Gadbois, William W. George, Gerald Goggins, Paula Green, S. Jane Griesbach, Mary Hanrahan, Bishop Timothy J. Harrington, Margaret Haverty, Jane Healey, Amy V. Heath, Dr. John T. Howard, Dr. Stuart R. Jaffee, Dr. Murray L. Janower, Dr. Daniel Kaplan, Dr. Stanley L. Kocot, Mary B. Lee, Dr. Gilbert E. Levinson, Arlene Lian, Robert C. Maher, Valerie T. Mancini, Dr. John J. Massarelli, Vera Massarelli, Rev. Francis D. McGrail, Margaret L. McKenna, Timothy J. Meagher, Viola Mish, Joseph Monroe, Dr. Mario F. Moretti, Dr. James M. Morrison, Dr. Leonard J. Morse, Jean McLaughlin, Owen Murphy,

Rev. John T. Murray, John L. Nespoli, Sister Mary O'Leary, Dr. Robert J. Phaneuf, Dr. Joseph A. Podbielski, Sister Kathleen Popko, Sister Mary Robert, Leslie Rutan, Tom Reid, Robert C. Reidy, Patrick J. Roche, Mabel A. Ryan, Rita Scanlon, Saul Seder, Dr. John F. Stapleton, Alan M. Stoll, Margaret Sullivan, Mary Swift, Monsignor Edmond T. Tinsley, Dr. Rudolf J. Utzschneider, Louise Ware, Clare Weeks and Elizabeth M. White.

Thousands of people contributed to the success of St. Vincent Hospital. Many of them are not mentioned by name in this volume, but their contribution is still recognized.

Contents

100 Years Ago

"Those attributes of man that seek to find expression in the Christian religion have provided the most powerful single stimulus to the development of the hospital. The character of the hospital today cannot be comprehended without an understanding of its Christian baptism and upbringing."
Dr. Edward D. Churchill, Harvard Medical School

*I*n an age of lasers and genetically engineered drugs, the bonds between health care and religion are less obvious than they were 100 years ago. A century ago, many people still believed that illness was a punishment for sin, and that spiritual care was more important to recovery than medical care.

Even today, the physician and the priest fight a common battle — the battle for life. As both a religious and medical institution, the Catholic hospital provides a fertile battlefield. With the physical and spiritual life of the individual at stake, the physician and the priest, as well as the nurse and the nun, struggle on a daily basis for the salvation of the patient's body and soul.

Given this natural link between spiritual and medical healing, it is no wonder that the link between health care and the Catholic Church is practically as old as Catholicism itself. In the spirit of Christianity, the Church resolved at the Council of Nicea in 325 A.D. to establish a hospital in every Cathedral city. Following through on this far-reaching goal, church-sponsored hospitals have since been established throughout the world to provide comfort, and medical and spiritual care for the sick and the poor.

Early Catholic hospitals may have provided healing for the soul, but they did little for the ills of the body. Through most of the nineteenth century, hospitals were little more than places where the poor went to die. Hospitals were, in fact, probably the most unhealthy place to be. The sick were cared for by other patients, so disease spread quickly. Few medications existed and physicians commonly used leeches to draw out what they believed to be contaminated blood. Conditions were so unsanitary that a physician often wore the same smock in an operating room for an entire year. And it was not unusual for a physician to examine a corpse and a living patient on the same table on the same day.

It is easy to see why hospitals terrified most people. Those who could afford medical care received it at home. Even surgery on the kitchen table was preferable to surgery in the hospital. For those unfortunate enough to be hospitalized, the priest, not the doctor, often offered the best hope for salvation.

St. Vincent Hospital is a few blocks up the street from what was once Dale Hospital, one of Worcester's earliest hospitals. Fourteen one-story wooden wards were erected at the site in 1864 to provide care for up to 1,000 Union soldiers at a time. But two months after the Providence Street hospital was dedicated, the Civil War ended. The hospital was dismantled a short time afterward.

Worcester's first medical school also was built on the site. Worcester Medical Institution didn't last long. In 1851, the same year that Dr. Calvin Newton moved his school to the site, he was expelled from the Massachusetts Medical Society for advertising the sale of an elixir. In an age when the medical profession offered little help to the patient, many chose to believe in the cure-all potions that were being peddled by unscrupulous practitioners. Dr. Newton died in 1853 and the school was closed. After the Civil War, Worcester Academy opened on the site and the building that housed the Worcester Medical Institution became Davis Hall.

Worcester's first Catholic hospital, and the city's first public hospital, also opened in 1864. The building of St. Elizabeth's Hospital on what is now Shrewsbury Street was spearheaded by the Very Reverend John J. Power, the pastor of St. Anne's Church and vicar general of the Springfield Diocese. The vicar general was second in command in the diocese and was always stationed in Worcester, the largest city in the diocese. Father Power, a Massachusetts native of Irish heritage, established St. Elizabeth's as a hospital for poor women.

Staffed by three nuns recruited by Father Power from the Sisters of Mercy in New York City, the hospital may have served as an early model for St. Vincent Hospital. Like St. Vincent, St. Elizabeth's did not discriminate in its admission policy. Its doors were open to people of all denominations and ethnic origins. St. Elizabeth's also adopted an early form of health insurance. By paying annual dues of $3 a year, a woman could avail herself of "all the privileges of the hospital board, nursing, doctor's attendance and medicine," according to Dr. Michael F. Fallon, the first chief of surgery at St. Vincent Hospital, who praised the "subscription" system in a 1923 address to the American College of Surgeons. Under the operation of the Sisters of Mercy, and with support from the community, St. Elizabeth's grew.

Two other hospitals soon opened to serve the growing city. Worcester City Hospital was created by an act of the state legislature and opened on Front Street in 1871. The Memorial Hospital, located on the former Samuel Davis estate on Belmont Street, was established the same year with a bequest from Ichabod Washburn, founder of the Washburn & Moen Manufacturing Company, though it did not begin operating until 1888. With the establishment of the two new hospitals, the Sisters of Mercy saw no further need for St. Elizabeth's and closed the hospital in 1872.

Had they waited a few years, the need would have been apparent. During the last half of the nineteenth century, Worcester's population grew rapidly, with most of the growth coming from Catholic immigrants. Worcester had only 2,000 residents in 1800, but by 1893, the year St. Vincent Hospital opened, the city had nearly 85,000 residents and was the thirty-second largest city in the country.

Not only was the Catholic population growing, but industrial development and technological change were transforming the city. Streets were lighted by electric lamps and telephones were being installed in private homes. Trolley cars, soon to be joined by automobiles, were making the horse and buggy obsolete. Some of Worcester's most successful companies today, such as Norton Company, the Paul Revere Insurance Group and Morgan Construction Company, were just getting started, but growing rapidly. Between 1886 and 1917, Norton Company expanded its manufacturing space from 17,000 square feet to a million square feet. Other companies, such as Washburn & Moen, Crompton Loom Works, and factories that manufactured machinery and wire, were already well established, but grew quickly and turned Worcester into a major industrial center. Responding to opportunities for employment, Irish, French Canadians, Swedes, Germans and other immigrants moved into the city in search of a better life.

With the growth in population came an increase in disease and a rising mortality rate. The city's Board of Health reported in 1892 that 200 city children died of cholera, and 190 city residents died of tuberculosis, 70 of diphtheria, 150 of pneumonia, 30 of scarlet fever and 30 of typhoid fever. As the demand for hospital services grew, the capacity of Worcester's existing hospitals was strained.

By the 1890s, there was a need for a new hospital, and it seemed particularly important to have a hospital specially suited to serve the needs of the city's growing Catholic population. Religion played an important role in the lives of most immigrants, especially the Irish. The Catholic Church, even more than their native country, provided their cultural and social identity. Bishop Thomas D. Beaven, an important figure in the founding of St. Vincent Hospital, recalled in 1907 that the people in his diocese had been treated with "chilling sufferance" by the non-Catholic hospitals in his diocese. With the mortality rate still very high in hospitals, Catholics wanted the ability to receive their last rites in their hospital beds. Protestant institutions like The Memorial Hospital or City Hospital were not receptive to priests.

Writing about discrimination in hospitals late in the nineteenth century, Paul S. Starr notes in *The Social Transformation of American Medicine* that "discrimination was a principal reason for the formation of separate religious and ethnic hospitals. Except against blacks, outright prejudice was rare, though the Massachusetts General Hospital initially refused to admit Irish patients on the grounds that their presence would deter other people from entering the hospital. The early moralistic aims of hospitals gave religious minorities reasons for anxiety. Catholics were afraid they might not be given last rites, and Jews feared they would have to eat non-kosher food and face ridicule for their appearance and rituals. Both religious communities worried that efforts might be made to convert some of their members in moments of personal crisis." Fear of being proselytized was nearly as strong as the fear of catching a dreaded disease. One of the greatest sins a Catholic could commit in those days was *Participatio in Divinis,* participation in divine worship with non-Catholics.

As insidious as hospitals seemed to the ethnic populations at the time, they would at least seem more welcoming if the hospitals were operated by people who shared their beliefs and heritage. That is why the wave of European immigration that took place in the eighteenth century was followed by tremendous growth in the founding of Catholic hospitals. By 1904, 442 ecclesiastical hospitals were operating in the United States, accounting for nearly a third of the country's hospitals. Approximately 80 percent of the Catholic hospitals operating in 1910 were established after 1880.

By the 1890s, hospitals had assimilated the advances in medical care that began during the Civil War. Largely because of the wartime efforts of Florence Nightingale, hospitals began to pay attention to cleanliness and order. Later in the century, Joseph Lister's work led to the understanding of asepsis, and surgeons were learning to make operating rooms sterile and germ-free. Anesthesia was widely used, and the autoclave, sterilized dressings and rubber gloves had been introduced.

Medical care had reached a point where it saved lives. Catholic hospitals were developing the ability to heal not just the soul, but the body. It was the ideal time for the opening of a new hospital.

CHAPTER ONE

Shaping the Work

"God is Charity."
St. Vincent de Paul

*T*he Right Reverend Monsignor Thomas A. Griffin is best remembered for something he never intended to do. His actions led to the founding of St. Vincent Hospital. But his role was accidental.

A century ago, Msgr. Griffin was the person Worcester's Irish Catholics went to when they wanted to get things done. By then, he already had accomplished much for the city's Irish Catholics. During the first three years of his 43-year service at St. John's Church on Temple Street, he oversaw the building of mission churches in Holden and Auburn, and began raising funds for a chapel in Shrewsbury. When St. John's pastor, the Reverend Patrick T. O'Reilly, was named the first bishop of the Springfield Diocese in 1870, Msgr. Griffin was left to run St. John's on his own. With more than 9,000 members at the time, St. John's was perhaps the largest Catholic parish between Boston and Albany. Just 34, Msgr. Griffin was considered too young and inexperienced to be a pastor, so he assumed the title of church administrator, even though he carried out the duties of a pastor. He also kept close ties with Bishop O'Reilly, serving as his chancellor and assisting him in overseeing a diocese that included all of western and central Massachusetts.

That Msgr. Griffin worked closely with the bishop is not surprising. In addition to working together at St. John's, both men were born in Ireland and trained at St. Charles College in Catonsville, Maryland, and St. Mary's Seminary in Baltimore.

They were also nearly the same age — Bishop O'Reilly, at 37, was just three years older than Msgr. Griffin and was the youngest bishop in the country when he was appointed. Throughout his life, Bishop O'Reilly remained Msgr. Griffin's "closest friend on earth," according to a history of the Diocese of Springfield written by the Reverend John J. McCoy, diocesan historian.

In his dual role as chancellor and priest, Msgr. Griffin achieved a great deal of success, judging by the brick and mortar he left behind. He founded two Catholic schools, Ascension for girls in 1872 and St. John's High School for boys in 1881. He also was responsible for starting three new parishes — the Immaculate Conception parish in 1873, Sacred Heart parish in 1880 and St. Stephen's parish in 1887. He served on the Worcester School Committee and was a library trustee. He raised funds for Ireland when the crops failed in the 1870s, and oversaw several renovation projects at St. John's. Given the buildings that were constructed during his tenure, he might have achieved a great deal of success in the private sector as a real estate developer. Indeed, he was lauded as a "Captain of Industry" by the *Boston Herald,* which hyperbolized more than a little in comparing him with John D. Rockefeller, Andrew Carnegie and J. P. Morgan. Still, Father McCoy's history may have been accurate in calling him the "hardest worker in the diocese."

Given his accomplishments and stature, he was the logical person to seek out when the people of his parish wanted to establish a home for the aged — specifically, according to one account, a home for aged women. The need for a home for the aged must have been apparent, as Worcester's Irish population was growing old. The first wave of Irish-Catholic immigrants came to Worcester in 1826, recruited by Irishman Tobias Boland to build the Blackstone Canal. The canal made Worcester a regional commercial center, because it allowed goods to be moved by water, which was a fraction of the cost and much quicker than moving them by land. The Irish stayed, despite local hostility toward immigrants. Soon after, they helped build the railroad through the Worcester area, again under the employment of Boland. Their ranks grew considerably in the 1840s, when the Great Famine hit Ireland, and continued to grow until the 1880s. Between 1880 and 1890, the city's population of Irish immigrants over age 65 nearly doubled, and many of the elderly Irish were forced to spend their waning years in the harsh surroundings of the community almshouse.

It was not unusual for ethnic groups to establish their own institutions. Worcester's Irish already had established their own churches, cemeteries and schools, including the College of the Holy Cross. Being from another country, with different customs, different values and a different religion, it was natural for them to prefer their own establishments to the existing Protestant institutions. Religion played a central role in the lives of the Roman Catholics immigrating to the Worcester area, and they feared that there would be attempts at proselytization if they went to Protestant institutions. Given that a home for the aged was a place where residents stayed until they died, it was critical to the Catholic immigrants that priests be available to administer their last rites.

When the idea of a home for the aged first arose is uncertain, but St. John's parish already had purchased the eight-acre Bartlett farmhouse at Vernon and Winthrop streets in December 1886 under the name of St. John's School, and presumably intended to use the site for the school. Msgr. Griffin had the home for the aged in mind when he instead built St. John's on church land on Temple Street in 1891. The old farmhouse was used for a short time to house the Christian Brothers, a religious order Msgr. Griffin recruited from Ireland to teach at St. John's School. The brothers, who had taught Msgr. Griffin in his native Ireland before he emigrated from Cork at age 16, left after a short time, perhaps because of a disagreement about how the school was being run, or possibly because of the dilapidated condition of their quarters.

Msgr. Griffin's first attempt to establish what was tentatively to be called St. Elizabeth's Home came in 1890. It failed, because he was "a bit too shrewd," according to *To Preserve the Flame,* a history of St. John's parish. He had the Ladies Charitable Society of his parish propose the idea and recruit a lay planning committee from all of the city's parishes. Presumably, all of the parishes were to contribute, even though the home was to be located to serve St. John's parish best.

His plans were rebuffed with opposition from the Reverend Richard S. J. Burke, pastor of St. Stephen's, who held a grudge against Msgr. Griffin for saddling his new congregation with a sizable debt and providing St. Stephen's with only a drafty school attic as its place of worship. Father Burke criticized the project in a series of sermons that were reported in the press. He argued that sons and daughters had a moral responsibility to care for their aging parents, and that the creation of a home for the aged would allow them to abdicate their responsibility. He also argued that the city's Irish Catholics, who already had invested much of their meager earnings into parish projects, could ill afford further debt.

After his local fund-raising effort failed, Msgr. Griffin approached the Sisters of Charity in Emmitsburgh, Maryland, for assistance in 1892. They rejected his request.

It may have been at the suggestion of Bishop O'Reilly that Msgr. Griffin approached a mission of nuns based in Holyoke, Massachusetts, in the Diocese of Springfield that also was operating under the name Sisters of Charity. Like the Sisters of Charity in Emmitsburgh, the sisters in Holyoke followed the teachings of St. Vincent de Paul. Historical accounts are unclear, but it appears that Msgr. Griffin made an initial request of support from the Holyoke mission and that his request was rejected. The Holyoke mission took its orders from a mother house based in Kingston, Ontario, and the Kingston mother house rejected Msgr. Griffin's request. Both the Kingston order and the Holyoke mission were operating under a "status quo" edict at the time, which would have prevented their involvement with a mission in Worcester.

However, circumstances soon changed. On his dying day in 1892, Bishop O'Reilly succeeded in obtaining a papal order that established the sisters in Holyoke as an independent diocesan community and allowed them to break away from their mother house in Kingston. The new congregation was later incorporated as the Sisters of Providence. Once the independent congregation was approved, Msgr. Griffin filed an early application with Mother Mary of Providence, the order's founder and Major Superior, and she tentatively gave her approval to make Worcester the new order's first mission. Final approval by Bishop O'Reilly's successor, Bishop Thomas D. Beaven, made the new Worcester mission official.

The Sisters of Providence gave Msgr. Griffin much more than he asked for. During a meeting in St. John's rectory with Msgr. Griffin, Bishop Beaven, a group of local doctors and the Sisters of Providence, a consensus was reached that Bartlett farm be used not only as a home for the aged, but as a hospital. They proposed that plans begin immediately for construction of a new hospital on the site, and that after construction of the new hospital, the existing farmhouse be used as an old-age home. They even looked ahead to the new building's conversion into a home for the aged, the razing of the farmhouse, and construction of a newer and larger hospital.

Although it is not well documented, the doctors probably played a critical role. In a history of Worcester's hospitals, Dr. Paul F. Bergin credits Dr. Thomas A. O'Callaghan, who first headed St. Vincent's medical staff, for working with Msgr. Griffin to establish the hospital. Most of St. Vincent's doctors were of Irish heritage and did not fit in at the existing Memorial or City hospitals — Yankee institutions where prominence eluded Irish doctors. The Irish doctors among the original staff of St. Vincent included Dr. Michael Fallon, who later played a key role in the hospital; Dr. John T. Duggan, who chaired the Worcester School Committee and later became mayor; Dr. Michael J. O'Meara; Dr. John J. Brennan; Dr. William J. Delahanty; Dr. P. H. Keefe; Dr. O'Callaghan and his sister, Dr. Mary V. O'Callaghan; Dr. John A. Carroll; and Dr. John Kelley.

In addition, there was a great need for a new hospital in the growing city. With a population of nearly 85,000, Worcester was an important industrial center. As the superintendent of City

Hospital noted in 1894: "Of all the cities and large towns in New England where hospitals are maintained, Worcester probably has the most meager and inadequate provision for the ordinary demands of the community, and is the least prepared to meet any emergency that may be thrust upon its hospitals by accident or public calamity.

"The seven largest cities in the country average one bed to every 300 of the population. Boston has one for every 244, and cities suburban to Boston provide one bed to every 600 inhabitants. Worcester, at a distance from any other hospital facilities, furnishes only one bed to 700 people, and, taking into account the 40,000 people in the immediate vicinity of the city, it provides only one bed to 900 inhabitants."

Given that hospitals were still largely feared and regarded as houses of death by many, Msgr. Griffin's proposal to build a home for the aged rather than a hospital was not necessarily the result of a lack of vision. But having failed at two attempts to establish the home for the aged, he would have been short-sighted indeed to turn down the offer from the Sisters of Providence to establish both a home for the aged and a hospital. The idea gained Msgr. Griffin's support. The first annual report of the House of Providence Hospital, as it was then called, shows Msgr. Griffin as the hospital's top contributor, having pledged $1,000 for the new endeavor — an amount equaled only by contributions from Stephen Salisbury III, the philanthropist who created the Worcester Art Museum and Institute Park, and Richard Healy, a successful retailer of furs and quality clothing, and founder of Bay State Savings Bank. Both Salisbury and Healy were members of the first Board of Trustees and its Executive Committee.

Granted that the Sisters of Providence paid St. John's $23,000 for the land, Msgr. Griffin's financial contribution showed that the Sisters of Providence had won his support for their hospital. Msgr. Griffin also said Mass at the opening of the hospital and served on its Board of Trustees. When he died in 1910, Msgr. Griffin's support for the hospital was noted in the annual report. In a eulogy, Local Superior Sister Mary

Isidore wrote: "We may even say that his zeal and charity were rewarded beyond his expectation, for while the original project of Msgr. Griffin, in bringing the Sisters of Providence to Worcester, was to establish a Home for Aged People, still, when opinion favored the foundation of a hospital, though on a very humble and modest scale, he made no demur, but allowed an overruling Providence to shape the work."

"Shape the work" they did. Arriving at the old Bartlett farmhouse with a dozen blankets, the desire to do God's work and little else, the Sisters of Providence encountered their first obstacle in the presence of "Mr. and Mrs. Butler," as they are identified in the writings of Mother Mary of Providence, the first major superior of the Sisters of Providence. Mr. and Mrs. Butler, tenants in the farmhouse who taught in Worcester's public schools, were allowed by St. John's parish to live in the farmhouse to keep it from falling into further disrepair. But when the sisters arrived, the Butlers were reluctant to leave and used one excuse after another to stay, keeping the sisters from giving full attention to their work.

The Butlers at first claimed that their new apartment was not yet ready for occupancy. When it was ready, Mother Mary wrote, the couple "would not move on Friday, because that was unlucky, nor Saturday, because 'flitting on that day meant a short sitting.' And, though the situation was vexing, there was nothing to do but await their good pleasure."

The Butlers soon ran out of excuses and left after 10 days, giving the sisters an opportunity to get to work. The Sisters of Providence not only ran the House of Providence Hospital, but kept the farm operating to provide meat, milk and vegetables. They raised funds to support the hospital by collecting door-to-door, occasionally working as private nurses, and even selling their sewing and paintings. They also renovated the farmhouse so that it accommodated not just 12 patients, but 20 patients.

Through hard work and resourcefulness, the sisters brought in $11,785.67 their first year, which, minus $5,685.43 for expenses, left $6,100.24 in a fund to build a new hospital. This fiscal achievement was reached even though only 30 of the hospital's 104 first-year patients paid the full price of treatment, and 43 received free care.

The medical staff also reported a successful year. Only three of the 104 patients treated died that year, and the hospital's first annual report notes that "one, a case of pneumonia, was in a morbid condition when brought to the hospital." The mortality rate was especially low, considering the meager supplies the staff had available. Supplies were so short that patients were moved to and from the operating room on an ironing board. And Dr. Thomas O'Callaghan notes in the first annual report, "In every surgical case, we have felt the need of a better surgery and a full line of instruments. The first need will soon be remedied — and it is hoped we will see our way towards securing a good supply of instruments — for it adds greatly to the labor of the surgeon to be obliged to bring his own instruments to every operation." The following year, the new hospital paid $1,000 for its first surgical instruments, "being of the latest pattern and purchased especially for the house by Dr. David Lovell on his recent trip to Europe," where the best medical schools, and the best medical supplies, were available at the time.

From the beginning, the Sisters of Providence complemented their willingness to work hard and long with considerable business acumen. Combined with the support of a growing community, the Sisters of Providence had the right formula for advancing St. Vincent's early success — a success so sweeping that two new hospitals were built in St. Vincent's first six years.

Who were these sisters who dedicated themselves so completely to a community that was foreign to them? What drove them to give of themselves so selflessly? And what brought an order of nuns from Canada to Worcester?

The Sisters of Providence is an offshoot of an order of nuns that was itself an offshoot of the Sisters of Charity of Providence. The Sisters of Charity of Providence was founded by Bishop Ignatius Bourget in Montreal in 1843. The first superior of the Sisters of Charity of Providence was Madame Emilie Eugenie Gamelin, a 43-year-old widow who dedicated herself to acts of charity after losing her husband and three sons all within a period of four years. The fortune left to her by the death of her husband was used to establish the order, and to provide care for the sick and the poor. Reflecting the loss of her family, Mother Gamelin dedicated much of her life to establishing refuge for the ill away from their homes, so, as the order developed, many of the sisters became trained in nursing.

After her appointment, Bishop Bourget sent her to the Sisters of Charity in Philadelphia and New York to learn the teachings of St. Vincent de Paul. St. Vincent de Paul, who lived from 1576 to 1660, is the patron saint of charitable works. A man of action, he worked for the poor and taught the meaning of charity to the rich. In an age when nuns were cloistered, the Daughters of St. Vincent de Paul walked among the sick and poor. As St. Vincent wrote, "the sick room is their convent cell, the parish church their chapel, the streets and lanes of the city their cloisters, and modesty their veil." St. Vincent was responsible for establishing seminaries, reforming preaching, rooting out scandals in the church and otherwise leaving his mark on Christianity. His motto, "God is Charity," was adopted not just by the Sisters of Charity of Providence, but by the Sisters of Providence and by the hospital that still carries the name of its patron saint — St. Vincent Hospital.

At the request of the Reverend Edward J. Horan, Bishop of Kingston, the Sisters of Charity of Providence sent four nuns to Kingston on December 12, 1861 to establish a separate English-speaking community.

In 1873, Sisters Mary Elizabeth and Mary de Chantel, representing the Kingston community, were visiting communities in New England and soliciting donations for their new mission. It was not unusual at the time for nuns to travel far away from home to solicit funds. In fact, after the Sisters of Providence became established in Holyoke, two of the sisters traveled throughout the country's mining district and into Texas and New Mexico, raising $2,000 for an addition to the sisters' new orphanage.

When they arrived in a new community, it was common practice for the nuns to approach the church pastors and seek permission to solicit funds from their parishioners. So when they arrived in Holyoke, the sisters approached the Reverend Patrick J. Harkins, who was then pastor of St. Jerome's Church, the only Catholic Church in the city. Father Harkins told the Sisters he would allow them to solicit his parishioners for contributions — but only if they considered making Holyoke their first mission.

The squalid conditions in Holyoke provided a convincing argument for the need to establish a mission. The population at the time included many immigrant mill workers living in over-crowded, unsanitary conditions. Typhoid fever and other dis-eases raged out of control. Holyoke had no hospitals or alms-houses, no homes for the aged or infirm, and no orphanages. Father Harkins convinced the sisters that there was a great need for a mission from their order. The sisters returned to Kingston with $1,500 and Father Harkins' message. Their message was compelling enough to initiate a visit to Holyoke from the Reverend Mother Mary John, head of the Kingston Community, and Mother Mary Edward, her first assistant.

Father Harkins and Dr. James J. O'Connor, a leading physi-cian in Holyoke who later became mayor of the city, followed the sisters' visits to Holyoke with a visit to Kingston on September 4, 1873, bringing with them a petition to establish the Holyoke mission. To the consternation of the still new and strug-gling Kingston order, which already had a shortage of nuns, Bishop Horan accepted it.

Two months after Father Harkins' visit to Kingston, four of the 25 sisters in the Kingston Community arrived in Holyoke and founded the House of Providence: Sister Mary Edward McKinley, Mary Mt. Carmel Byrne, Mary of the Cross Keating and Mary Patrick McKinley. When they saw the large Catholic population in Holyoke, they realized it was the ideal city for a mission, because it would give them an opportunity to attract new vocations.

Immediately, the sisters set about caring for the poor, sick and orphaned, many of whom were referred to them by the city almoner. The house provided to the sisters for performing their work filled quickly. The sisters also went into the homes of the sick and poor, nursing the sick, spending nights with the dying and preparing the dead for burial, a role they played for several years until an undertaker was available to serve Holyoke's Catholics. To support themselves, the Sisters of Providence sold altar breads and other goods they baked, and the church linens, vestments and burial robes they sewed. By 1873, they had established the first Catholic hospital in western Massachusetts, which later became Providence Hospital.

In 1875, Father Harkins again petitioned the Kingston Community, this time for teachers for his school for boys. The Sisters of Notre Dame de Namur already taught the girls in his parish, but were prohibited by their order from teaching boys. He employed lay teachers at the school, including his sister, but as Mother Mary of Providence wrote in a history of the order, "discipline had been neglected . . . truancy tolerated . . . and the general standard of the school was low." Teaching was not intended to be among the functions of the Kingston order, and the order still did not have a large enough base of nuns to support the project, so at first the sisters resisted his petition. But Father Harkins was insistent and eventually his petition was answered favorably. On August 12, 1875, Sister Mary of Providence, the former Catherine Horan, arrived in Holyoke with five others to take teaching assignments at St. Jerome's School for Boys. A year later, Sister Mary of Providence was appointed principal of St. Jerome's school.

One reason for the increasing support from Kingston was the appointment on April 18, 1875 of Bishop John O'Brien to replace the deceased Bishop Horan. Bishop O'Brien, who had been Father Harkins' professor at Regiopolis College in Kingston, pledged to "support and encourage" the Holyoke mission.

In 1878, the Holyoke mission purchased "the Parson property" from St. Jerome's and used a building on the property for Providence Hospital. Soon after, they built an orphanage in the Ingleside section of Holyoke on land that initially was purchased by the sisters with the assistance of Dr. O'Connor. According to legend, the orphanage was built from plans sketched in pencil by Sister Mary of Providence and Sister Mary John, the Mother General of the order.

The sisters found the Catholic community in Holyoke to be supportive of its work. The city was developing rapidly, and workers were beginning to earn good wages, Mother Mary of Providence wrote, "but spending freely and living chiefly in tenement houses, not having yet turned their attention to becoming owners of their own houses, consequently not hoarding their savings."

As the work of the sisters became known throughout the diocese, Bishop O'Reilly became interested in establishing the Sisters of Providence as an independent diocesan order, rather than a mission of Kingston. According to the history of the Springfield diocese, "He felt that the round-about way of reaching the headquarters in Canada was unbusiness-like, and not at all suitable to the direct American method." Perhaps Bishop O'Reilly believed that if the sisters did not have to report to Kingston, they could perform their works of charity more efficiently, but it also was natural for him to want control of an order of sisters that was growing steadily within his diocese. More specifically, if the Sisters of Providence were going to raise funds to support their efforts in his diocese, he wanted those funds to be under his direction. He did not want to see funds raised in the Springfield diocese diverted for the benefit of a Kingston order.

In addition, as *Can Spring Be Far Behind?* recounts, "Most Bishops preferred their own diocesan congregations, and just as every pastor wanted to build a church . . . so every Bishop wanted to be the founder of a congregation of religious . . . And every Bishop thought he knew more about structuring the private lives of women religious than St. Vincent de Paul did. God bless him. Bishop O'Reilly was probably no exception."

Bishop O'Reilly had the Reverend Thomas D. Beaven of the new Holy Rosary Church in Holyoke apply to Rome on his behalf for permission to grant the Sisters of Providence independence from Kingston. Most of the nuns in Holyoke favored the split from Kingston, but many in Canada opposed it, including Mother Mary Edward, who had devoted many years to developing the Holyoke mission. Initially, Rome rejected the request, but Father Beaven appealed on behalf of Bishop O'Reilly, declaring that he would take the cause to "the Holy Father himself, if need be." Bishop O'Reilly and Father Beaven pushed for the split for two years and finally, on Bishop O'Reilly's dying day in 1892, the separation was granted. Bishop O'Reilly was unconscious when the papers granting the separation arrived and was, therefore, unable to sign them. As his successor, Father Beaven had, of course, already worked on the issue from the beginning and was ready to sign the papers on the day he officially became bishop.

While little is written about Bishop Beaven, Father McCoy's history describes him as "a dynamo at organization and administration (who) worked indefatigably to develop and enhance the diocesan school system and to place all the temporal affairs of the diocese on a sound business basis." A newspaper of the day adds this odd description: "His eye is his best feature. It is large and full and open, much like the eyes we see in young Augustus, that kind of eye with which a man looks sideways and back as well as straight ahead, and which is always an index of strength of character. He looks like the Bishop."

Bishop Beaven's life as a priest began at Our Lady of the Rosary Church in Spencer, where he served for three years as a curate and 10 as pastor before moving on to become pastor of the Holy Rosary Church. He was known as a devoted but conservative bishop, who believed that nuns should remain cloistered rather than operating hospitals and schools. While such thinking was common among bishops at the time, it is ironic considering his role in the founding of the Sisters of Providence.

Because of his role in establishing the new diocesan order in Holyoke, "The announcement of the appointment of Rt. Rev. Thomas D. Beaven as successor to the late Rt. Rev. P. T. O'Reilly automatically severed the connection between the

Mother House and the mission at Holyoke, and an immediate withdrawal of the sisters kept us practically stranded," Mother Mary of Providence wrote in her history, "especially as no advance measures had been taken in anticipation of the proceedings."

The break between Kingston and Holyoke created sadness and hard feelings among some of the sisters. Those who wished to, answered the call to return to Kingston, leaving 30 sisters to operate the new order. None of the four original arrivals was among the sisters who stayed. One died and the three others already had returned to Kingston by the time of the separation. Many of the sisters who joined the Holyoke mission were from the Holyoke area. Others, like Sister Mary of Providence, were of Irish heritage and perhaps felt comfortable working with Holyoke's largely Irish immigrant population. Sister Mary of Providence was named the first major superior of the new order and became Mother Mary of Providence. Sister Mary Ursula Nixon, a devoted friend and confidante to Mother Mary, returned to Holyoke from Kingston to join the new order as first assistant.

Symbolizing their break from Kingston, the Sisters of Providence of Holyoke adopted a new name for a short time, calling themselves the Sisters of Charity. Soon after, for legal reasons and to gain tax-exempt status, they incorporated as the Sisters of Providence of Holyoke.

They also adopted a new garniture, but, perhaps signifying their common mission, the garniture remained very similar to that of the Kingston community. The new garniture of the Sisters of Providence covered all but the facial features of the sister, coming in close to the eyes and mouth, but the pointed pleat at the top of the Kingston community's garniture was rounded into a kind of bonnet. When Bishop Beaven told the Sisters of Providence to choose their own garniture, Mother Mary was surprised to find that they chose a design so similar to that of their former order.

On the day he was consecrated, Bishop Beaven bought property in the Brightside section of Holyoke, and handed it over to the Sisters of Providence, paying off $21,000 of the $41,000 mortgage for the land and an additional $20,000 for repairs to buildings on the property. The sisters used the property not only for their mother house, but to establish an orphanage for boys and a home for aged men.

In the 15 years after the order was established as a separate diocesan community, the Sisters of Providence established 20 works of charity, including several hospitals, an orphanage, nursing homes, a residence for working girls and a home for unwed mothers.

The nuns in the order who were most important to the initial success of St. Vincent Hospital were Mother Mary of Providence and Sister Mary Ursula.

Although Sister Ursula served as the superintendent of the hospital for its first 10 years, the influence of Mother Mary of Providence extended much wider and for a longer period. Reports conflict about whether she actually came to the hospital to oversee its initial operation, but it is clear that she played an important role in everything the Sisters of Providence did.

In her memoirs, Mother Mary says that she knew by the age of 11 she wanted to be a nun. Her sister, Elizabeth, was just the third postulant in the Kingston order, joining in 1862 and becoming Sister Mary of the Seven Dolors. Mother Mary was accepted into the Kingston order as a postulant in 1869. Her rebellious nature was apparent from the beginning. Adjusting to a diet so meager she barely sustained herself, she once sneaked two ears of corn into her room, a severe transgression from the obedience that was required of all nuns. She was slow to be accepted, but she finally made her profession in 1872.

The first hint of the greatness she was to achieve came during her naming ceremony. Most nuns, in receiving their religious names, have "no more freedom of choice than an infant in baptism," according to *Can Spring Be Far Behind?*, and typically, as with Sister Mary of the Seven Dolors, they are given the name "Mary" to grant them the protection of the Blessed Virgin, the Mother of Christ, along with the name of "some obscure saint under whose patronage the vow-sister is placed for life." To the surprise of Kate Horan, the name Sister Mary of Providence, invoking the name of her religious community, "was bestowed on her like an accolade."

Three years later, just a month after being named Secretary General of the Kingston order, she was assigned to the Holyoke mission to teach at St. Jerome's School for Boys. She wrote that her assignment "was somewhat of a disappointment to me, as I had been wooed to my vocation by a great sympathy for the poor, and an ardent desire to relieve them in their sufferings. . . . However, I was consoled by the circumstance that my charges were of lowly condition." In her second year, "stir," as her young charges called her, abbreviating "sister," was named principal.

When Bishop O'Reilly sought independence for the Holyoke mission, Sister Mary of Providence was torn between following her major superior, Mother Mary Edward, who strongly opposed the break, and the Vatican decision to allow independence to the mission. She risked excommunication by defying Mother Mary Edward and declaring that she would abide by the decision of Rome.

Under her leadership, the Sisters of Providence became a formidable order, operating Providence Hospital and the Mount St. Vincent Orphanage, and founding not just St. Vincent Hospital, but Mercy Hospital in Springfield and Farren Memorial Hospital in Montague City. In addition, they founded the Holy Family Institute, Bethlehem at Brightside; the Beaven Kelly Home for Aged Men and Harkins Home for Aged Women, both in Holyoke; St. Luke's Home for single, unemployed women in Springfield, and Greylock Rest in Adams. Despite her heavy administrative load, Mother Mary still found time for manual labor, and could be found in the laundry room of the mother house every Monday.

Alfred "Pop" Logan, an orphan who lived with the sisters his entire life and, as an adult, performed odd jobs at St. Vincent Hospital, wrote that when he was a boy in 1925, Mother Mary enthusiastically joined the orphaned boys in their play: "Mother enjoyed the ball games with the boys. She could bat and run for bases, so the boys claimed her to be tops. One time, Mother joined the children on their sleds and tore her habit. We kids had about fifty cents and we wanted to pay for it. Instead, mother treated us to candy."

Mother Mary of Providence tended to do things her way, and, although Bishop Beaven chose her to run the new order, he sometimes found her independence disconcerting. He was the ruling authority of the diocese and expected Mother Mary of Providence to obey him, as the hierarchy of the church demanded. So imagine his reaction to the likes of Mother Mary. When seeking bids for the construction of Mercy Hospital in Springfield, she chose a non-Catholic contractor without consulting anyone. Her explanation, according to *Can Spring Be Far Behind?*, was that "bricks and mortar don't know the hands on them are Catholic or Protestant — (William J.) Burnham was the low bidder."

Over the years, Bishop Beaven grew increasingly critical of the independence shown by the Sisters of Providence. He sent them missives criticizing their reading of non-Catholic, non-religious texts — especially books about the subject of obstetrics, which was forbidden, even though many of the nuns were nurses. He also criticized what he believed to be their intemperate indulgence in tea and coffee, and their use of the telephone.

Although Bishop Beaven and Mother Mary of Providence had different ideas, they admired and respected each other and, for the most part, got along. But by 1910, with the Vatican dictating complete obedience from its nuns, Bishop Beaven forced Mother Mary to step down from her position. While the sisters were supposed to be free to elect their major superior, and they unanimously cast their support for Mother Mary, Bishop Beaven required them to reconsider. Mother Mary removed her name from the ballot and Bishop Beaven required the sisters to choose between Sisters Mary Fidelis and Mary Vincent. They chose Sister Mary Vincent. Still, 10 years later, when Bishop Beaven died, Mother Mary mourned, and said, "Our founder. My friend. Now I have no one left to tell me my faults."

Mother Mary of Providence served the order for 35 years, 18 as major superior, then 16 as councilor and treasurer general. She was instrumental in establishing the New England Catholic Hospital Association in 1923, and served as its first president for seven years. In 1926, she became superior of St. Luke's Hospital in Pittsfield, where she remained until retiring in 1932. She suffered a stroke in 1936 and never fully recovered. She died in 1943 at the age of 93.

Father McCoy describes her as "a marvelous woman, small of frame and delicate appearing, low voiced, with an almost hesitating manner, yet with the mind of a man fit to direct armies." The *Holyoke Transcript,* at her death, recalled a conversation that took place after she opened a new hospital: "'She has the mind of a man,' said the grizzled old contractor. 'You're wrong, man,' said the clergyman. 'I've been meeting men all my life and I could count on the fingers of one hand all the men I ever met who could match her.' "

Sister Ursula was Mother Mary's greatest supporter. During her years as the hospital's superintendent, she oversaw the work of the other nuns and inspired them to work as hard as she did. Her duties included fund raising, approving admissions, overseeing expansion of the new hospital and ensuring the financial stability of the new institution. Although born in the United States, she was trained in Kingston and was serving there when the Sisters of Providence split from their mother house. She came to Holyoke to be close to Mother Mary.

The Catholic Free Press describes her as a diplomatic administrator who could "with casual facility handle a professional situation with consummate diplomacy, cordially greet a high-ranking dignitary or lend a willing ear to the plea of the indigent."

But even her diplomatic skills did not save Sister Ursula when, in 1910, she attempted to negate Bishop Beaven's decision to replace Mother Mary of Providence with Mother Mary Vincent. Sister Ursula stood up for what she believed in, and she believed the election broke the rules of the church. With Sister Genevieve, Mother Mary's first assistant, Sister Ursula attempted to travel to Washington, D.C. to state her case before the apostolic delegate. Their limited funds took them as far as New York, where they took their case to the cardinal.

After hearing them, the cardinal contacted Bishop Beaven by telephone. At the end of his telephone conversation, he relayed the bishop's advice to Sister Ursula — that she seek a dispensation from her vows and leave the order.

She followed the bishop's advice, but years later, after the bishop's death, she returned to the order.

Organizing a new hospital would be a major undertaking for a group of 30 ordinary people. For the 30 Sisters of Providence, it was just one of many projects. In 1893, when the sisters agreed to open a hospital in Worcester, they already were busy preparing the construction of Providence Hospital in Holyoke, in addition to settling into their mother house in Brightside, operating an orphanage and a school, and performing other acts of charity throughout the Holyoke and South Hadley area. This tremendous workload was made all the more difficult, because even lending institutions had a shortage of money. In 1893 and 1894, according to Mother Mary's journal, "Banks were unwilling to lend any considerable sum, under mortgage security, lest there might be a general withdrawal of deposits, and where the Mother Superior made application for a loan, she was courteously met with a refusal."

On August 31, 1893, Sister Ursula arrived in Worcester with four assistants — Sisters Mary Andrew Proulx, Mary Agnes Walsh, Mary Christina McMahon and Mary Fidelis Quirk. Mother Mary could spare only five sisters, but they soon had other help to rely upon, as well.

"With compassion," *Can Spring Be Far Behind?* notes, "the General Superior stripped her convent of the best workers, sending them for a time down to Worcester to help arrange the furniture, and she slipped in as a bonus, one of the older girls from Mt. St. Vincent's Orphanage to assist in the domestic work, and even one grown boy for general services. But though there were only five nuns regularly assigned to the Mission, the community had 268 devoted women volunteers and a small crew of doctors struggling valiantly to break down the truly deep opposition of the majority of skilled medical practitioners who opposed this wild, twelve-bed, harum-scarum so-called Hospital."

The 268 women established a tradition of volunteerism that continues today at St. Vincent Hospital, and played an important role in transforming the "wild, twelve-bed, harum-scarum so-called Hospital" into a true healing institution.

When they came to Worcester and took their first look at the old Bartlett farm, the sisters must have considered the eight-acre lot on top of Vernon Hill ideal for a new hospital. As Dr. Duggan, president of the medical staff, noted in 1900, the site was far enough from the "neighboring nuisances" of the center of the city, and its high elevation provided an abundance of fresh air and sunshine — practically the only medical remedies available in 1893. At the time, the wealthy typically built their homes on top of the city's many hills, away from the sooty air of the tenements of factory workers. George Crompton, owner of Crompton Loom Works, the city's largest employer, built his famous 37-room Mariemont estate next to the Bartlett farm in 1865, because his physician recommended the fresh air of a high elevation to help suppress his cough. Dr. Duggan also noted that the subsoil of rock on the site reduced the likelihood of damp walls, and the high elevation provided excellent surface drainage.

Whether the sisters thought it was coincidence or divine intervention, they also must have found it wondrous that the land was next to Providence Street, a street named for an old route to the Rhode Island city.

While the location was ideal, the farmhouse was not. Mother Mary of Providence wrote, "Not only the patients sought admission, but even the elements vied for entrance in the House of Providence, and frequently, the Sisters enjoyed the luxury of a canopied bed at night — an umbrella serving to ward off the rain seeping through a leaky roof." And the farmhouse was so congested, that "when overnight guests arrived unexpectedly, a Sister, dispossessed of her bed, was forced to make up her couch on a table." They didn't even have pillows, and had to bundle the tops of their blankets under their heads for comfort.

With $2,000 in borrowed funds, the sisters set about converting the farmhouse to a hospital, furnishing it with beds and supplies. By September, the hospital was ready to open for business. On September 8, Msgr. Griffin officially opened the new hospital by saying Mass, setting up a chapel with the altar left behind by the Christian Brothers. By October, the sisters had established a medical staff and formed a Board of Trustees, which was assembled with the help and influence of Msgr. Griffin.

Reflecting a desire that the hospital serve all of Worcester's citizens, regardless of their religious beliefs or ethnic origins, the first board and medical staff included a fair representation of the community, including clergy, prominent Yankees, and representatives of the Irish community. Board officers were Bishop Beaven, who chaired the board, Mother Mary as treasurer and Sister Ursula as secretary. The Executive Committee included Salisbury, Healy, Matthew B. Lamb, Denis C. Leonard, James H. Mellen, David F. O'Connell and Daniel Downey. Clergy on the board included Msgr. Griffin, Father Power, Rev. Denis Scannell, Rev. Thomas J. Conaty, D.D., Rev. D. H. O'Neill, Rev. Robert Walsh, Rev. Joseph Brouillette and Rev. Burke. Mary C. Crompton, whose family played a key role in the hospital's history, was the only lay woman on the board. Other board members included Elijah B. Stoddard, Charles A. Chase, Andrew Athy, Eugene M. Moriarty, George F. Bayle, William Hart, Frank J. Houston, Thomas Barrett, John J. Riordan, John Timon, George A. McAleer, Patrick Power, David F. Fitzgerald, John B. Simard, James A. McDermott, John A. Kennedy and M.J.P. McCafferty. Having representatives of the local Yankee elite on the board, such as Salisbury, Chase and Stoddard, was in line with the hospital's philosophy of serving the medical needs of everyone in the community, regardless of background. It also helped when it was time to raise funds for the hospital.

At the time, a typical doctor's practice ran the gamut of general medical and surgical practice, but the St. Vincent staff showed some breakdown by area of specialization. The surgical staff included Dr. Thomas O'Callaghan, first chairman of the medical staff, and Drs. Homer Gage, P. H. Keefe and Joseph Kelly.

Dr. Fallon joined the staff as a pathologist, though he later earned his reputation as a surgeon. Dr. Michael J. O'Meara was the obstetrician, Dr. William J. Delahanty was a family physician who also served as the hospital's orthopedist, and Drs. David Lovell and David Harrower were aurists and oculists, ear and eye doctors. Drs. George F. Francis and Leonard Wheeler were listed as consultants. The medical staff included Drs. Mary V. O'Callaghan, John J. Brennan, John T. Duggan, John A. Carroll, Joseph E. Gendron and M. J. Halloran.

The doctors on the St. Vincent staff were among Worcester's most noted and respected citizens. Dr. Gage served at all three of Worcester's hospitals, but was most often associated with Memorial Hospital. It was said that no one, with the possible exception of founder Ichabod Washburn, had done as much for Memorial as Dr. and Mrs. Gage. Over their lifetime, they contributed $1,130,655 to the hospital. Dr. Gage also served as medical director of the State Mutual Life Assurance Company for more than 40 years, and in his later years as president of Crompton & Knowles Loom Works.

Dr. Wheeler, who became superintendent of City Hospital, was "naturally a student and educated in the best schools," according to Dr. Bergin's history of Worcester hospitals. His work "showed in marked contrast to the older members of the staff who did not believe in records, and whose method depended on personal experience rather than on scientific research, and we note that in 1872, during his service, for the first time in the history of the hospital, the diagnosis of pneumonia was made on physical signs, and not on cough and rusty sputum."

Dr. Delahanty, a well-liked family physician who was known as "Handlebar Hank" because of his bristling mustache, was, according to Dr. Bergin, "an acute diagnostician, who relied not on ancillary aids for making the correct diagnosis, but upon the five senses endowed to him, and on experience and intuition." Dr. Delahanty was the quintessential family physician, who in more than 50 years of service cared for several generations in the same families. Dr. Fallon called him "the best beloved doctor in Central Massachusetts."

The inclusion of a woman, Dr. Mary O'Callaghan, on the St. Vincent staff was not unusual. She was one of several women on the hospital medical staff during the early years. The Worcester District Medical Society began admitting women in 1873, although with some reluctance and much debate.

With their staff in place, the Sisters of Providence were ready to begin their work.

Building a Hospital

"Everything in the management of the institution was placed on a business basis, and its humble beginning directed to safe and steady growth."

Sister Mary Ursula, first superintendent of St. Vincent Hospital

For the first few months, the sisters had difficulty attracting patients. As Mother Mary tells it, "Few seemed to know of the existence of the new Establishment, known as the House of Providence; fewer still were interested."

But just eight months after the hospital opened, with seven sisters on staff and beds for 20 patients, Sister Ursula wrote that the hospital's accommodations "have at times been taxed to the limit," and "new buildings must be built if its full measure of work is to be performed."

With well-known and respected citizens on its medical staff and Board of Trustees, the local community must have recognized that the hospital provided a quality of care at least equal to that available at other area hospitals. But it also was apparent to everyone involved that, even with the best doctors of the day, the hospital could not survive for long in the drafty old farmhouse. Even as the sisters were treating their first patients, they were planning the construction of the new hospital.

The strategy adopted by the Sisters of Providence was both practical and clever. A new, small hospital would be built immediately, and the old farmhouse would become Msgr. Griffin's home for the aged. Once the patient load outgrew the small hospital, a larger permanent hospital would be built, the home for the aged would move into the small hospital building and the farmhouse would be razed. By starting small, Stephen Salisbury later noted, the sisters were able to determine what their needs would be in a larger hospital. Starting in a small building also gave them an opportunity to expand their patient load gradually as they became more well known in the community.

Among the 104 patients treated during the first year, typhoid fever was the most common disease, striking 12 patients. According to the hospital's first annual report, four women were treated for "carcinoma of breast," and three were marked cured, one improved. Five patients were treated for melancholia, three for alcoholism, five for dysmenorrhea and six for appendicitis. Of the 104 patients, 43 were treated without charge, and 31 were treated at reduced rates. Until recent years, it was common at St. Vincent and other hospitals to charge on a sliding scale, with the wealthy paying more for medical care. The basic charge at the time was just $1 a day in the hospital ward, or $10 a week and up for a private room. But the average wage was, of course, much lower than it is today. A typical Worcester man at the time earned less than $500 a year.

Paying patients provided the hospital with nearly $4,000 during that first year, but money raised from medical treatment was generously supplemented by community donations. The hospital's annual report notes private donations of everything from flowers to underwear, in addition to cash donations. The sisters also did their own fund raising, earning, during their first year, $268.62 from their sewing and painting, $1,000 from "entertainments," and $3,540 from subscriptions to the building fund. That the sisters understood fund raising is apparent in the early annual reports, which include a "Form of Bequest" for raising funds for the new hospital. The form notes that a $25 donation provided a bed in the hospital ward, while a $50 donation furnished a private room.

The Washington Social Club sponsored the hospital's first major fund-raising effort, which was called the Midway Plaisance after the section of a park in Chicago that was used for an amusement midway at the Columbian Exposition of 1893. The Washington Social Club, named after the Washington Square neighborhood where its earliest members came from, was founded in 1882 as an outgrowth of a sandlot baseball team, but by 1894 its members represented the most successful of the city's Irish immigrants. The Washington Social Club, like other clubs of the day, was known for its showy balls, which featured formal dress, orchestra music, midnight banquets, and halls decorated with canaries in gilded cages and Turkish-rug wall hangings. The Midway Plaisance raised $4,000 for the hospital — more than was raised from patient care in the hospital's first year.

Most of the money went into the hospital's building fund.

Today, building a new hospital takes many years of planning. From determination of need procedures to the drafting of architectural plans, from choosing a general contractor to obtaining financing, the steps to building a modern hospital are painstakingly long.

When the Sisters of Providence set out to build a new hospital, they just went ahead and built it. In spite of the order's early financial difficulties, Bishop Beaven readily gave his approval.

From the beginning, the old farmhouse was seen as temporary quarters. The building was so decrepit that the Christian Brothers, who were invited by Msgr. Griffin to teach at St. John's school, apparently refused to live in it, and the condition of the building may have influenced their return to Ireland. The Sisters of Providence renovated it and lived through an entire New England winter there.

But by June of the first year of operation, the Board of Trustees recognized that, even with an addition, the Bartlett farmhouse would be inadequate to serve as a hospital for very long. The board approved construction of a new 35-bed hospital, retaining Earle and Fisher as the architectural firm and Thomas Barrett as the contractor. In November 1894, ground was broken for a two-story, wood-frame building on the Bartlett farm site. It was 35 feet wide and 75 feet long with four wards — a surgical ward and a sick ward for each sex. The building was completed and blessed on September 9, 1895, and the new hospital opened on October 9, 1885. The new hospital cost $17,455 to build — $22,214 including furnishings and equipment.

With the opening of the new hospital, Msgr. Griffin at last was able to establish his home for the aged in the old Bartlett farmhouse. The hospital already had begun to treat a few aged, chronically ill women, and they remained behind when the other patients transferred to the new hospital, giving the home for the aged its first tenants.

The new hospital was named St. Vincent Hospital after the patron saint of the Sisters of Providence. The House of Providence name was dropped from the first hospital, perhaps because the sisters already operated a Providence Hospital in Holyoke. Providence Hospital also had been named the House of Providence when it opened. Among the speakers at the dedication ceremony, Rev. Thomas J. Conaty, a hospital trustee, said, "The sisters have won not only the respect of the Catholic people, but non-Catholics as well, and they have succeeded in winning the undivided support of all classes. They have not been limited by any religious feeling, neither is their hospital limited to any creed or race. They have opened their doors to all, regardless of creed or color. It stands for a hospital for the sick and the suffering, and no question of creed or color will debar anybody from this institution."

In line with the nonsectarian mission of charity that the sisters had embarked upon, hospital records show that, from the beginning, the hospital treated a cross-section of the Worcester area's citizens. In 1896, St. Vincent's patient population was demographically similar to the population of Worcester as a whole, and included 120 people of Irish origin, 164 people who were born in the United States, 32 natives of Canada and a scattering of patients from other countries. Patient occupations included 48 laborers, 25 mechanics and three merchants. Patients were treated for a wide range of illnesses, including 10 cases of neurasthenia, seven of influenza, five of dyspepsia, nine of pneumonia, nine of rheumatism, 13 of adenoids and 18 of cataracts. Dr. O'Callaghan reported that 200 operations were performed that year with "a mortality almost nil."

After the new hospital opened, business picked up immediately, and so did the hospital's revenues. For the year 1895, St. Vincent Hospital treated 144 patients, with 85 paying full cost and only 34 receiving free treatment, while for 1896, 331 patients were treated — a 125 percent increase — and 209 paid at full cost. Much of the early growth was aided by the non-Catholic doctors on staff, who were treating an increasing number of patients at the new hospital.

As the hospital grew, so did its expenses. "Though somewhat embarrassed by the burden of unpaid balances on contracts and incidental expenses," Sister Ursula and Mother Mary wrote in 1895, "we are not disheartened, for the Treasurer's Report proves that if our expenses have increased, our receipts, without any unreasonable drain upon public charity, have been in fair proportion to our growth."

By the following year, all expenses were paid off, and the sisters ended the year in the black — with a positive balance of $1.12. The expense of building the new hospital was paid by January 1, 1897, just 15 months after the hospital opened.

"In addition to paying off the balance of the $6,359 due on the new building and $545 for grading, also current expenses," the sisters wrote, "we have improved our surgical department by putting in a sterilizing apparatus at a cost of $461, and adding several pieces of aseptic furniture to the operating room." The hospital also added two small wards in 1896, allowing the medical attendant to separate "his noisy and delirious patients from his convalescents."

With a rapidly growing patient load, no debt except the original mortgage on the land, and an able and hard-working staff of physicians and sisters, it was already time to replace the wood frame hospital with a new, larger brick-and-mortar structure. The sisters no longer had to wonder whether their hospital would succeed. It already had.

Mother Mary of Providence and Sister Ursula wrote in their annual report that year, "Bear in mind that this has been all paid and we have a cash balance above written, then judge whether this gives us sufficient encouragement to undertake more, or whether we should rest content, perhaps losing opportunities by delay."

By 1897, Dr. O'Callaghan and Dr. Fallon noted, "In our second annual report, we wrote: 'Today we occupy a house which in neatness and convenience is a modern hospital.' Compared with our old quarters, the new St. Vincent Hospital was a palace, and when we first occupied its cheerful and roomy wards, we firmly believed we were equipped to respond to every call on our charity, for several years to come.

"The members of the Board of Trustees of St. Vincent's have taken such an interest in the daily doings at our Hospital, that many of them are less surprised than we, that less than two years after we wrote the above self-congratulatory report, we are again asking for more room."

While the Sisters of Providence lived by the slogan, "God is Charity," that does not mean they were willing to give away the services of the hospital. On the contrary, they recognized that if they provided free care to someone who could afford to pay, they might have to deny care to someone who could not afford it.

In the 1899 annual report, Sister Ursula and Mother Mary note that in 1898 the number of patients increased to 436, up by 96 from the previous year, but, "The income has not increased proportionately because there are among those 109 who have failed to remunerate the hospital for the care given and, as much of the money will never be paid, that number became practically free patients, but stringent measures in regard to the payment of hospital dues have never been enforced as such would not be in keeping with the spirit of the institution."

The Sisters of Providence were clearly forgiving when necessary, but they also looked to the future, recognizing the need to save for yet another new hospital; to replace wood with bricks. In just two years, the new hospital had become old. While structurally it was a great improvement from the old farmhouse, it already was filled to capacity.

With the wounded from the Spanish-American War adding to the patient load, the tiny hospital was taxed beyond its capabilities. The war victims came home in wretched health and required intensive medical treatment, according to "A New Era in Medicine," an essay by Dr. Fallon.

"Although they had been only a few months in Cuba," he wrote, "malaria, yellow fever, typhoid fever, yes, even the infected food provided by the government, had all taken their dread toll so that when these poor fellows on their return home marched, or rather tottered through our streets, they were nearly all of them mere skeletons, yellow from disease. Their appearance was a harrowing one; and even strong men wept at the sight of them, and all this disability and suffering were the result not of bullets, but rather of disease contracted in the Tropics."

While the Spanish-American War created terrible health problems for the American soldiers, it provided a tremendous windfall for the Sisters of Providence, who were by then trying to prove themselves with three new hospitals — St. Vincent Hospital, Providence Hospital in Holyoke and Mercy Hospital in Springfield. With the casualties of war filling all of the local hospitals, those who still had reservations about the sisters' abilities put aside their doubts. They quickly found that the care provided by the sisters and their medical staff was second to none.

With the debt paid off on the new hospital, the Sisters of Providence were ready to move ahead again and Boston architect C. J. Bateman was hired to design a new hospital. His design included a 100-foot tower with a gilded cross on top, clearly and proudly identifying St. Vincent as a Catholic hospital.

Also prominent were the sun parlors that protruded from the building. At the time, the sun was considered perhaps the best medicine available for healing the sick. Dr. Fallon wrote as chief of surgery in 1911 that fresh air and sunshine are "two of God's best medicines," and that they helped patients build up resistance against typhoid fever, septicemia and puerperal fever. "These, indeed are true stimulants," he wrote, "just the opposite of alcohol." Because sunshine was practically the only medicine available at the time, the entire building was designed so that the sun dispensed its medicine as widely as possible in every room.

At the annual meeting on January 26, 1898, all debt had been erased and a cash balance of $2,162 was available. The sisters were assisted in their fund-raising efforts by the creation of the St. Vincent Hospital Aid Association, a forerunner of today's Guild of Our Lady of Providence. Association members not only made sheets and pillowcases, and other items for the patients' comfort, but also held fund raisers. Under the leadership of its first president, Dr. Fallon's wife, Ella, the association raised $3,500 in its first year with the help of a calendar party. The four seasons of the year and each month were represented by appropriate costumes, and foods representing every holiday were served.

Additional funds were raised by the association's annual dues of $1. Always with a mind toward business, the sisters encouraged the association to increase its ranks. "Members may also give very efficient aid by inducing their friends to join the society," the sisters recommended, "thus giving to its treasury the membership fee to increase its fund." The Sisters of Providence, in turn, promised to pray daily for their benefactors, offer a Mass for the association on the first Friday of every month and offer a Mass on the death of a member.

Active members of the St. Vincent Hospital Aid Association met at the hospital on Tuesday and Friday evenings to assist in sewing, and much of the sewing was sold to raise funds. Whist parties and lectures also were held to raise money for hospital beds.

"Its object," according to association bylaws, "is to assist in providing money to aid the works conducted by the Sisters of

Providence. Saint Vincent, who founded a similar association, called the 'Ladies of Charity,' is patron of the society, and they adopt his favorite motto, 'The charity of Christ presseth me.' The holy thought embodied in this motto will always stimulate the members to zeal and generosity in the beautiful work in which they are engaged."

After seven years, the association had 400 members and had raised nearly $11,000 for the hospital. Perhaps because of the association's help, the hospital seemed to have little trouble raising money, despite the continuing poverty of much of the population it served. "It is a generally accepted fact that Roman Catholics are as liberal supporters of their churches, their clergy, their church institutions and bazaars as any religious body in the world," an *Evening Gazette* of the time notes, "and Protestants often express their well-founded amazement at the sums of money their Catholic brethren raise without apparent effort."

Of course, it also should be noted that some of the hospital's biggest financial supporters were Protestants. The hospital's financial supporters, like the hospital itself, knew no religious boundaries.

"The word hospital has a chilly sound," an anonymous writer notes in a 50th anniversary history of St. John's parish written in 1896. "To the Irish heart, in times past, it has been synonymous with poor house, and enough of that feeling still lingers to make the children of Erin willing to bear suffering and risk death rather than seek relief in the public ward of a hospital."

And yet just two years later, 5,000 people, including many "children of Erin," gathered of their own free will on the top of Vernon Hill, despite dark skies, to witness the laying of the cornerstone for the new St. Vincent Hospital.

By October 9, just 21 working days after the laying of the foundation, the structure already stood five stories tall, as though it had grown impatient waiting for the cornerstone. Bishop Beaven led a procession that included the Hibernian Rifles, the

Garde Lafayette, 60 altar boys and others. They marched in formation from the old hospital to the new hospital as the Worcester Brass Band played the march processional. During the ceremony, Bishop Beaven placed a copper casket into the cornerstone. The casket included photos of many of the people who played key roles in the founding of the hospital, including Msgr. Griffin, Bishops O'Reilly and Beaven, and Sister Ursula. Before the ceremony ended, the crowd of 5,000 joined the United Catholic Choirs of Worcester to sing, "Te Deum" and "America."

In June, with construction of the hospital virtually completed, the St. Vincent Hospital Aid Association held a four-day bazaar to raise the $6,000 to $7,000 needed to furnish the new building. The bazaar featured music, refreshments, a fortune-telling booth and more. But the greatest attraction was the hospital itself. An admission price of 15 cents was charged for those who wanted to see the new hospital, and "season tickets" were made available for 50 cents.

Another attraction was the hospital's new 750 lb. bell, which was donated by Peter Baker, owner of the Baker Lead Manufacturing Company, a manufacturer of pipes for plumbing. The bell, which was cast at the Meneely Bell Foundry in Troy, N.Y., was so popular, the hospital charged a separate admission of a nickel a person to see it during the bazaar. This netted the hospital "many dollars," according to *The Boston Post*.

On November 8, 1899, the crowd gathered at St. Vincent Hospital again, this time to dedicate the completed building. "Catholics and Protestants attended the dedication, and showed the best of feeling," according to Father McCoy's history of the diocese.

A separate dedication ceremony also was held for the hospital bell — the only piece of equipment from the hospital still being used regularly today. The bell was of great significance at the time, and its dedication ceremony, according to newspaper accounts of the day, was "one of the most imposing of the Catholic Church." Comparing the "baptism of the bell" to the baptism of a child, the newspaper describes the seven-part ceremony, which included cleansing the bell with holy water to make it "a pure agency in the worship of God." The role of the bell, according to the translation from the Latin, is to "praise the Lord, summon the laity, assemble the clergy . . . bewail the dead, dispel the tempest, honor the feast." The bell is inscribed with chapter xvii, verse 18 from the Book of Ecclesiastics: "The alms of a man is as a signet with God" in reference to the charity of its donor.

James Baker, grandson of Peter Baker, grew up on Vernon Hill and recalls that when he was a child, his mother had some regrets about the gift of the bell. It always seemed to toll just as she was putting him down to sleep.

Conscious of the value of a positive public image, the Sisters of Providence conducted press tours of the new hospital. In a lengthy and detailed article, *The Boston Post* on June 24, 1899, described the new St. Vincent Hospital, as "one of the finest buildings of its kind in the country. Resting upon a beautiful hill where a magnificent view of the surrounding country is to be had, and erected at a cost of over $80,000, it surely stands as a monument to the pluck, perseverance and business capacity of the Sisters of Providence who have charge of the work and who have, almost unaided, completed this great task."

Each floor had its own dining room, and private bathrooms and toilets were available — a breakthrough in patient care at the time.

The new hospital featured some of the amenities associated with today's hospitals. A "specially constructed elevator," operated by pulleys, took patients to the upper floors. Private rooms were available for one or two patients, while the general wards contained nine beds each. Unlike most hospitals of the day, St. Vincent's wards were spacious. The *Post* notes that "an electric bell at the head of each bed connects with a room for the nurse on duty, and if a patient cares for anything, all that is necessary is to touch the button and the sister is summoned to the bedside."

Perhaps confusing the staff, but befitting a Catholic hospital, "The rooms are not numbered, but named after saints, so they can be easily designated, as St. Theresa, St. Anthony and so on."

The *Post* describes the operating room of the new hospital as being "as fine as anything of its kind in the country. The operating room is perfectly lighted, and is two stories high with a gallery surrounding it from which the nurses may watch the operations. This room is finished in white marble and will indeed be the joy of the surgical staff of the hospital. The flooring of the rooms . . . is of Terrazzo, which is small bits of marble in cement, rubbed to a smooth finish."

The *Post* reporter also writes: "In the surgical flat is the operating room, and a truck is used to bring the patients in. The room is supplied with a number of white painted tables of iron with glass tops. Large glass bowls for disinfectant solutions stand about the room on iron frames, and a glass case holds the shining instruments. A cupboard nearby is filled with a curious collection of enameled vessels, each for its special purpose when an operation is in progress.

"The sterilizing room is reached by a few steps leading up from the operating room, and contains all the modern equipment for sterilizing. The nickel sterilizing oven is fitted with a wire cage, something like an old-fashioned rat trap, and into it is put all the sponges, bandages, cottons and the like used in an operation."

Continuing his description, the *Post* reporter also notes that patients marked the passing of time by changes in the patterns on their dishes: "Each patient has his own tray, small coffeepot and dainty dishes, which go a long way toward making things taste good to a sick person. Now and then the patterns of the dishes are changed for the patient who has been in the hospital some time and no one better appreciates a variety in that line."

As impressed as the reporter was with the hospital itself, the work of the 22 Sisters of Providence who operated the hospital at the time also caught his attention. "One sister has charge of the kitchen, superintends the cooking and is assisted by two young girls who come from an orphanage under the patronage of the order." One of the sisters was the pharmacist and prepared all of the medicines needed.

He also writes that "the sisters dress alike and it is hard to pick out the nurses from others. The costume is a plain black gown, with a deep circular collar about the neck. A black veil, coming from the white linen garniture, which forms a white roll, flaring a trifle about the face, falls to the waist. A smooth, wide band of white linen passes about the forehead, with the ends confined by the white garniture."

He notes that while the sisters' life was hard and never idle, "it is one of the laws of the order to cultivate all tendencies to art, literature and a sense of the beautiful which may exist in the different personalities who come under its care." Two of the sisters painted on china and another was a florist. The sisters also embroidered, and maintained the vestments of the priests.

Observing the work of the Sisters of Providence, the reporter concludes: "Nothing can exceed the care and attention the sisters as nurses bestow upon their patients. They suffer with them, they are sympathetic and thoughtful, anxiety is depicted on their countenances when their patients are dangerously ill and joy pervades their life at the recovery of those who come to their hospital for treatment. It is their life work, with no remuneration but their living and the knowledge that they are doing good to suffering humanity."

With the opening of the new hospital, the farmhouse was razed and the wood-framed building became the St. Vincent Home, serving the needs of the aged for a number of years, even though it again became overcrowded. The hospital's 1902 annual report notes that the house was so crowded, "not only are we unable to admit the number who apply, but on account of the dilapidated condition of the premises and the crowded quarters, the inmates are subject to many inconveniences which are a trial to those afflicted with the infirmities of age."

However, the sisters found that the home provided not only an additional source of revenue for the hospital, but a source of labor. The 14 "inmates" of the home helped the sisters whenever possible. One old man did the gardening, while the women who were able to helped with the hospital's sewing and mending needs.

At about the time the new hospital was built, the structure of the hospital's management also changed. The Sisters of Providence conducted the affairs of the hospital on their own until January 1899, but at that time the hospital was incorporated as St. Vincent Hospital, with Bishop Beaven as president of the Board of Trustees.

Explaining what amounts to a change in ownership, Father McCoy writes in his history of the diocese, "The Bishop believed that the sisters might show the world an example of extraordinary unselfishness if they agreed to put the hospitals raised at Worcester and Springfield, principally by their own endeavors, into the hands of corporations made up of priests and laymen of each city."

CHAPTER THREE

Doctors and Nurses

"The exceedingly large number of eleven hundred admissions during the year which has closed (1903) warrants us in the assumption that those prejudices and feelings of aversion to hospital treatment, which have existed in days gone by, are fast dwindling away under the riper knowledge and sounder judgment of an intelligent people. They are becoming more fully enlightened to the fact that the combined efforts of the physician and the nurse, in battling with the ills to which humanity is prone, are productive of far better and more satisfactory results than when either the one or the other enters the contest single-handed and alone."
Dr. John T. Duggan

Even working 16 hours a day, seven days a week, by 1897 the Sisters of Providence could no longer handle all of the nursing duties by themselves.

As the public began to overcome its fear of hospitals, the work load at St. Vincent increased to the point where the sisters needed help.

In the typically practical fashion of the Sisters of Providence, instead of simply hiring a staff of lay nurses, Mother Mary of Providence hired Emily Stoney, former Superintendent of Nurses at the Carney Hospital in Boston, to train the sisters to instruct lay nurses. At the time, nursing was developing as a popular potential career for young women. By establishing a nursing school at the hospital, the sisters supplemented their staff without the expense of hiring nurses. At the same time, they provided a needed service to the community and assured themselves that the nurses were trained to act with the discipline the sisters demanded.

In the early days of hospitals, the nurses were practically as decrepit as the worst patients. They were, in the words of Florence Nightingale, "generally those who were too old, too weak, too drunken, too dirty, too stolid, or too bad to do anything else." But, through her efforts, nursing began to change after the Civil War, and by the 1890s it was an established profession — one of the few that was socially acceptable for young women.

The growing popularity of nursing as a career is evident in the growth of schools for training nurses at the time. In 1890, there were only 35 hospital-based nursing schools in the United States. In 1900, when the St. Vincent School of Nursing was founded, it was one of 432 nursing schools across the country. Ten years later, the number of hospital-based schools tripled, and, at their peak in the early 1930s, there were 1,844 nursing schools based at American hospitals.

Nursing training at St. Vincent, as at hospital-based schools throughout the country, was intensive and hands-on. Like joining the Sisters of Providence, nursing was not just a job, it was a vocation. Practically from the first day of training, nurses worked with doctors on life-or-death cases. The nurse in training was able to determine quite quickly whether the exhilaration of helping to save a life offset the tediously long hours and constant exposure to the dead and the dying. The nurse served as an assistant, organizing the surgeon's bundle, making certain the instruments were in proper order, both before and after an operation. She applied dressings, and assisted in the dispensing of medication and anesthesia. With the link between cleanliness and good health having been established, the nurse had to make certain the hospital rooms were spotlessly clean at all times. The nurse also served as the intermediary between the doctor and the patient. She explained procedures to patients, calming their fears, and discussed patient complaints and symptoms with the physician. Sometimes the nurse provided the companionship that served as important therapy to lift the patient's spirits and assure the patient that everything would, indeed, be all right. It was the nurse's duty then, as it is today, to ensure that doctor's orders were carried out and that patient care met the highest standards possible.

But nursing then was primitive by today's standards. Asked what she learned in Miss Stoney's nursing classes, Mother Mary gave a one-word answer: "Charts." While other responsibilities were, of course, learned, Miss Stoney, and the nuns she taught, placed a great deal of emphasis on their patients' charts.

Still, graduates of the nursing school seem to agree universally that nursing training by the sisters was exceptional. "We thought they were very strict," said Mildred Collins, a nurse at St. Vincent Hospital for 50 years. "They didn't put up with any nonsense. The nuns gave us the fundamentals of nursing that we never forgot."

The St. Vincent Hospital School of Nursing opened with Sister Mary Carmelita as its first director. Appropriately, Dr. Duggan served as president of the medical staff at the time. Dr. Duggan's praise of the nursing staff was often effusive. He supported the nurses at a time when many doctors believed that they did not belong in the hospital. "There was a time, not many years ago, when members of the medical profession looked upon the nurse with disfavor," he wrote in 1911. "They could not at all understand when she was in the least conducive to the best interests in the province of medicine. They thought she should be enrolled in a sphere more suitable to her own proper calling. She received the appellation of a busy-body interesting herself in a profession that belonged only by right and title to the learned sons of Aesculapius. But most frequently the mist and gloom of the past are dispelled by the light of common sense of the present, and today, in all the hospitals of the land, as well as in private practice, the members of the medical profession recognize no more necessary and highly useful assistance than that which is rendered by the trained and efficient members of the nursing profession."

Befitting the importance of the first graduation ceremony for the School of Nursing, blue-and-white streamers, ferns, palms and pink roses lent color and fragrance to the St. Vincent Hospital chapel for the occasion. A full program of speakers and music, pomp and circumstance was prepared. The first graduation ceremony for the St. Vincent Hospital School of Nursing was a typical graduation ceremony except for one thing. There was only one person in the graduating class.

The graduating class consisted of one Cecilia Mary Fair Morrilly of Fitchburg, who bore the distinction of completing the three-year course of training in two years. Along with her diploma, Miss Morrilly received a gold pin with the hospital's motto: "Deus Est Caritas," or "God Is Charity." A few months later, Eva Gallagher became the second graduate.

In 1911, the nursing school was still graduating only three or four nurses a year. While nursing candidates were not required to join the Sisters of Providence, the annual report for 1911 explains, each nursing candidate had to be between 21 and 35, and present "a letter from her pastor as to moral character." Training included a three-month probationary period, during which the senior nursing students required the "probbies" to perform an extra measure of work. Nursing students took courses in ethics, bacteriology, dietetics and other medical subjects, and received additional practical instruction in everything from bed making to care of the dead.

Throughout its existence, the School of Nursing never graduated a large number of nurses. In fact, just over 1,000 nurses graduated from the school during its first 50 years and 3,402 before it closed in 1988. But many of the nurses who are still alive today, some of whom attended the school as early as the 1920s, say they received a nursing education unlike any other. They say that once a nurse was trained by the Sisters of Providence, she was trained for life.

By the early part of the century, some patients were coming home from hospitals legitimately cured. This raised the social status of doctors, but especially of surgeons.

"There was very little medical treatment prior to World War II," according to Dr. John J. Massarelli, a senior physician on the staff of Fallon Clinic. "Supportive measures, like digitalis for heart failure, came about in the late '30s. Before that, patients were treated mostly with fresh air and sunshine. But the appendectomy and gall bladder operations had reached a level not much different from what it is today, so the surgeons were very well respected. The surgeons were looked at as being a step above everyone else. The only people who got better in the hospital were those who were operated on."

As Paul Starr notes in *The Social Transformation of American Medicine,* "It was not actually until the 1890s and early 1900s that surgery began to take off. Then, in a burst of creative excitement, the amount, scope, and daring of surgery enormously increased. Improvements in diagnostic tools, particularly the development of X-rays in 1895, spurred the advance."

Before these advances, surgery was regarded as the lowest form of medical practice and was limited primarily to amputations and minor operations. When surgeons did perform serious operations, the patient's chances of survival were low. In an essay on surgical history, Dr. Fallon records the experience of Dr. Samuel D. Gross, who is regarded as the father of American surgery. Dr. Gross recorded 296 deaths out of the 622 hernia operations he performed in the mid-nineteenth century — a mortality rate approaching 50 percent. But that was before surgeons learned how to control bleeding and prevent infection. By 1907, even Dr. Duggan, who was a medical doctor, believed the surgeons should be entitled to special status. As he wrote in the annual report that year: "The rapid progress made in the domain of surgery during the past ten years has made it possible to prolong the lives of many who would undoubtedly have succumbed to maladies which were considered fatal in days gone by. The successful work done by surgeons in hospitals entitles them to the fullest measure of respect by every member of an enlightened community. The fear that took possession of the poor stricken sufferer in former days when the hospital was mentioned is fast giving way to the implicit trust and confidence which took place in the successful operator and his assistants."

✣ ✣ ✣

Undoubtedly one reason Dr. Duggan accorded such respect to surgeons was that his own chief of surgery was Dr. Fallon, whose skills quickly became well known throughout the Worcester area and beyond.

Dr. Fallon's start in medicine is linked with the closing of Dale Hospital, Worcester's Civil War hospital. Without Dale Hospital, his parents never would have been able to afford to send him to medical school, let alone sending him to the finest medical colleges in the world.

Dr. Fallon's father, James Fallon, emigrated from Ireland in the 1840s. After arriving at Boston harbor with $5 in his pocket, he bought a meal of bread and cheese and sat down in Boston Common to eat. A tall man — about six-and-a-half feet tall, according to legend — he attracted the attention of a well-dressed man with a silk hat and inverness cape.

"What is a man like you doing on a work day, sitting here and not working?" the man asked.

"I've just arrived off the boat from Ireland," James Fallon replied, "and I'm needing a job."

"Well, what can you do?" the man asked.

"I know pigs . . . and cows," said Fallon, who, like most of his countrymen, had been a farmer.

"I need a gardener," the man said. "Do you want a job?"

"Why, yes sir," Fallon answered. "But what is your name?"

"John Quincy Adams," the man replied.

While working for the Adams family, James Fallon married the milk maid, an odd match, perhaps, considering that Mary Fallon was just four feet, 11 inches tall. Not one to stay in one place for too long, James Fallon took his wife to Worcester, where he worked as a foreman for the Boston & Albany Railroad. While in Worcester, the Fallons started their family, and as the family grew, Mary became determined to raise her children in Worcester and to see that they were well educated.

After the Civil War, James Fallon's restless nature drove him to seek work making shoes in Brockton. Mary stayed in Worcester and not only raised the children, but earned the money for their education.

When the federal government was ready to tear down Dale Hospital, she submitted the winning bid for the work. She hired carpenters, bought a parcel of land next to St. John's Church and used the wood from Dale Hospital to build several three-deckers. With the money she collected for rent, she was able to put her son Michael and three of his four brothers through the College of the Holy Cross.

Dr. Fallon was born in Worcester in 1863. After graduating from Holy Cross, he attended Harvard Medical School, one of only three reputable medical schools in the country at the time. After graduating in 1887, he spent two years studying in Europe in the world's finest medical schools — in Vienna, Heidelberg and London — before entering private practice in Worcester.

In the late nineteenth century, at the time he attended medical school, the social status of doctors reflected the whole of society. Doctors who were well educated and attended to the medical needs of the upper class typically were themselves members of the upper class. Doctors who attended to the medical needs of the middle and lower classes were themselves middle class.

Medical training among physicians varied widely. Boards of medical examiners were being established at the end of the last century and qualifications, such as a degree from a reputable medical college, were just beginning to be required. Internships and residencies were still a new idea. Doctors typically went right from the classroom to the operating room and Dr. Fallon was no exception. Study in Europe was the best training available and was a prerequisite for the most successful doctors of the day. Despite his European training, Dr. Fallon joined the staff of a hospital that was created to treat anyone — regardless of class, creed or color. He became an original member of the House of Providence staff, joining as chief of pathology in 1893.

At the time, medical treatment was still very generalized, but surgery was beginning to become an area of specialty. From

1902 on, Dr. Fallon devoted his practice exclusively to surgery, and in 1908 he became the hospital's first chief of surgery, a position he held until his death in 1939.

The importance of that position increased dramatically in 1910, when the sisters announced a change in the hospital's surgical service. By limiting surgical service only to those surgeons elected by the Board of Trustees, the board essentially was making Dr. Fallon the hospital's only full-fledged surgeon, giving him a great deal of power. This change was so "radical," Mother Mary and Sister Mary Isidore, who replaced Sister Ursula as local superior in 1903, wrote in the annual report, that they had "some anxiety and misgivings," and were concerned that "there might come a withdrawal of patronage."

The change ended the practice of rotating surgeons. Previously, many of the city's most prominent physicians — notably Dr. Gage and Drs. Samuel B. and Lemuel Woodward — were able to establish busy practices by rotating between St. Vincent, Memorial and City hospitals at three-month intervals. At the same time, Dr. Fallon practiced almost exclusively at St. Vincent, except for a brief service on the visiting staff at City where, being a devout Irish Catholic, he perhaps was not made to feel welcome. Despite their misgivings, the sisters believed that a dedicated surgical staff would improve the quality of health care at St. Vincent and decrease the work of the nursing staff.

The change in surgical services may have decreased the surgical staff, but it increased the number of surgical cases and helped establish St. Vincent as a widely respected surgical hospital — a status it still holds. Dr. Fallon, his associate, Dr. J. Arthur Barnes, and Dr. William F. Lynch, the house surgeon, operated on 1,546 patients in 1910, performing 781 operations of a magnitude where etherization of patients was required. For the hospital as a whole, the sisters' fear of losing patients proved groundless. The number of patients for the year was 2,244, an increase of 213 from 1909. Among the patients, only 374 were treated by medical doctors and several hundred additional patients were treated for specialized ailments, including diseases of the ear, nose, throat and eyes. Nearly three patients out of four were surgical patients.

✤ ✤ ✤

As an Irish doctor, Dr. Fallon's decision to practice at St. Vincent Hospital is not surprising. Even though his education qualified him for work at the well-established hospitals of Boston, or for treatment of upper-class patients, his working-class, Irish-immigrant roots must have made him feel both comfortable and appreciated at St. Vincent.

Instead of treating the wealthy, Dr. Fallon chose to join the Sisters of Providence in treating people of all classes, and he developed a reputation for being sympathetic and helpful to the poor. As one newspaper account puts it, "It made no jot of difference to him whether a patient ranked low on the social scale and was penniless, or whether he was an important and affluent figure in the community."

In a letter to Dr. Olier L. Baril, a biochemist who established the Fallon Clinic's first laboratory, Dr. Fallon's son John wrote about the 20 years of free medical care his father gave to the Congregation of the Little Franciscans of Mary, the "Gray Nuns" who established an orphanage in Worcester and who later established the St. Francis Home for the elderly. "His idea was that they were immigrants one generation behind him," Dr. John Fallon wrote. "He had seen as a boy the difficulties his family had as immigrants. He wanted to do what little he could — from the high eminence of one generation's difference! — to ease their way."

Like most other offspring of Irish immigrants, Dr. Michael Fallon was a devout Catholic. It must have pleased him greatly when his work with the poor was recognized by the Vatican, and Pope Pius XI honored him with the title of Knight Commander of St. Gregory.

The importance of the Catholic Church to the Fallon family is self-evident. Three of Dr. Fallon's brothers became priests, and an adopted sister became a nun. Dr. Fallon also was active in the church. According to his obituary, "It was his practice to assist at daily mass, and before a major operation he invariably sought the help and spiritual assistance of Divine Providence to strengthen him in the tremendous tasks before him. For years he was seen in pious supplication at the 8 o'clock mass in the chapel of St. Vincent Hospital as a humble communicant of the church." He was active in the Worcester community as well, serving as a School Board member for six years and as a library director.

Although he abandoned his work as a pathologist, he approached his surgical work and, indeed, his entire medical career, in the reflective and probing manner that might be expected from a pathologist. He was driven by the desire to learn the causes of disease because, he wrote, "Celsus said that to find out the cause of a disease often leads to its remedy." Reflecting the emphasis his mother placed on education, Dr. Fallon furthered his medical training throughout his life, always devoting time to learn the latest medical breakthrough. He was both a diligent reader of medical journals and a prolific writer, contributing frequently to the journals of the day. His range of knowledge and interest is apparent even in the titles of his works, a few of which include "The Heritage and the Reckoning of the Surgeon," "What Should Be the Attitude of the State Toward Hospital Standardization?," "Cesarean Section After the Death of the Mother" and "Sepsis."

During his first few years as a surgeon, he traveled to Boston evenings to study at the laboratories of the Harvard Medical School and to practice his surgery on cadavers. Today we can only imagine what it must have been like, being a busy young doctor, yet still making time to travel at night into Boston. How long would the trip take, during the turn-of-the-century horse-and-buggy days?

Although he practiced at St. Vincent Hospital for his entire professional life, he took several weeks every year to study at a medical center, most often the Mayo Clinic in Rochester, Minnesota. Sometimes he left his practice behind for longer periods. In 1900, he spent nine months working and learning in New York hospitals, and in 1902 he performed experimental surgery with Dr. Harvey Cushing at Johns Hopkins University in Baltimore.

Dr. Fallon's long hours of study and work reflected his adherence to the principles of his greatest role model, Louis Pasteur, whose discovery that diseases were spread by germs made the successful practice of surgery possible. Pasteur was passionately devoted to his work, to God and to his wife. His favorite phrase, according to Dr. Fallon, was "Let us work!" Pasteur died with one hand holding a crucifix and the other in the hand of his wife. This romantic and religious scene is idealized in Dr. Fallon's writings. Like Pasteur, Dr. Fallon was passionately devoted to his work, to God and to his wife, Ella.

Ella Fallon, in turn, was ever supportive of both Dr. Fallon and St. Vincent Hospital. She served as the first president of the St. Vincent Hospital Aid Association, which proved to be as important to the hospital's early success as her husband's surgery, and she later played an important role in raising funds for an addition to the hospital.

Dr. Fallon liked to tell the story of the time that a man with an advanced case of smallpox stumbled into his office. By treating his patient, Dr. Fallon exposed himself to the deadly disease and had to seek isolation. As he prepared to leave for the Home Farm, a quarantine shelter known facetiously as "the penthouse," he found Ella waiting for him in the buggy. He told her to get out of the buggy, but she would not budge. She was determined to go with him. She was willing to risk her life for him, just as he had risked his life for his patient. Fortunately, Dr. Fallon contracted only a mild case of smallpox and Mrs. Fallon was unaffected.

When Dr. Fallon decided to become a surgeon, it was not enough for him to read the medical journals and attend classes. He had to learn by doing. And Mrs. Fallon was, as always, ready to help. She even taught him an important skill he could not learn in medical school — she taught her husband how to sew. She chose fabrics for him that best simulated human flesh and helped him establish conditions imitating those of an operating room.

A newspaper account says Dr. Fallon had "a small butter firkin with narrow mouth, and thrusting his fabric down into it, sewed under blind and trying conditions. It was his custom in those eager days always to keep a hank of fabric and needle in a convenient drawer of his office desk, and to practice between consultations. The moment a patient left the room, out would come the 'sewing,' to be as quickly whisked out of sight with the arrival of another."

Dr. Fallon was a pioneer in the use of rubber gloves, calling them "the greatest blessing ever conferred on surgery," and he wrote in his paper on sepsis, "I would not put my finger in the mouth of a patient to examine a tooth unless I had a pair of rubber gloves." Human hands could never be made completely free of bacteria. They could not be boiled, but rubber gloves could. The use of rubber gloves meant a loss of feeling and a new clumsiness in his now-nimble fingers, so he resumed his sewing practice, and added "other exercises which approximated the use of the fingers in the course of major operations," according to the newspaper account. "Throughout his career, Dr. Fallon's work was based upon such scrupulous attention to seemingly small things."

This streak of perfectionism extended even to his use of catgut, which was then used for stitching wounds. He was not satisfied with the catgut that was then commercially available, so he made his own. The records fail to explain where he purchased the raw materials, but he did, and he developed a method of sterilizing the gut with the assistance of Mrs. Fallon.

"They worked out a way to maintain a constant water heat from the boiler of the kitchen range," according to a newspaper account, "and Mrs. Fallon and a woman who lived with them stood watch through the night to insure that the gut was perfect in its sterility."

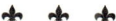

Despite St. Vincent Hospital's growth, the surgical staff remained a three-man staff for many years. Except for doctors who served on the staffs of both St. Vincent and the Fallon Clinic, a group practice started by Dr. Fallon in 1929, the only surgical appointments made during Dr. Fallon's tenure were the 1933 appointments of Dr. Eugene Richmond and Dr. John B. Butts.

Even though the staff was small, it was clearly divided into rival camps. The Dr. Barnes camp included Dr. Richmond and Dr. Butts. Dr. Fallon supporters included, of course, the Fallon physicians. Dr. Lynch initially worked closely with Dr. Fallon, but a rivalry later developed with him as well. Dr. John J. Dumphy, a general practitioner, worked closest with Dr. Fallon, meeting with him at his home for an informal Sunday dinner every week, where they discussed their upcoming cases.

Despite the rivalry, it was clear at St. Vincent that Dr. Fallon was by far the most powerful, and most respected, member of the medical staff. His position on the staff was reinforced daily by the formal processions that accompanied his medical rounds.

When Dr. Fallon arrived at the hospital in his horse and carriage, all activity ceased. The sister in charge rang a bell and an entourage assembled immediately to attend to his needs — one nurse with towels, another with a bowl of water, others to follow his orders, whatever they might be. Staff and nurses dressed in stiff, clean aprons and always wearing their caps, silently accompanied Dr. Fallon, taking notes and following his instructions. Dr. Fallon himself dressed in an immaculate white uniform. A full report, including typed histories of each patient, was expected to be ready and waiting for Dr. Fallon by the time he left the hospital for the day.

Dr. Fallon's procession is remembered by one doctor as being "like a Roman phalanx," with Dr. Fallon at the head of it, and other doctors and staff following behind in descending order of importance. The house officers who accompanied Dr. Fallon hung on his every word. No one dared question his opinion.

The special attention accorded to Dr. Fallon reflects not just a feeling of awe and respect, but the strict sense of professionalism instilled in the staff of St. Vincent. It also reflects social differences that existed in the early part of the century, when people who attained social or professional positions with a great deal of power were accorded a greater degree of respect and special treatment.

As chief of surgery, Dr. Fallon wrote extensively in the hospital's early annual reports. His writing provides insight not only into the medical treatment of the day, but into his own personal philosophy.

Not surprisingly, the largest number of operations in 1910 were for appendicitis, which accounted for 234 operations. At the time, appendicitis was one of the few ailments that could be cured by surgery. Dr. Fallon attributes the low mortality of just two deaths from the 234 operations to the promptness with which physicians sent their cases to the hospital. He also notes, "It is now generally recognized, even by the layman, that the risk in appendicitis is not in the operation, but in the delayed operation."

As if seeking a genetic cause for appendicitis, he notes that 24 of the patients operated on that year had other family members who previously had been operated on. "One patient, a college boy who had appendicitis, said that six members of his family — two of them physicians — had been operated on for appendicitis."

While many patients were being cured of appendicitis at the time, many others were being treated unnecessarily. Since it was one of the few operations surgeons performed successfully, it is easy to see why some doctors may have found cases of appendicitis where it really did not exist. Dr. Fallon noted in 1911 that "successful surgery depends quite as much in refraining from operating on unsuitable cases, as it does in selecting suitable cases for operation."

One problem is that many other ailments at the time created some of the same symptoms as appendicitis, including hernia, cancer of the bladder, pneumonia and even lead poisoning. "Patients having lead poisoning with abdominal symptoms are apt to come from certain communities," Dr. Fallon wrote in 1911, "and the interns, knowing this, are on their guard, so as not to be deceived by them.

"The custom still obtains, strange to say, in some towns of Massachusetts, of using lead pipe for drinking water, and some of the users of this water develop abdominal symptoms that mimic appendicitis. One such patient after examination was sent home. She improved rapidly with treatment, and after the lead pipes in her house had been removed. Another member of her family with similar symptoms went to a distant hospital where a diagnosis of lead poisoning was also made. It was learned that lead pipes were quite commonly used in the town in which they lived, and that a surprisingly large number of the residents of that town had had their appendices removed."

In 1910, Dr. Fallon also performed 42 operations on the gall bladder, another common operation at the time, but one that patients nonetheless were reluctant to receive: "At this writing a patient with cholangitis lies dying in the hospital, seeking relief when it is too late. He was advised by his physician two years ago to have an operation, but refused. In common with all hospital surgeons, we regret the postponement of timely operation in troublesome gall stone cases, and this, often, by the patients themselves."

Dr. Fallon's surgical work went well beyond the standard appendicitis and gall bladder operations. His case load in 1910 included 109 operations for hernia, 18 hysterectomies, nine kidney operations and two cases of Cesarean section, about which he comments: "The operation was attended with less mutilation to the mothers, and with less disturbance in the convalescence than if the delivery had been done with high forceps, or with death dealing instruments. The writer reiterates his expressed opinion concerning this operation: I believe that a timely Cesarean section, properly done, is not attended with much more danger to the mother than is an interval operation for appendicitis; and it offers life to the child. In reality, it is an endeavor to save two lives instead of one."

He reports a 1910 operation in which he removed an ovarian tumor that "looked like a football" from a 77-year-old woman who recovered and was in good condition two months later. And he includes the following report accompanied by a black-and-white photo of a kidney split into three pieces:

"This was in the case of a man, a farmer, who, while picking apples from the top of a 6 ft. ladder, fell and became 'doubled up' with the ladder." After his accident, the man walked several hundred feet and up a flight of stairs before collapsing. The next day, he was driven 24 miles to the hospital. During the fall, the man tore his renal blood vessels in such a way that a "spontaneous closure" of the blood vessels took place "so that in removing the kidney, it was not necessary to tie the renal blood vessels." Had the blood vessels not closed up, the patient most likely would have bled to death. Instead, he recovered after the removal of his kidney.

✤ ✤ ✤

At a time when much of the fundamental medical information available today was still unknown, Dr. Fallon saw the hospital as a "clearing house" for new medical and surgical techniques. Much was learned on the job by trial and error, and there was a great deal of uncertainty about treatment.

In many cases, it appears that some doctors obtained positive results from their treatment based on short-term observations, and that, in some cases, the patients were not actually cured. For example, the early annual reports list many cases of patients allegedly being cured of various types of cancer. Dr. Fallon notes in 1911: "When it is considered that almost one third of all cases of cancer in the human body affect the stomach, it is a lamentable fact that surgical relief is not sought sooner. Cancer of the stomach in the beginning is always a surgical case, and not a medical case, and at times even when it is apparently advanced — even when a tumor is palpable — it can be cured by operation."

He also writes that pneumonia patients, especially young and middle-aged people, responded well to "the open-air treatment," accounting for a "reasonably low" mortality rate of 20.6 percent.

In obstetrics, he notes mixed results from patients with convulsions, and concludes, "It appears to us that excellent results would be obtained if the patients, before convulsions had taken place, were transferred to the Surgical Service for Cesarean Section."

Hernia, he writes, typically was treated with an "astringent injection." Cases where the injection method is used, Dr. Fallon notes, "try our patience and skill more than all the other hernia operations combined." In one case, this treatment so badly damaged a patient's intestine that part of the intestine had to be removed.

In 1911, Dr. Fallon writes that St. Vincent treated 40 typhoid patients during the typhoid epidemic of 1910 and 1911 with a mortality rate of only 2.3 percent. The outbreak was traced to a dairy owner, who unknowingly contaminated his milk with typhoid bacteria. He attributes the mildness of the epidemic in the city "in great measure, to the method of feeding."

"While it is probably true that liberal vicarious feeding in typhoid is more popular today than ever," he writes in the 1911 annual report, "many excellent practitioners still cling to a milk diet. We have been more conservative this year than last, and have used for the most part a more limited liquid diet. The chief objection to milk seems to be that it does not provide sufficient calories. This objection may be met, we think, by giving more milk than is usually given. We gave most of our adults eight ounces of milk every two hours, day and night, and this amounted to three quarts in twenty-four hours. When it is remembered that a normal average adult can maintain body weight on four quarts of milk per day, that given our typhoids can hardly be called 'starvation diet.' The milk was alkalimated with a tablespoon or two of lime water. Between the milk feedings, the patients were given broths, tea, coffee, chocolate, lemonade or water, six or eight ounces. . . . Our patients did not waste, as we have seen many typhoid patients on other diets, and the food described provides sufficient variety for the average sick typhoid case."

The conclusion was that water washes the system of toxins, and that delirium "is some index of toxemia."

Dr. Fallon did not take his surgery lightly. As he notes in the 1911 annual report: "We believe that it is not alone necessary that the patient should be alive after the operation, but also that he be benefited by the operation. An operation is a serious thing — the patient surrenders himself wholly; he allows himself to be made unconscious; to be as putty in the hands of the surgeons and their assistants; fathers give up temporarily their means of livelihood, mothers the care of their families, in the hope of being restored to health. Hence, from the time the patient enters the hospital until he leaves, his welfare and betterment are, and should be, the cause of the greatest solicitude from all who in any way have to do with him. He should be safeguarded by a careful diagnosis; his physical and mental health should be carefully looked into; the surgeon should, after proper study of his case, decide whether he can be benefited by the operation or not."

✢ ✢ ✢

At the turn of the century, as health care was undergoing a tremendous transformation, there was still much disagreement about the cause of and cure for disease. Many people still believed in the magic elixirs available on the market, the nostrums and tonics that purported to cure everything from balding to typhoid fever.

Even among physicians there was much disagreement. One popular alternative to the "regular" medical practice of St. Vincent Hospital was homeopathic medicine, which was founded by Dr. Samuel Hahnemann, a German physician. Homeopathic physicians prescribed to a "law of similars" and maintained that disease was primarily a matter of spirit. They believed people were cured by drugs that produced the same symptoms in healthy people as in sick people, that the effects of drugs were heightened when administered in minute doses, and that nearly all diseases were a result of a suppressed itch.

In 1896, a homeopathic hospital was founded in Worcester and named Hahnemann Hospital after the founder of homeopathic treatment. Despite its openness to all types of patients, St. Vincent Hospital was reluctant to open its doors to homeopathic physicians. As a way to raise money, the hospital's board considered allowing physicians who were not on staff to use the hospital, but it balked at the idea, because open staffing would have allowed homeopathic physicians to practice at St. Vincent Hospital.

"The hospital authorities are frequently asked by members of the medical profession, who are not associated with its staff, if some means could not be devised by which they might send patients to the hospital and have them come under their own direct supervision," Dr. Duggan writes. "This is a matter of very serious consideration on the part of the corporation, and due care should be exercised before answering the question. It must be looked into both from a financial and from a physician's viewpoint."

With a limited means of financial support and no endowment, Dr. Duggan concludes, the opening of services to non-staff physicians might be favored by the hospital board. "On the other hand," he continues, "you must ever remember that all members of the medical profession are not practitioners of the same school. The homeopath and the regular have different systems, and it is oftentimes embarrassing for both to be called into consultation, and which might frequently occur in a hospital, over a patient who was admitted and who would expect all the rights and privileges that the institution should afford."

Homeopathic care soon fell out of favor, as "regular" medical care increasingly succeeded in curing people.

The most important advance in health care in the last half of the nineteenth century was the development of aseptic medical treatment, which recognized the need for a sterile, germ-free environment to prevent the spread of disease and infection. By 1893, many cities were beginning to sand-filter their water and regulate the supply of milk, helping to control typhoid fever and decrease infant mortality. Asepsis affected everything from the milk people drank to the way they dressed. In *The Story of Worcester, Massachusetts,* authors Albert Farnsworth, a teacher at Worcester Academy, and George B. O'Flynn, assistant principal of Providence Street Junior High School, wrote, "As the new century dawned a new attitude toward dress took place, largely instigated by the medical profession, which was turning its attention toward prevention rather than to the cure of ills. It saw in the tight, restricted dress of the day much harm to the body's delicate organs and in the trailing skirts of women, gathering grime and dirt from the city streets, carriers of germs of serious diseases. Likewise, better sanitation in the home was encouraged and hardwood floors with art squares and scatter rugs took the place of the heavy, tightly-tacked carpets. . . . More air, greater light, and better plumbing were advocated. With more comfortable clothing, women began to take greater interest in sport and exercise. . . . The mustache and 'side burns' or whiskers of the men began to disappear because they, too, were unhealthy, and hygiene rather than physiology was taught in the schools."

The need for cleanliness, of course, meant more work for the Sisters of Providence and their student nurses. As Dr. Duggan wrote in 1907: "In the hustle and bustle of the active pursuits of life, one seldom finds time to fully realize the great amount of work that is performed within the walls of a hospital. The strict exactions in the preparation of food for the sick rooms, the absolute degree of cleanliness demanded in the laundered material for use in the wards and private rooms; the careful and painstaking preparation for operations and the complete sterilization of everything that might act as a positive agent in the transmission of poisonous germs; the administration of medicines and the attendance that must be given to the manifold other wants of the patient form only a small part of the daily routine and the performance of which means constant and incessant toil."

For the first time, physicians were taking great care in preparing patients for operations. Preparation for an operation included a tub bath, shaving the area to be operated on, and scrubbing with benzine and iodine. As Dr. Fallon notes, "Patients frequently were wont to say that the preparation for operation was more unendurable than the operation itself."

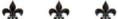

As St. Vincent Hospital grew, so did the services it offered. In 1903, an outpatient department was added to treat the poor. Gynecologists, oculists and aurists participated, charging patients only a small fee for medicine. The following year, the department expanded to include free treatment of the poor in their homes. Eighty-four people were treated the first year — twice that number if people who only had their dressings changed are included.

In 1904, St. Vincent Hospital's first ambulance was donated by Charles Crompton. The ambulance was a sign that the new hospital had come into its own, both financially and as part of the community. The hospital deferred the expense of a new ambulance for many years by using an ambulance owned by the city, but the sisters realized that a growing hospital needed its own ambulance.

"No hospital is complete in its appointments without a proper conveyance for the sick and injured," the sisters note in the 1904 annual report. "The growth and progress of the city, in the last twenty years, has been a source of surprise and wonderment to all of her inhabitants, and, in the minds of thinking men, the question, no doubt, has often arisen as to what would be her resources in the event of any calamity, for the conveyance of those whose condition might demand their expeditious removal to a hospital.

"It is evident to all that the ambulance service of the city would be entirely inadequate to the task."

The new ambulance, which was drawn by two horses and carried a driver, a surgeon and an attendant, made its way up and down Vernon Hill 175 times during its first year. The clatter of the horse hooves on the cobbled streets beat out "the unrhythmical notes of a weird symphony" that caught both the attention and respect of all who heard it, according to *The Catholic Free Press,* which reminisced about the ambulance in 1951, reporting, "It sent first a thrill, then a shudder through everyone who heard it, its effect being much the same as a police car weaving its speedy way through traffic today." The ambulance "spelled esteem, maturity, solvency," according to the account, providing an important sign that the 12-year-old hospital was financially sound.

But the syncopated clatter of hooves on cobblestones was short lived. In 1915, an ambulance was purchased that required no horses to pull it.

Nearly as important as the ambulance to the future status of the hospital was another Crompton family gift — the donation by George Crompton in 1907 of $600 for an X-ray machine. Mother Mary spurred the gift when she wrote in the 1906 annual report, "An X-ray machine would be a valuable aid, but we dare not incur this expense so long as we find the hospital income barely equal to the current expense."

The X-ray machine was a Waite & Bartlett coil-operated machine. It had no meters. Voltage was estimated by the distance the high-tension current jumped across a spark gap. And X-ray penetration was judged by changes in the appearance of a gas tube during operation of the machine. Long exposures were necessary — eight seconds on the hand from 17 inches, 20 seconds on the shoulder and 30 to 60 seconds on the urinary tract. In 1910, the addition of a counterbalanced tube stand, stereoscopic apparatus and intensifying screens reduced exposure time to a tenth of what it had been.

The largest number of the 307 X-ray admissions in 1910 was for fractures. The X-ray machine also was used therapeutically for treatment of skin lesions and skin cancer. Dr. Andrew E. O'Connell, one of the first Fallon Clinic doctors, ran the X-ray department from its inception until 1946.

With the addition of an ambulance and an X-ray machine, it must have seemed at the time that the hospital had everything it would ever need.

A Growing Hospital

"With no compensation other than the bare necessities of life for the exacting and arduous duties which encompass their daily labors, with all these personal sacrifices and more, they surrendered their lives to that great and noble principle, 'For God and Charity.'"

Dr. Duggan on the Sisters of Providence

The Sisters of Providence, the medical staff and the nursing students had become very busy, indeed. Each year, the number of patients at the hospital increased — 1,315 patients in 1906, 1,705 in 1907, 1,712 in 1908. By 1913, St. Vincent Hospital's annual patient load increased to 2,500.

At the same time, the home for the aged was fully occupied, with about 90 patients. The scope of services provided by the hospital also was increasing. By 1906, some women were even going to the hospital to give birth — a previously unheard-of idea. The hospital records note 40 cases of child birth that year. The same year, 31 patients were treated for alcoholism, an interesting note, given that the medical community did not begin regarding alcoholism as a disease until the 1950s.

By 1908, 40 sisters were running St. Vincent Hospital. They were stationed in practically every corner, from the basement to the attic, which served as their sleeping quarters. They truly ran the hospital and expected everyone, including the medical staff, to heed their orders.

Dr. Duggan wrote about the sisters that year, "While some are performing their allotted duties out of vision of the public

eye, in the kitchen, preparing some delicate morsel for this convalescent; in the laundry, whitening the linen for the comfort of
some fever-stricken sufferer; in the pharmacy, dispensing some
potion for the mitigation and assuagement of pain, others are
equally doing their chosen work in the ward, the operating and
sick-room, all united for the accomplishment of the same benefi-
cent end. While in the possession of health and strength it is the
work of their lives."

The public's increasing acceptance of medical treatment, the
reputation of the St. Vincent medical staff and the growing population each played a role in the hospital's success, but the high
regard accorded to the Sisters of Providence also contributed
greatly. The motto "Aegroti Salus Suprema Lex," "The welfare
of the patient is the supreme law," was taken to heart not just by
the medical staff, but by the sisters.

That the sisters were held in high regard is apparent in the
writings of noted Worcester author S. N. Behrman, who grew up
on Providence Street. Behrman, who wrote many Broadway
plays, also wrote a book called *The Worcester Account* about
Worcester during the early part of the century.

Behrman makes note of the "castles" on the top of Vernon
Street, including Worcester Academy, the Crompton estate and
St. Vincent Hospital. After describing Worcester Academy, he
writes: "There was one other great demesne at the top of the hill
— St. Vincent's Hospital. St. Vincent's was not walled. The
great central red-brick building was set in a park. We saw the
nuns scurrying about in this park and they were very friendly.
My mother was always being hospitalized in St. Vincent's and
she died there. She never could say enough in praise of the nuns.
Though my mother spoke very little English, she managed to
become firm friends with many of them. Whenever she came,
they welcomed her. It was a charming consideration on the part
of the nuns that they veiled the holy pictures on the walls — the
Virgins and Crucifixions — to spare the religious sensibilities of
their orthodox Jewish patients."

This religious and ethnic tolerance was echoed by Dr.
Duggan in the 1913 annual report when he wrote, "We have

noticed the son of the Emerald Isle, the Frenchman, the Swede, the Italian, the Englishman and the Polander, the Grecian, Austrian, Hungarian, the Turk and American, the Scotchman, the German and the far off Russian lying side by side in the wards of the hospital, moving us to higher and nobler action in the thought that sickness brings us all down to the same common level of human equality."

Getting patients to come to the new hospital for treatment was one thing. Getting them to pay for treatment in those pre-insurance days was another.

Yet the Sisters of Providence knew how to run a hospital as a business and paid strict attention to cash flow. They understood that to sustain the hospital's growth without the benefit of an endowment, they had to pay attention to collecting revenues and holding down expenses.

The issue of free care and bad debt, which is still so important to hospitals, was addressed frequently by Mother Mary and Sister Isidore in the hospital's annual reports during the early part of the century. In 1906, despite the growth of the hospital, the sisters were finding it difficult to pay off their debts. While Mother Mary strongly believed that God would always provide for the sisters when His help was needed, she also felt compelled to do what she could on her own to control the accounts receivable. She and Sister Isidore wrote in 1906, "Notwithstanding our reluctance to dwell persistently upon our debt, we feel compelled to remind you again that the limited resources of the hospital so cripple our management that the administration of our institution imposes much anxiety and fruitless uneasiness, but we indulge the hope that in the current year an effort may be made to ease the situation, by some means that will reduce the debt, for unburdened by the heavy interest that must be met semiannually, we could make those repairs and add those improvements to the equipment of the hospital, that would enable our medical staff to keep pace with the highest attainments of the profession."

The same year, Dr. Duggan departs from his annual opportunity to praise the sisters and the nurses, and uses his message in the annual report to appeal for aid from the state legislature. His appeal proved fruitless. St. Vincent continued to support itself with assistance from the community.

By 1911, the sisters' tone was less polite and more critical: "In the past year, we have had a very considerable shortage in receipts. The deficit, on account of charity for free and partly free patients, amounted to $2,086. There are worthless bills due the hospital by persons who were admitted at regular rates, but who failed to meet their obligations to the hospital.

"We lay stress on this feature of our resources, because members of the Corporation may sometimes hear that the management of St. Vincent Hospital always exacts payment, and that little, if any charity is extended, but we assure you that it is a governing principle with us, that no worthy person is to be refused, because of inability to pay; that for any who present fair and reliable representation that they cannot pay in full, either on entrance or at the time of discharge, due consideration is made, but we have had experience of a class of persons who seem to study ways and means to elude payment of their obligations to the hospital."

Then in 1913, under somewhat better circumstances, they wrote that among their 2,500 patients "there were many who could not or did not remunerate the hospital for services rendered either in whole or in part; still, this has been compensated for in a measure by the fact that each year the Treasurer's Report has shown a balance on the right side of the ledger."

Almost from the moment the hospital opened, its staff moved from one health crisis to another. The Spanish-American War ended the nineteenth century and gave the hospital a steady clientele of injured soldiers to treat. A diphtheria epidemic hit Worcester in 1906 and the typhoid epidemic followed in 1910. Then came World War I in 1914. Much of the nursing and medical staff contributed to the war effort, leaving the hospital severely understaffed. On the heels of the war came an influenza epidemic that struck in 1918. No wonder there was such a growing demand for the hospital's services!

It was, in fact, World War I that turned public opinion in favor of hospital care. While war ends many lives at too young an age, it also teaches those who participate in it a great deal about life and death. As if to make up for the casualties of war, balancing the scales of life and death by divine intervention, every war seems to end with a giant step forward in medical care. World War I brought doctors from all over the world together on the battlefields of Europe, and they shared their technical knowledge and training. For the sake of efficiency and timely treatment, the doctors fighting in Europe divided into multispecialist groups. After the war, this more efficient, more practical approach to medical care was brought to American hospitals. Medical supplies, many of which were imported from Europe before the war, had to be manufactured domestically during the war because of the unavailability of European goods. American industry responded to the demand. The nursing profession also grew as a result of the war. Nursing schools and government recruitment programs made it clear that patriotic young women should choose a career in nursing. The military mobilization of medical forces that was practiced during World War I was put to effective use at home during the influenza epidemic of 1918. The public observed the progress of America's hospitals and most concluded that hospitals had developed the power to heal.

According to Dr. Fallon, health care during World War I was markedly improved from what it had been during the Spanish-American War. "This was truly a campaign for health," he wrote, "and nearly all of those who were returned to their homes were in far better health than when they enlisted: and they became missionaries for spreading the knowledge of how to acquire and keep good health."

In addition to the constant crises in the world and the community, the early part of the century was a turbulent time in the management of the hospital. The Sisters of Providence, like other religious orders, reassigned the sisters quite frequently, often with no apparent reason or logic. Sister Mary Fidelis Austin followed Sister Isidore as superintendent of St. Vincent in 1914, during the early days of World War I, but held that position for only a short time. Her commanding presence contrasted sharply with that of Sister Mary Agatha McKenna, who managed the hospital from 1915 to 1917. According to Mother Mary, Sister McKenna's "genial, happy disposition and infectious laughter brightened the oft-times overshadowed atmosphere of the hospital."

Sister Mary Consilii, a registered pharmacist and a "live wire" with strong executive abilities, served as superintendent from 1917 to 1926, a time of relative calm, during which the hospital expanded and matured. Like many of her predecessors, she was recognized for her abilities, and she became the third sister superior at St. Vincent to be named mother superior of the order.

Although sometimes stern, Mother Consilii was also diplomatic. Despite the bitterness between Holyoke and Kingston over the split in the order, Mother Consilii managed to reestablish communication with the Canadian order in 1927, 35 years after the Sisters of Providence of Holyoke established their independence. She also approved the return to the order of Sister Ursula. Sister Mary Consilii was replaced at St. Vincent by Sister Mary Leocadia, who served from 1926 to 1937.

Over the same period, management of the School of Nursing was equally tumultuous. Sister Mary Carmelita was replaced as director by Sister Mary of the Immaculate Heart in 1901. Two years later, Mary Clare of the Cross was named director, but in 1905 Sister Mary Carmelita returned to the position, serving until 1909.

The school's most well-known director, Sister Mary Angelica, took over management of the school in 1909, serving until 1916. Sister Mary of the Sacred Heart served from 1916 to 1923, when Sister Mary Angelica returned to the position, serving another six years until 1929, when she was replaced by Sister Mary Camilla. Alumnae of the school created a scholarship in memory of Sister Angelica after she died in 1950, during the 50th anniversary of the School of Nursing. In a 50th anniversary eulogy, she is described as "a well-beloved preceptor" and a pioneer of nursing education. "Unassuming, devoted to her work, and withal, possessing a keen sense of humor and a vibrantly youthful spirit, Sister Mary Angelica was the ideal nurse and teacher," according to the eulogy. "Her sympathy and kindness in the various crises that beset the path of the nursing student are especially remembered by those whom she taught and guided in the arduous tasks of nursing."

The medical staff, meanwhile, held steady with Dr. Duggan serving as president until 1921, when Dr. Fallon added the title, serving as president until his death in 1939.

Changes were taking place within the administration of the diocese as well. In 1920, Bishop Beaven died after leading the diocese for 28 years. The Vatican appointed Thomas Mary O'Leary — a pious, formal, somewhat regal figure — to replace him. The choice pleased most of the nuns.

"He was not a tall, commanding man, like their late bishop," according to *Can Spring Be Far Behind?* "but he had great suavity, the fresh complexion of a child, and he covered a slight lisp by a deep and totally episcopal basso profundo. Of course, most of all, he was known to be for them indeed partial to the Sisters of Providence. His great personal friend was Sister Mary Consilii, a very able woman indeed."

Bishop O'Leary established the practice of maintaining a special suite in the hospital for his overnight use on visits from Springfield, which was not the one-hour trip that it is today. Bishop O'Leary was less involved with the operations of the hospital than his predecessor had been. Perhaps because he realized that the hospital was in capable hands, he did not visit often. With the seat of the diocese in Springfield rather than Worcester, it also is probable that Bishop O'Leary considered Worcester as being a distant second in importance to Springfield and less worthy of his attention. He might come to the hospital three times one month and then not return for a couple of months. But, like Bishop Beaven, he chaired the Board of Trustees, and the sisters always had to be prepared, just in case he dropped in unexpectedly.

A visit from the bishop was always an important event. He was God's representative on earth, and was treated as such. When the bishop left the diocese offices on his way to Worcester, the sisters at the hospital received a call from Springfield, alerting them that Bishop O'Leary was on his way. They prepared as if for a visit from any important dignitary. Everything was clean, and the nuns and nurses were immaculately dressed. The hospital elevator was locked in place as long as a half hour before his arrival, waiting to whisk him up to his suite. The well-polished silver was brought out to serve him his meals. Working in the kitchen, Sister Mary Anna spent much of her time during the winter searching frantically for fresh grapefruit, because she knew the bishop expected it when he came to visit. The grapefruit had to be pink — never white — with slices of onion placed between the sections.

As the bishop walked through the hospital corridors, the sister superior heralded his coming with a bell. The nurses, and even the doctors, were expected to kneel to him and kiss his ring. A retired nurse who was a student during Bishop O'Leary's tenure remembers passing Bishop O'Leary on the way to deal with a medical emergency. She was reprimanded by her superior for failing to stop on the way to kneel to the bishop.

"I figured the patient's life was more important," she said.

Jeanette Couillard, a 1939 School of Nursing graduate, was often on duty on the bishop's floor and had to heed a sign reminding her to be quiet when the bishop was in. She lived in fear that any noise would wake the bishop, and when her bell rang, she answered it immediately.

"He carried quite a bit of authority," Mrs. Couillard said. "Even the priests were afraid of him."

✤ ✤ ✤

In those days, Vernon Hill must have been an impressive sight. Walking up the hill, past the three-deckers and tiny shops, two buildings were certain to stand out. St. Vincent Hospital, with its 100-foot tower and protruding sun porches filled with hospital beds, had become a social center, a source of community pride and a place of awe. But standing nearby, another center of influence and even more a place of awe, was Mariemont.

Mariemont was the home of the Crompton family, owners of what by then had become the Crompton & Knowles Loom Works, a company that was world famous for its looms at a time when the textile industry was thriving. William Crompton patented the Crompton loom in 1837, and his son, George, renewed the patent in 1851 and established the Crompton Loom Works in the area that became Worcester. In 1862, with a growing family and a thriving business, he purchased 11 acres of land on Providence Street from Darius Rice, a descendant of Jonas Rice, the first permanent settler in Worcester, and hired Elbridge Boyden, architect of Mechanics Hall and St. Paul's Cathedral, to design Mariemont. Mary Crompton, the namesake of Mariemont, asked the architect to model the home after Holland House, a famous Elizabethan home in England. Mariemont became the site of many of Worcester's most magnificent social gatherings of the day. Because of their success, the Cromptons were accepted into Worcester society at a time when other Catholics were scarcely allowed to live in the city.

Inside, Mariemont was adorned with marble busts, Indian teakwood furniture and Chinese vases. The grounds included a rose garden with a fountain, croquet grounds surrounded by Chinese lanterns, and a tennis court. Those who grew up around Mariemont especially remember its colorful gardens. The Cromptons were entitled to indulge in a bit of eccentricity, and one section of the grounds became a cemetery for the family dogs. A 1946 article in the *Worcester Telegram* notes five engraved tombstones, dating back to 1899, that mark the graves of Dion D'Or, Spice, Lovelace, Sparkles and Spangles. Some of the gravestones include brief epitaphs. Sparkles', for example, reads: "With my hand upon thy heart, I my benediction said, therefore and forever."

"Walking by it as a little girl, I used to think it was a castle," Miss Collins said of Mariemont. "It was a beautiful place."

Author S. N. Behrman also refers to Mariemont as a castle, and recalls it as a place of great mystery, which, although a central focus of the neighborhood, was still very detached from the neighborhood. Unlike at St. Vincent Hospital, the boys of Providence Street had no idea what went on inside Mariemont. Behrman writes: "Providence Street was crested with castles. One of these was the twelve-acre estate of the Cromptons. It was surrounded by a gray stone wall. Just inside the wall was an unbroken line of tall hemlocks. Above the trees we could see the great central tower of the mansion. The Crompton house was one of the first Elizabethan houses to be built in this country. Its wall braked the teeming life of our street, which came to a dead halt there."

In contrast to the opulence of Mariemont, many of St. Vincent's future doctors were growing up in the early 1920s as the sons of immigrants in Worcester's less prosperous neighborhoods.

Drs. Robert A. Abodeely and Raymond W. Gadbois grew up driving the horse-drawn delivery truck for the Bolduc Market at Suffolk and Wall streets. In addition to their payment, they received the lamb organs that the grocer otherwise would have discarded. They grew up eating sweetbreads.

The neighborhood was not safe, and there were "gangsters on the roads," according to Dr. Abodeely, so he stayed indoors most of the time and read books. Dr. Abodeely recalls that many of the boys he grew up with in "the Worcester slums" became doctors, lawyers and successful businessmen, proving, he believes, that success depends "not on where you come from, but on who your parents are."

✤ ✤ ✤

As Catholics and neighbors of St. Vincent Hospital, the Cromptons were active in the hospital's affairs from the beginning. Mary Crompton, who became president of Crompton Loom Works in 1886 when George Crompton died, was the only lay woman on the first board. Her eldest son, Charles, who was the first person in Worcester to own an automobile, became president of Crompton Loom Works when his mother died in 1895. He donated the hospital's first ambulance. Another son, George, became vice president of the hospital's board and donated funds for the hospital's first X-ray machine.

In 1919, George Crompton proved for St. Vincent Hospital that he had the Crompton family's flair for business. He chaired a fund-raising drive that in a single week raised enough money to pay for a 60-bed addition to the hospital, which was added in 1919.

Although historical accounts provide little detail, the brick hospital built in 1898 was designed to be added onto in stages and was supposed to have a total construction cost of $250,000. Perhaps because of the interruption of World War I, the only addition ever made to the 135-bed "1898 building" was the 60-bed wing.

The crowded hospital apparently tried to expand into Millbury before settling on the construction of a new wing. In the *History of Worcester and Its People* published in 1919, newspaper publisher Charles Nutt wrote, "The work of the hospital has been extended by the purchase of a farm at Millbury, where provision will be made for maternity cases, and for others preferring a hospital in the country. It is known as St. Joseph's Institute." But a separate account, *The Story of Holyoke,* refers to St. Joseph's Hospital in Millbury, where the Sisters of Providence provided care for unwed mothers from 1915 until 1920, when it was destroyed by fire.

To raise funds for the new hospital wing, a 150-person advisory committee was assembled and divided into teams. The committee included many of the Worcester area's most prominent citizens, including local industrialists and clergy. Mrs. Fallon was placed in charge of the women's teams. Taking time off from their jobs from December 1 through 7, the team members canvassed people throughout Worcester County, in some cases starting out at 6 a.m. and not returning until 12:30 a.m. Each day, results of the fund-raising effort were chronicled in local newspapers.

"Worcester folk will sleep sounder at night when they know that sick and injured, who now must be placed in corridors if they are not to be turned away, are to be comfortably cared for because of the additional room made available by the new wing," one newspaper account notes.

While the fund-raising drive was expected to net $100,000, it instead raised more than $150,000. Despite the success of the drive, Crompton remarked, "This campaign was probably more difficult than previous drives, because you did not have behind it the glory of a great war."

The new wing was designed by John William Donohue of Springfield and built by M. J. Kane. Construction was completed in 1921 and more than 600 people came to the opening ceremony for a tour of the new facilities. The opening was celebrated with a whist party and an afternoon tea.

"The rooms are like hotel suites and are richly and tastefully furnished," according to a newspaper account of the day. "Visitors were amazed at the splendor of the interior. It is said there is no hospital in this part of the state that is more modernly equipped. All through the corridors and in the rooms, flowers of the season added beauty." The addition included three third-floor operating rooms finished in Vermont marble, an X-ray department, a pathology department, an obstetrics department, and the capacity for 60 more beds.

The *Sunday Telegram* described the wing down to the most minute detail, including information about the "walnut and bird's eye maple dressers," and the color code by floor for hospital china. "Each floor has a rest room for visitors or patients," the *Sunday Telegram* reported. "The rooms are furnished with dark leather lounging chairs, the walls tinted in rose and gray while artistic paintings adorn the walls. The lights throughout are unique and have been designed after special drawings. Each floor has its serving room, a chart room and a rest room for nurses, as well as ample cupboard rooms, blanket warmer closets, supply rooms and baths."

With the new wing in place, St. Vincent Hospital accommodated up to 180 patients — 15 times the number that the House of Providence could accommodate when it opened just 28 years earlier. But the building continued.

The Human Touch

"I've always been grateful I was a nurse. Those were the happiest days of my life."
Mildred Collins

*M*any of the people who grew up on Vernon Hill in the 1920s and 1930s remember St. Vincent Hospital playing a central role in the neighborhood, rivaled only by the Cromptons' Mariemont mansion.

James Baker, whose grandfather donated the bell for the hospital, got to know the hospital from the inside as well as the outside when he was growing up on Vernon Hill. In 1925, he suffered from a ruptured appendix and peritonitis. He was unconscious for a week and in the hospital for six weeks, and Dr. Fallon gave him "an incision like the Callahan Tunnel." "They thought I was going to die," he said. He was given a room second in size only to the bishop's suite, and he had wheelchair races in the corridor with the other young patients.

Mary Swift, who was born at St. Vincent Hospital in 1914, grew up on Vernon Hill and was trained at the St. Vincent Nursing School from 1934 to 1937, remembers watching the ambulances rushing into and out of the hospital grounds when she was a child. She enjoyed eavesdropping on the St. Vincent nursing students at the neighborhood drugstore when they talked about their work. The hospital itself was a central site, and neighborhood kids used to have their pictures taken next to the statue of St. Vincent.

Like Mrs. Swift, Mary Hanrahan used to watch and listen to the nurses — and fantasize about becoming a nurse herself. "I had only one wish when I was about eight years old," she recalls. "I saw the nurses and I said, 'That's what I'm going to be when I grow up.' " Her wish was fulfilled, and she became one of the most well-known nurses at the hospital.

Another neighborhood girl, Sister Mary Francis, used to have picnics on the lawn at Mariemont after the house was abandoned by the Crompton family. She went to the School of Nursing, decided to join the order after two-and-a-half years of training, and graduated in 1927.

It's not surprising that so many of the Vernon Hill girls grew up to become nurses. At the time, most women had two careers to choose from — teaching and nursing. While the Worcester area also produced a number of women who became doctors, including Drs. Mary O'Callaghan and Clara Fitzgerald, who both served early on St. Vincent's staff, nursing was by far the more typical path to a medical career for a woman.

As the number of student nurses and nuns at the hospital grew, the need for a dormitory and a convent on the hospital campus became apparent. While St. Vincent finally seemed to have ample space to accommodate its growing patient population, many of the Sisters of Providence were still confined to the attic of the hospital. Living conditions were so cramped, many of the sisters and nursing students were forced to live in the Home for the Aged. About 100 nuns and student nurses served at St. Vincent Hospital at the time.

Driven forward by its success, in 1922 St. Vincent undertook another fund-raising effort, resulting in the building of the St. Camillus Home and Our Lady of Perpetual Help Convent behind the hospital at Winthrop and Providence streets. In addition to living quarters for the sisters and nursing students, the new building featured an auditorium, classrooms, a library and laboratories. It was dedicated by Bishop O'Leary on January 22, 1925.

✤ ✤ ✤

From the opening of St. Camillus until the 1950s, the routine for nursing students, and the relationships between doctor, sister and nurse, remained practically unchanged.

The School of Nursing grew, but still remained small enough so that the sisters ran it the way they wanted to run it. With 25 to 50 students at a time in the three-year program, the sisters could train their students carefully, according to the standards of the Sisters of Providence.

There were three types of nurses at the hospital — the sisters, nursing students and private-duty nurses. Until the 1940s, no lay nurses were employed by St. Vincent. Ironically, the students who were training to be lay nurses filled in any gaps in staffing and made it possible for the Sisters of Providence to operate the hospital without the expense of hiring lay nurses. The sisters held all supervisory positions and ran the hospital, even maintaining supervisory control over the medical staff. Detailing the power struggle this relationship sometimes created, *Can Spring Be Far Behind?* recounts: "While the Sisters must recognize what was due to the dignity of the medical profession, they must also, as quietly as was possible, but as firmly as was sometimes necessary, maintain the fact that they, the Sisters, were the owners and administrators of their own hospitals.

"They had particular trouble with the doctors who had worked in public hospitals, and who seemed to have the erroneous notion that they should have some voice in the government of private institutions. They certainly didn't know how to deal with Sisters. They had no idea what the prerogatives of the nuns really were. Gradually, the foundress became convinced that a religious (a nun) must train the physicians to confine their attention to the care of the sick. Beyond that, doctors must not intrude into administration."

The nursing students, the second group of nurses, held only nonsupervisory, nonadministrative positions. They received much of their training on the job and began caring for patients from their first day as students. Classes were secondary and were attended only when the daily hospital work was completed. Some believed that the student nurses were exploited by the nuns, because they were required to work such long hours, and because much of their work was routine and contributed little to their education. But the nurses themselves, while emphasizing the strictness of the nuns, also believed that their on-the-job training provided them the best possible education. While some might argue that emptying bedpans and cleaning the rooms contributed little to their medical knowledge, they also received firsthand experience they could not have gained in the classroom. They learned to be nurses by actually being nurses.

The private-duty nurses were self-employed nurses, who paid dues to have their names listed on a register. When a doctor needed a nurse's assistance, he consulted the register to see who was available. Many doctors had favorite private-duty nurses they became accustomed to working with. Dr. Butts, for example, often called upon Mrs. Swift. Like substitute teachers, the nurses waited to be called. If they were not called, they had no work.

Private-duty nurses were a throwback to the days when people were treated at home instead of in the hospital. They typically stayed with their patients, sleeping on cots in the same room, and gave full attention to their needs until they recovered and were able to fend for themselves. Wealthy patients might even hire more than one nurse if they desired. For example, Cora Crompton, the last of the Crompton family to live at Mariemont, retained two private-duty nurses to care for her. In the mid-1930s, private-duty nurses were paid $35 a week for 12-hour-a-day, seven-day-a-week duty and $42 for 24-hour-a-day duty.

"I did private duty all my life," said Miss Collins, who began her career during the Depression. "You'd do 24-hour duty. I'd be on call for 21 hours, and have three hours off in the afternoon. A medical man would call, you'd come in and sometimes you'd stay for two or three days." She stayed as long as 13 weeks with one patient. Antibiotics were not yet available, so it took much longer for patients to heal. But the lengthy recuperation periods had their advantages, too.

"It was a marvelous opportunity to get to know the patient; to recognize their problems so that I could help the doctor," Miss Collins said. But she also learned to keep the information she learned about her patients confidential. "Whatever you learned at the bedside stayed there."

Despite their differences, the three groups of nurses worked together with the same objective — providing the patient the best health care possible. But there was one type of patient that neither the lay nurses nor the nursing students were allowed to treat. In a Catholic hospital, only the sisters were allowed to provide nursing services to priests and nuns. Student nurses were not allowed to enter the bishop's suite or the room of a priest who was a patient, although, out of necessity, the religious were treated by lay physicians. Each room in the hospital had a light over the door. If the light was on, it meant a religious figure was being treated in the room and that the lay nurses were not allowed to enter.

This taboo caused a dilemma for Mrs. Swift one night when she heard a priest screeching in his room, obviously in great pain. Mrs. Swift couldn't find a nun to help him, and there was no paging system at the time. The priest continued to scream for help, so finally she took a deep breath and entered the room.

At the time, hospital beds did not have crib sides, and patients were pinned into their beds to keep them from falling out. The priest was literally pinned into his bed, with a pin sticking into his side. Mrs. Swift removed the pin, swore the priest to secrecy and made a hasty departure.

While the sisters, private-duty nurses and student nurses worked together, they did not socialize with each other and rarely even carried on casual conversation, even though the sisters and nurses lived in the same building. The sisters, being "in community," were expected as part of their devotion to remain silent whenever possible. Except while instructing or supervising the students, the sisters typically spoke to them only in whispers.

The private-duty nurses were isolated from the student nurses, too, because they spent all of their time with their patients. The student nurses also were allowed only very limited socialization, but typically became close companions among themselves.

Despite their closeness to each other, there was a strict hierarchy among the student nurses. The nurses judged each other by the number of bands on their caps. Three bands, for example, meant a student was in her third year of study. The new students did not wear caps. Probationary students, or "probbies," were at the bottom rung of the nursing hierarchy and were treated with little respect by their fellow nursing students. They were given the worst assignments, and they had to hold open the doors for the "three banders." They had to be subservient to everyone — doctors, nurses, priests and sisters, as well as fellow students. Probbies who managed to last through six months of training traveled to the Sisters of Providence Mother House in Holyoke for a traditional picnic, where they received their caps. The handing out of the nurse's cap is a ritual that some nurses wish had remained part of the hospital.

"It was a big event," according to Mrs. Swift. "When I became the acting director of nursing in 1968, some of the students were removing their caps. We worked so hard to get them, I hated to see it. I told one nurse that a woman patient asked me if she was a maid or a nurse. Nowadays, nurses are wearing everything. Interns come in wearing blue jeans."

The original St. Vincent nurse's cap, which had four corners that stood for faith, hope, charity and pride, was replaced in 1930 by a simpler cap that was easier to launder. At the same time, the traditional blue-and-white-striped uniform, which included a white apron and bib, was replaced by a one-piece white uniform with the hospital's insignia on the left sleeve.

The hierarchical nursing system also changed.

"The 'probbie' system went out when I became a senior," according to Jean McLaughlin, who graduated from the School of Nursing in the 1940s. "We realized it didn't pay to treat them shabbily."

✤   ✤   ✤

The sisters worked hard and expected the nursing students to work hard as well.

"When they got up, they said their prayers, ate breakfast and went to work, and stayed until 9 or 10 p.m., seven days a week," according to Dr. Stanley L. Kocot. "Individuals today don't ascribe to a lifestyle so disciplined in their dedication to their goal. A nurse today typically works 40 hours a week. There was no such time commitment from the Sisters of Providence. It's not what time allowed, it's what they felt that they had to do. The Sisters of Providence set objectives for themselves, then set about meeting those objectives."

The students also were required to work a very full day with almost no time off. They had to rise early in the morning and report to the superintendent of nurses' office "with your cap on straight" by 6 a.m., according to Mabel A. Ryan, who began her nurses' training in 1921. Before reporting, they had to have their rooms immaculately cleaned. Mrs. Couillard remembers losing her privileges a couple of times for having a single piece of paper in her wastebasket.

The day began with 15 minutes of prayer and it was not uncommon for the students and even the nuns to become drowsy from overworking and to fall asleep. The penalty typically was lost time off for the students. The nuns were expected to report their transgressions even if they were not caught. As punishment they typically were required to say extra prayers.

After the morning meditation, they ate breakfast. Lining up for breakfast, they had to pass inspection from Sister Camilla. If a nursing student was wearing lipstick or if she was not wearing a hairnet, she was scolded, and might be required to roll bandages or lose time off as punishment. Day nurses began the day's work by 7 a.m. Twelve-hour shifts were typical. The 7 a.m. shift typically extended until 7 p.m., "and you would be on call until 11," according to Marjorie Sullivan, a nursing student in the 1940s. The 11 p.m. to 7 a.m. shift, likewise, extended until about 8:30 a.m. while the sisters checked to ensure that everything was in order. Training extended practically year round for three years, and students who took sick days had to make them up before graduating. Lights were out at 10:30 p.m. every night "and that was it," said Jane Healey, another early nursing student.

The nursing students received a half day off each week, during which they could spend time with their families. But if a student did something to displease the sisters, she was "campused" and lost her half-day privilege. Even when a half-day privilege was not lost, it was not unusual for a nurse to still have to work until 8 p.m. and she was always required to return to her dormitory by 9:45 p.m.

It was quite easy for a student to displease the nuns and lose her time off for the week or receive some other punishment, like being assigned to roll bandages, or writing, "I will not talk during class" 50 times. Mrs. Ryan recalls one incident when she was campused: "Once when I poured medicine I got some over the label. I had four or five half days taken away."

Nursing students were required to show the utmost respect to the doctors. One student said she was reprimanded because a doctor, who was a neighbor, called her by her first name. The nurses were supposed to rise from their seats when a doctor entered the room. One nurse who went to work at The Memorial Hospital rose from her seat when the doctor entered the room, and she remembered him laughing and saying, "You can sit down. You're not at St. Vincent now."

Recalling that she was once disciplined for returning a half hour late from the White City Amusement Park in Shrewsbury, Sister Mary Francis said, "The Sisters were strict, but still had a sense of humor. As you get older, you realize that to accomplish the things they did, you had to have some discipline."

The nurses rarely were allowed to leave the hospital campus, and when they did, they had to return by 9:45 p.m. at the very latest. The one exception was during the annual alumni ball, when they were allowed to stay out until midnight. Sister Camilla waited for their return and smelled their breath for signs of alcohol when they returned. Anyone who arrived even a minute after midnight lost her privileges for the week.

A nurse's shift was typically filled with work, and the students had to follow the sister's orders to the letter. Mrs. Sullivan said, "When the sisters told you, 'Go down and have lunch, but be back in five minutes,' you only took five minutes."

Like any other group of people, the personalities of the sisters varied widely. Some were very strict, some were more easygoing. The nuns were frequently reassigned, so the nursing students kept a close watch on who was coming and who was going. Every summer the nuns went away on religious retreats, and when they returned, they were given their assignments.

"July 19 was the biggest day in our lives, because that was the day the nuns would be changed," Mrs. Swift said. The nuns were not asked where they wanted to be assigned. One of the administrators in the order simply gathered everyone together, stood on a chair and read off the list of assignments. The nuns carried out their assignments, like them or not, without complaint.

According to Dr. Lambi Adams, the doctors had a great deal of respect for most of the nuns. One nun he remembered was so knowledgeable, "she could pass for a doctor. When she called me and told me there was something wrong with a patient, I came right away."

Nursing was simpler then, but the scope of work was wider. The emphasis was on practical training, not education. Nurses had to complete their morning work before attending class, and quite often it was completed on time, so they missed at least part of their afternoon classes.

Mrs. Swift remembers that the sisters expected everything to be kept clean and free of dust. When Sister Mary George inspected the rooms, she inconspicuously placed a hand on top of the bed frame to see if it was dusty. Even the walls had to be washed by the nursing students.

"We did the spring cleaning, too," Mrs. Healey said. "In those days, you didn't have building service people. We cleaned utensils. We cleaned and sterilized the bedpans, too. And when a patient was discharged, two of us would carry the mattress to the back porch and air it out."

Many of the labor-saving devices that are taken for granted today were not available in the early days. Elevating beds, for example, did not exist, and the nurses had to prop up patients on pillows to make them comfortable or help them to breathe.

Nursing students also had to spend much of their time cleaning and sterilizing supplies so they could be reused. From the beginning, the Sisters of Providence learned to use their limited financial resources wisely.

"We reused everything," according to Clare Weeks, also a nursing student. "It was the saving generation."

Old bed sheets were torn up and made into bandages. Hot-water bottles were patched and reused. The sisters mixed all of their own solutions and medicines whenever possible. Gauze was washed out, resterilized and folded for reuse. Every floor had two syringes and needles, which were sterilized and reused. As a private-duty nurse, Miss Collins recalls that as the needles became dull, they were resharpened on soapstones.

"Almost everything was reusable," added Elizabeth M. White, another nursing student. "We strung catgut for sutures in surgery, and made all of our own dressings. Everything was literally homemade."

Linen was in short supply, so the nurses hid sheets under a mattress to make certain they had enough for their patients. Rubber gloves also were in short supply in the '20s and '30s, so the nurses had to work without them. Instead, when they were working in the operating room, they had to scrub their hands for 20 minutes under barely tolerable hot water. Little money was wasted on medical supplies, but even less was spent on material goods. When it was time to redecorate the nurses' dormitory, the nuns turned the old curtains inside out, resewing them so that previously covered material was exposed, giving the illusion that the curtains were new and clean.

Nurses were taught to use supplies wisely, but they had a further incentive — if a nurse broke anything, she was required to pay for it. The nursing students recall paying for eggcups, syringes, thermometers and other supplies. A couple of the doctors, Drs. Arthur FitzGerald and Raymond Gadbois, were especially good to the nurses and sometimes took the rap for broken or missing equipment, according to Mrs. Swift. Miss Collins recalls an anxious moment when she tripped and broke the glass top on a table. She nervously measured the glass and had her father replace it. "You foolish girl," her supervisor told her. "I was anxious to get rid of that table."

One reason the nuns did not allow the nurses to be wasteful was to teach them a lesson. Dr. Kocot remembers seeing Sister Mary Denise with a team of nurses looking for a missing thermometer. "I asked why they bothered looking for a thirty-cent thermometer. 'That's part of the discipline,' she said. 'We can't afford to make mistakes when we're treating human beings.' "

Mary Darcy, director of public relations at the hospital, said of Sister Mary Denise, "If you threw away a paper cup, you'd have to account for it." It was not parsimony. They wanted to make certain all resources were put to their best use. And, according to Dr. Kocot, they believed that waste was sinful.

During the 1920s, they had to be especially frugal and save to pay off the debt on the new hospital wing, and the new dormitory and convent. From 1926 to 1930, the sisters received assistance in paying off their debt through the formation of a new fund-raising group called the Society of Patrons of St. Vincent Hospital. The society was formed for the sole purpose of paying off the debt, and members were required to pledge $25 a year to become curates and $50 or more a year to be listed as hospital patrons.

The sisters' frugal use of resources served them well long after the debt was paid off. Through the Great Depression and World War II, despite difficult financial times, they saved enough money so that by the end of the war, they were able to plan for a new building. They knew how to save well and invest well, and by the 1950s they saved up $2 million toward financing the new hospital. In those days, $2 million was a very hefty down payment.

What was considered so new at the turn of the century already seemed old and overcrowded by the 1930s. But as crowded as it became, many of the nurses who trained in it recall the old hospital with fond nostalgia. By the very nature of the hospital's crowded condition, the nurses say they were brought together. Ask any nurse who trained in those days and, chances are, she'll refer to the people she worked with as "family."

"Everyone knew each other very well," according to Mrs. Healey. "If there was a function and you had 46 people in your class, 46 participated. That's the way it was then. We did everything together. We were very close."

Although some of the nurses who lived in the neighborhood were allowed to stay with their families overnight, most lived on campus, so the same student nurses were together almost constantly for three years. They had little choice but to do everything together. In addition, they often had to cover for each other and help each other. It was sometimes the only way they could finish all of their work. For most, it was the first time away from their families. They spent every waking hour together, from morning prayer to evening prayer, sharing the events of a new career, sharing the birth of babies and the death of incurable patients. They were, the nurses say, as close as sisters.

Some of the closeness that was part of the old hospital seemed to be lost with the evolution of medical technology and the changing treatment of patients. In the 1930s and 1940s, Dr. Stephen Bergin used to keep his maternity patients confined to bed for two weeks. Today new mothers are typically home a couple of days after giving birth. Patients stayed in long enough for doctors and nurses to get to know them, and the "bedside manner" was as much a part of the treatment provided by some physicians, like Dr. John Meyers and Dr. FitzGerald, as any medication.

"The camaraderie was very good," according to Mrs. McLaughlin. "Now there's a little more freedom, but the new technology has gotten the nurse away from the bedside too much. We rely too much on machines rather than the human touch. We have to get back to the idea that there is a person in that bed who means something to someone. Computers are wonderful, but they can't take the place of the human touch and the human heart."

As the century progressed, requirements for nurses became more stringent, and opportunities increased for trained nurses. In 1911, 39 sisters were admitted to the Massachusetts Board of Registration in Nursing under a waiver, and in 1916, St. Vincent Hospital became a member of the newly formed Catholic Hospital Association. In 1921, the hospital was accredited by the American College of Surgeons. In 1931, the School of Nursing obtained registration with the Board of Regents of the State of New York. In 1936, the School of Nursing affiliated with Worcester State Hospital to provide psychiatric training for its students, and in 1940, it affiliated with St. Luke's Hospital in New Bedford to provide pediatric training.

Although there were no active efforts by the sisters to recruit novices from among their students, some did join the order. Etta Hayes graduated from South High School in Worcester, worked for three years as a telephone operator and began her nurses' training in 1929 with the idea of becoming a secular nurse. After a year of training, she decided to join and became Sister Mary Robert, because, she said, "I saw what dedicated people they were and I was attracted to them."

Doris E. Harrington of Holden, the eleventh child in her family, attended the School of Nursing from 1926 to 1929, then worked for two years as a private-duty nurse. She was often called by Dr. Dumphy. On Christmas Eve in 1931, she accepted Dr. Dumphy's recommendation and went to work for Dr. John

M. Fallon for six months, taking care of his two young children, John Jr. and Michael. Dr. Fallon, the son of Dr. Michael Fallon, was a fellow at the Mayo Foundation from 1927 to 1929, after which he came to Worcester to help his father establish the Fallon Clinic and to work as a surgeon at St. Vincent Hospital.

At the end of her stay, she decided to join the Sisters of Providence. Although she already had a natural sister in the order, "I had no idea at all of entering," she said. She recently celebrated her 60th year in the Sisters of Providence "community."

Although there was never any aggressive soliciting to get lay nurses to join the order, those nurses who spent longer than the required time at chapel might at least be asked it they were interested in joining. Mrs. Swift used to say the Stations of the Cross every day when she was a nursing student. One of the sisters noticed her religious dedication and approached her, suggesting that she consider joining the order. She stopped saying the stations after that.

Because they were granted few privileges, the nurses made their fun wherever and however they could. They enjoyed showing off Dr. John Fallon's specially ordered size 13¹/₂ shoes when he was not around, and some of the nurses were even brave enough to try walking in them. Other nurses sneaked soap to give to Dr. Meyers, who used to sculpt it into animals and figures for them.

But the big thrill for the nurses was the formidable challenge of seeing what they could sneak by the nuns. It was so rare for the nuns to miss anything, the ability to get away with any small pleasure was especially cherished. Finding a way to sneak off campus was always a rare and special thing to do. One trick was to wear street clothing under a nurse's uniform, and to hide the uniform in the bushes around St. Camillus. Many of the nurses seemed to spend a lot of time doing laundry or giving confession — two acceptable reasons for going off campus.

The doors were locked early at St. Camillus, and getting back into their rooms was as difficult as getting out. Mrs. Ryan used to bribe the night security man with snuff to get him to unlock the door for her.

Sneaking out at night also made it difficult to report for the 6 a.m. roll call the following morning. Mrs. Ryan and another student used to answer for each other during roll call so they could take turns sleeping in, but only until they were caught.

Miss White recalls that the nurses used to have to wear bandannas to cover their hair and they were not allowed to wear their hair in pincurls. She tried wearing her hair in pincurls under her bandanna, leaving the few locks that were exposed uncurled, but she was quickly found out. "We tried to outfox them," she said, "but they outfoxed us."

"We were all scared to death of the nuns," added Mrs. Swift. "They got plenty of respect." The first nun she met was Sister Camilla, who served as superintendent of nursing from 1929 to 1936, when she was replaced by Sister Mary Anthony. "Nobody got away with anything with Mary Camilla. I had to do night duty on Thanksgiving, because I didn't go to Mass that morning. I couldn't go to Thanksgiving dinner. But she was an excellent teacher and very fair. You had to respect her. You had to like her."

The nurses were fed little, and what they did eat was not very good, according to Mrs. Couillard, so it was a common practice for them to sneak food into their rooms. Mrs. Ryan's father owned a meat business, and she sometimes used to sneak food in to her room. She was never caught with her extra food, but she did get caught with two food trays, and she lost a half-day off as a result.

"The sisters were very strict," Mrs. Ryan said, "but you learned, and they saw to it that you did."

Mrs. Ryan had particular respect for Sister Mary of the Sacred Heart, who served as director of the School of Nursing from 1916 to 1923. One thing she learned from Sister Mary was the dignity of her profession.

Once, while working as a private-duty nurse, she was called to the home of a member of the Whitin family from Whitin Machine Works, because a family member had become ill with a rare disease and she was one of the few nurses in the area who had experience with the disease.

"In those days," she said, "we were taught by the sisters to take the task at hand, whatever it was." When she arrived at the home, "there were servants of all descriptions. They said, 'You have to use the servants' entrance.' I said, 'I'm a professional. I'll use this door, or I won't go in.' Sister Mary of the Sacred Heart taught me that."

Surviving the Depression

"Three basic principles characterized this foundation: unfaltering trust in Divine Providence, unselfish devotion to the sick, and systematic organization."
Dr. Paul F. Bergin

*E*ven more than today, doctors and nurses during the first half of this century put themselves at risk while treating infectious diseases. Polio, mumps, whooping cough and tuberculosis were still common, and both the defense against them and medical weapons to fight them were paltry by today's standards. Sister Mary Adrianella, who developed tuberculosis while working as a lab technician in the 1940s, considers herself fortunate, even though it took her 10 years to be cured. She realizes that if she had contracted the disease in an earlier day, she would have suffered the fate of many of her fellow Sisters of Providence and died from it.

Diseases like polio and typhoid fever were still quite common, according to Sister Mary Denise, a 1929 graduate of the School of Nursing, but "you never thought about catching it. It didn't bother you."

Even when the nurses were safe from infection, they often suffered socially. People who knew they worked with infectious patients often avoided them to ensure that they were not infected themselves. "I was working with people with TB and no one wanted to be with me," Mrs. Ryan said. "The only one who would be with me was the man I eventually married."

Despite the dangers and the social difficulties, the medical staff went about its work, taking safety precautions, but otherwise giving little thought to catching disease. The staff seemed always ready for the next crisis and willing to offer assistance wherever it was needed. In 1928, when an epidemic of septic sore throat infected practically the entire population of Lee, Mass., many of the students and graduates of St. Vincent made the trip to Lee and offered their help.

In 1927, the School of Nursing affiliated with Belmont Hospital, Worcester's hospital for infectious diseases. The affiliation was discontinued in 1934 but resumed in 1947. In 1935, the school affiliated with Charles Chapin Hospital in Providence, R.I., another communicable disease hospital. The following year, Mrs. Swift was among the St. Vincent students who went to Chapin Hospital. At Chapin she learned a thorough procedure for avoiding infection. The procedure called for careful removal and laundering of contaminated clothing, elaborate scrubbing, and avoiding contact with contaminated items.

"The first lecture we got," Mrs. Swift said, "was, 'If you come down with any disease, it's your own fault. You weren't following our technique.'"

Rubber gloves were becoming more widely used and helped prevent the spread of disease. Clare Weeks, who would become a scrub nurse for Dr. Paul F. Ware, one of the hospital's most renowned surgeons, said that the early "wet gloves" were difficult to use. The gloves were sterilized in boiling water and reused. Even though they were cooled in cold water after sterilization, she said, "sometimes you'd put them on and you got burned."

If, as Sister Denise believes, hospital personnel never thought about catching the diseases they were treating, it may be because they were occupied with other worries. The financial ills of the day spared fewer people than the medical ills of tuberculosis and polio. When the Great Depression struck in 1929, it had a huge impact on both the hospital and its patients.

Virtually all hospitals relied on private donations, so they were hit hard by the Depression. From 1929 to 1930, average hospital receipts per patient in the United States fell from $236.12 to $59.26. Average occupancy fell from 71.28 percent to 64.12 percent, and average deficits as a percentage of disbursement rose from 15.2 to 20.6 percent. With no endowment to fall back on, St. Vincent Hospital had a particularly difficult struggle. The Society of Patrons of St. Vincent Hospital, which was organized in 1926, fell victim to the Depression and disbanded in 1930.

"The Depression was hard, hard times," according to Sister Mary Devota, who was in charge of admissions and billing at the time. "No one could pay their bills. People had victory gardens, and they used to bring in produce to pay their bills."

St. Vincent Hospital weathered the Depression better than many other hospitals, according to some of the nurses who were students there at the time, because the hospital was accustomed to operating on the tightest of budgets. The sisters and students did almost all of the work for no pay, providing a huge savings in labor costs, while supplies and medications were used sparingly.

Sister Mary Leocadia O'Connor advanced from surgery supervisor to superintendent of St. Vincent in 1926, and weathered the Depression in that role until 1937, when Sister Mary Loreto Donovan took over. Sister Leocadia is remembered as being nice to the nursing students, but strict, not unlike many of the other Sisters of Providence. Under Sister Leocadia, St. Vincent faced its greatest challenge. The hospital had survived bouts with typhoid fever, influenza, tuberculosis and other diseases. It had healed the wounded during two wars. But, like hospitals across the country, St. Vincent had to fight hardest for its survival during the Depression.

Despite its own financial hardship, St. Vincent Hospital remained faithful to its motto: "God is charity," and whenever anyone entered its doors in need of medical treatment, the patient was treated. With a sense of pride, Sister Mary Devota, who began working in admitting in 1933, said, "We never refused anyone."

At the time, St. Vincent charged a flat fee of $10 for the use of a room, $5 for anesthesia, $3 for lab work and $2 for medicine, "but people couldn't pay it," according to Sister Devota.

Throughout the country, use of hospital services dropped dramatically; many people simply remained in ill health, because they could not afford medical attention. With less money coming in, hospitals could no longer afford to provide free services to the poor, so they sought reimbursement from welfare departments in what was the beginning of state-subsidized health insurance.

One positive impact of the Depression was that it created a great deal of cooperation between the city's hospitals. By then, Worcester's hospitals included Doctors, Belmont, Memorial, City, Hahnemann, Fairlawn and St. Vincent. They shared many of the same physicians, and "if we didn't have a bed for a patient, we'd call them." They exchanged blood and supplies, and "it was like one big family," Sister Devota said. "Everyone was struggling to survive. It brought everyone together."

Patient bills continued to go unpaid even into the 1940s, although the creation of Massachusetts Blue Cross in 1937 and Blue Shield of Massachusetts in 1941 eventually helped to stabilize health-care financing, for the mutual benefit of both hospitals and patients.

"I don't know how we existed, but we did have food on the table," Sister Devota said. "I remember one poor man was in the office telling me about his bad luck. I said, 'I'll make a deal with you. Give me 50 cents a week.' He said he would give me $1 a week. He was so faithful in paying, when the bill was half paid, Mother Loreto canceled it. There were thousands of bills she canceled."

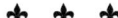

A report from the hospital's annual meeting in January 1936 shows that, despite the Depression, the hospital admitted 5,370 patients in 1935, compared with 5,011 patients in 1934. The total number of hospital days was reported as 61,300. Given that there were 210 beds in the hospital at the time, the occupancy rate for the year was about 80 percent — much higher than the national average. But, as Sister Devota said, the hospital did not turn people away.

The newspaper account of the meeting does not give many financial specifics, but says, "Besides the charity extended to worthy cases, which amounted to $21,467.07, the hospital had a loss much larger than in preceding years, because many patients were unable to pay when discharged." Actual annual reports and records from the era no longer exist, so it is difficult to measure just how deeply in debt St. Vincent Hospital was at the time.

The newspaper account shows that St. Vincent, like other hospitals around the country, was adapting the latest scientific and organizational advances. The hospital installed a central solution room in 1935, where all intravenous solutions were prepared; a central dressing room, where all supplies were sterilized and distributed, and a central linen room. Centralization of these functions freed up the nurses, allowing them to perform their nursing duties more efficiently, according to the newspaper report. Also in 1935, the hospital added its third oxygen tent and a diathermy machine, a physical therapy device that used high-frequency electromagnetic waves to generate heat in body tissue. In addition, the hospital was planning the installation of a deep-therapy X-ray machine for cancer treatment and a cystoscopic table for urology cases.

The medical staff of the day combined many of the hospital's old-time doctors with a number of newer staff physicians who made their mark on the hospital in later years. Drs. Michael and John Fallon were the dominant surgeons on the staff, but the hospital was again allowing consultants to practice at St. Vincent, including Drs. Gage and Lovell from the original St. Vincent staff, and Drs. T. E. McEvoy and David Harrower. Joining the Fallons as full-time surgeons were Dr. Barnes and Dr. Lynch, who replaced Dr. Michael Fallon as staff president in 1936, as well as Dr. James Cole McCann.

Others on the 56-doctor staff included old-timers like Dr. Delahanty and Dr. Brennan, and a number of doctors who are still well remembered today, including Dr. Dumphy; Dr. Richmond; Dr. Thomas C. McSheehy, a general physician; Dr. John W. O'Meara, an orthopedist; and Dr. Gadbois, who was new to the surgical staff that year. In addition to surgeons and general physicians, the staff included obstetricians, a gynecologist, ophthalmologists, pediatricians, neurologists, orthopedists, urologists, a cystoscopist, a roentgenologist, a pathologist and five dental surgeons.

Despite the increased specialization, many of these practices were still fairly new, not too sophisticated and not widely used. Most doctors were still general practitioners. Recalling her work as a nurse in obstetrics, Mrs. Ryan said, "We didn't have many deliveries, because there was no money to pay for deliveries in the hospital and it was not covered by insurance. It was usually done at home by general practitioners. There were not many obstetricians then."

Sister Mary Robert, who started training at the School of Nursing in 1929 and decided to join the order a year later, became an X-ray technician first at Providence Hospital in Holyoke and later at St. Vincent. In her early years, she said, roentgenology was a new science. X-rays were primarily used for the colon, stomach and kidneys, and they were just beginning to be used widely. At the time, the dangers of exposure to radiation were not widely known, so "there were no precautions taken. The only precaution we had during the early days was lead glass around the control room. There were no rubber aprons."

The Great Depression created financial hardship not only for the hospital, but for the Worcester area's first group medical practice, the Fallon Clinic. The clinic was started in 1929, at the beginning of the Depression, by Dr. Michael Fallon. From the beginning, the clinic formed a strong relationship with St. Vincent Hospital. When it started, the Fallon staff was made up of several of St. Vincent's most prominent doctors — Dr. Dumphy, Dr. O'Connell and, as its surgeons, Drs. McCann and

Lynch. Dr. Fallon also convinced his son, John, to cut short his training at the Mayo Clinic to join the new clinic and the St. Vincent staff.

A doctor earned about $3,000 a year during the Depression, which even then was not a rich man's salary. As the Depression worsened, Drs. Dumphy, Lynch and McCann left the clinic to go into private practice, where they had a chance to earn more money. The group was suddenly more like a family, with just the two Fallons and Dr. O'Connell on staff.

The clinic remained small for many years, but did occasionally add to its staff. Dr. James T. Brosnan joined in 1930 and Dr. John Meyers joined in 1936. Both played prominent roles in the history of Fallon Clinic and also left their mark on St. Vincent Hospital.

As with other group practices sprouting up around the country at the time, the model for the Fallon Clinic was the Mayo Clinic in Rochester, Minnesota. Started when William and Charles Mayo joined their father's practice in the 1880s, the brothers later built a huge practice that was successful enough for them to create and endow the Mayo Foundation for Medical Education and Research. Dr. Michael Fallon spent several weeks practically every year studying with the famous Mayo brothers, and his son, John, studied at the Mayo Foundation and was "Dr. Will" Mayo's last assistant before his death. John Fallon even photographed Dr. Mayo's final operation.

The Mayo Clinic's history has strong parallels with the history of St. Vincent Hospital and the Fallon Clinic. The parallels are not entirely coincidental. Dr. Fallon was learning as much about the structure of a medical clinic as he was about medicine from the Mayo brothers. In an essay on the Mayo Clinic's history, Dr. Lynch writes about Dr. William Mayo's support and lengthy relationship with an order of nuns in Rochester, Minnesota. With Dr. Mayo's support, the nuns were able to found St. Francis Hospital.

"The Sisters wished to show their respect and gratitude to Dr. Mayo for his long and valuable service to them and to the community," Dr. Lynch wrote, "so they supplied the funds and the building, and with these went the assurance that they had implicit confidence in his integrity and ability, for they at once appointed him Chief-surgeon, in complete charge of the hospital."

The Mayos became so influential in their community, they even dictated the fares charged by cab drivers, preventing them from taking advantage of doctors who were visiting the clinic.

The Mayo Clinic became not only a model for Fallon Clinic, but a source of new additions to the Fallon and St. Vincent medical staffs. From its origins to today, Fallon Clinic has had a high percentage of Mayo fellows on staff. When Dr. Fallon wanted to add to the clinic's staff, it was not unusual for him to contact the Mayo Clinic to find out who might be available to fill an opening.

After beginning the Fallon Clinic, Dr. Fallon wrote a booklet of instructions for the clinic's house officers, outlining everything from his advice on narcotic dosages to patient diet. His desire to put the patient above all else is evident in his instructions.

"Introduce yourself to the patient," he wrote. "He wants to know who you are as much as you want to know who he is. No vaginal examinations are to be done in unmarried women. Otherwise, feel free to examine the patient to any extent you wish. The only limiting factor is the patient's wish not to be examined. The stated, or even implied, wish of the patient not to be examined is final."

Managing a hospital successfully during the Depression required an even greater than usual adherence to procedures. The procedures existed, as far as the sisters were concerned, to keep the hospital operating as efficiently as possible, and, therefore, as cost effectively as possible.

The medical staff didn't always see it that way. Relationships between physicians and the sisters were almost always professional, and most of the physicians have nothing but praise for the nuns' work. But when the nuns' rules intefered with the physicians' work, the physicians sometimes tried to find ways around the rules, testing the will and the wits of the nuns.

Working in the admitting office from 1933 to 1951, Sister Devota was among those who had to be most wary of the doctors. Admitting, discharging, billing and the telephone switchboard were all in the same area at the time. Sister Devota watched the doctors carefully, even memorized which car belonged to which doctor, so she could look out on the parking lot and be able to tell who was in and who was not in.

From the 1930s on, doctors had an increasing amount of paperwork. It was Sister Devota's responsibility to ensure that doctors who were negligent in keeping their records up to date be kept "in the dog house." They were not allowed to admit new patients. Being a skilled physician or surgeon did not ensure that a doctor also was proficient at keeping patients' records. In fact, some of the busier doctors saw the paperwork as more of a nuisance than a medical necessity. Rather than reform their ways after being turned down by Sister Devota, they sometimes turned their attention to finding ways around her.

"They would deliberately wait until I was gone, and say they had to admit a patient because it was an emergency," Sister Devota recalls. "I used to tell whoever was relieving me not to admit patients of certain doctors, no matter what, but they'd always say it was an emergency." Once a patient was admitted, there was little that Sister Devota could do about it.

Some of the senior doctors often tried to use their seniority. One doctor complained that he could never get a bed for his patients. But his patients, many of whom were highly paid professionals, had many outstanding bills.

Supervising the operating room, Sister Mary Clare also had a challenge keeping the doctors in line. A petite wisp of a woman, she did not back down for anyone. She even stood up to Dr. John Fallon, a huge man with an equally huge practice. It was not uncommon for Dr. Fallon to receive a telephone call after he began scrubbing for an operation. When he returned, she reminded him with a "Scrub 15 minutes!" that he had to prepare for his operation all over again to ensure the safety of the patient.

She scheduled the use of the operating rooms strictly and did not allow the surgeons to deviate from her schedule. She also was strict about not allowing surgeons to schedule "dirty" cases, those in which the patient might spread an infection, early in the morning, because it took too long to clean up afterward, and she did not want to risk spreading an infection from an operating room that was improperly cleaned.

"I had to tell the doctors the rules and the regulations," she said. Even if they already knew them.

As difficult as the Depression was, it did have one positive by-product — the widespread use of group health insurance. The Depression exposed the volatility of the existing health care system, and the financial dangers it posed both to hospitals and patients. Patients could not afford to pay their bills, so hospital revenues dropped dramatically, bringing many hospitals close to bankruptcy.

Before the Depression, health insurance was available to very few people. Insurance companies reasoned that if they offered health insurance, only sick people would buy it. That would drive up the cost and make it prohibitively expensive. In 1929, Baylor University Hospital in Dallas created a group health plan that is credited as being the precursor to Blue Cross. Baylor began by offering 1,500 teachers up to 21 days of hospitalization for a $6 annual premium and soon expanded the program by offering it to other groups in the area. Banding various groups into a pool not only increased Baylor's total premiums, it also spread the risk over a larger pool of people. Recognizing the success of Baylor's insurance pool, other Dallas hospitals formed their own group plans. In 1932, a group of community hospitals in Sacramento went even further and banded together to offer a single group-health-insurance plan.

The American Hospital Association put its support behind the concept of community-wide plans that were underwritten by hospitals and began calling such plans "Blue Cross" plans. In 1934, New York passed a law allowing hospital service plans across the state that were exempt from the reserve requirements of other insurance programs. By 1940, 39 Blue Cross plans insured more than 6 million Americans. By then, millions of Americans were insured by other types of health insurance as well, including group health insurance offered by commercial insurance companies.

In 1939, medical societies in California and Michigan began offering physician-sponsored health insurance through their statewide medical societies. Other states followed suit, forming their own "Blue Shield" plans, usually in association with Blue Cross. Blue Shield was created to provide coverage solely for low-income individuals. In the 1930s and 1940s, physicians still charged patients for their services on a sliding scale. A rich man paid much more to have his appendix removed than a poor man. Blue Shield provided a social program for low-income individuals, while preserving the sliding-scale payment system.

If Once I Fly

"I never did anything to deserve this."
Mother Mary Loreto, on the naming of a shelter for
homeless women and children in her honor

$\mathcal{W}$hile the decade was financially difficult, many of St. Vincent's most well-known and well-respected doctors and administrators served at the hospital during the 1930s. Among the most widely known and remembered was Dr. James Cole McCann.

Born in Bangor, Maine, the son of Dr. Daniel and Mary Cole McCann, James McCann was an accomplished violinist and debater during his high school years, and he served as president of his class for four years. He attended what was then called Georgetown College in Washington, D.C., finishing the four-year premedical program in three years, even though he took time out to be commissioned as a second lieutenant in the Army reserves. He then attended Harvard Medical School and served as an assistant professor of anatomy after graduating in 1924. After completing his surgical internship at Carney Hospital in Boston in 1926, he served as a fellow in surgery at the Mayo Clinic from 1926 to 1929, and at the same time earned his doctorate at the University of Minnesota. During his surgical training, he researched peptic ulcers and the physiology of the stomach.

While at the Mayo Clinic, Dr. McCann accepted Dr. John Fallon's invitation to join him in practice at the Fallon Clinic and he naturally joined St. Vincent's surgical staff at the same time. He stayed at the Fallon Clinic for only a short time, but he remained on the St. Vincent staff for many years. In 1936, he received a medal of honor for his medical contributions from Georgetown University, which was celebrating its 175th anniversary.

While at St. Vincent, he was appointed to the council of the Massachusetts Medical Society and, as a council member, he organized Massachusetts Blue Shield in 1941. Dr. McCann served as the first president of the organization, filling the post until 1953. He became a nationally known expert on Blue Shield, and presented papers on the organizational problems of Blue Shield before state medical societies in Maine, Connecticut and California. He also was appointed to the National Committee on Medical Service Plans to advise the AMA, which was establishing a permanent organization for medical service plans.

He was appointed an assistant surgeon at Tufts Medical School in 1949, and he established an affiliation with Tufts that became one of the first fully approved four-year surgical residency programs in the New England area. Serving as chief of surgery at St. Vincent from 1954 to 1963, Dr. McCann was instrumental in transferring the affiliation to Georgetown University in 1954. He also was a cofounder of *Worcester Medical News.*

A skilled researcher, Dr. McCann published numerous papers on phlebitis, peritoneal diseases, and diseases and surgery of the stomach. His most well-known research was on the physiology of a patient's respiration while under anesthesia. His work on the subject was presented at three successive meetings of the International Congress of Anesthesia in New York and before the scientific section of the California Medical Society.

Although his organizational and research skills were considerable, Dr. McCann is best remembered for his surgical skills. A technically accomplished surgeon, he pursued his profession with a passion. According to Sister Devota, Dr. McCann "had the most skillful hands God ever made." Once he had a patient with a tumor that accumulated 32 pounds of fluid. If the tumor broke, the patient would have died. "He removed the tumor without breaking it. It was marvelous." The tumor became something of a local attraction, wondrous to behold, and people came from throughout the hospital to see it.

His hobby was sailing and he spent most of his free time at the Corinthian Yacht Club in Marblehead. Those who knew him say he applied the same sense of balance and care to his surgical and administrative responsibilities that he applied to steering his sailboat.

"He was in the forefront when it came to reviewing your work," Dr. Robert Blute, who joined the St. Vincent staff as a urologist in 1955, said. "He brought new standards of quality control to the hospital. He established a tissue committee, so that every tissue removed was examined by a pathologist to determine whether the surgeon had made an accurate diagnosis."

Dr. McCann "was not fearful of having his work examined minutely," according to Dr. Blute. "He had that confidence."

Mrs. Swift remembers Dr. Richmond as another skilled surgeon who took his work seriously. Dr. Richmond began operating during the early days of St. Vincent and stayed for many years, becoming president of the medical staff in 1954 when the new St. Vincent Hospital opened. "He used to wear leather heels, and you could hear him coming down the corridor," Mrs. Swift said. "Everyone would dive when they heard him coming. He was a very, very strict person, but a tremendous man. I idolized him." The thick leather heels that were a trademark of Dr. Richmond may have been worn to make him appear taller.

During an operation, Dr. Richmond maintained total silence — and he expected everyone else to as well. He believed that an operating room was not the proper place for conversation of any kind, even if the conversation related to the work at hand. When he wanted a certain instrument, he let the nurses know which instrument he wanted by using a special sign language he developed, and God help the nurse who mistook the sign for an "alice" clamp as the sign for a "kelly" clamp.

Being a Catholic hospital in a community with a large population of Irish immigrants, it is not surprising that, during the 1950s, St. Vincent had several doctors from Ireland on staff. Culture and language differences sometimes caused miscommunication. One Irish doctor drove down the wrong side of Vernon Street, though it was not the wrong side to him. One day while Dr. John T. Howard was on duty, Dr. Richmond called with a very sick patient. An Irish doctor told Dr. Richmond that Dr. Howard was "at the theater."

"What do you mean, he's at the theater?" Dr. Richmond replied, none too calmly. The Irish doctor explained that "the theater" is what he and his fellow Irishmen called the operating room.

Dr. James M. Morrison, an internist who came to St. Vincent after World War II, recalls Dr. Dumphy as having the respect and admiration of the entire medical staff. The library in the current hospital is named in his honor. With his soft-spoken, unassuming manner, those who didn't know him wouldn't know that he was considered to be among the city's best doctors.

Dr. Morrison recalls hearing how one night when Dr. Dumphy was on call, he went to the home of a patient who had pain in her legs. The next morning, the patient's husband called his regular physician, and said, "I think that doctor who went out to see my wife really didn't know what he was doing. All he did was take out a tape measure and measure her leg." The doctor's reaction was "Look, you had the best damn doctor in Worcester examining your wife." Dr. Dumphy had silently measured the patient's leg, because that was the common test for phlebitis.

Dr. Lynch, who served as president of the medical staff from 1936 to 1943, is remembered for testing the nurses and keeping them attentive. After an operation, when the nurses had to account for every piece of equipment to make certain nothing was sewn up inside the patient, it was not uncommon for him to hide a sponge by stepping on it, making it difficult for the nurses to account for everything.

His strictness in the operating room was balanced by the warm feelings he held for the sisters. Sister Mary Denise, who trained in the School of Nursing from 1926 to 1929 before entering the order, recalls that Dr. Lynch was especially fond of the nuns and brought them each a bag of penny candy when they left for their religious retreats in June and July.

Like his father before him, Dr. John Fallon is the most well-known and widely remembered St. Vincent doctor of his day. The only child of Dr. Michael Fallon, he was in many ways a reflection of his father. As a child, John Fallon sometimes followed his father during his rounds. He witnessed his first operation when he was nine, and, according to legend, already decided by then that he would be a doctor.

John Fallon never attended grammar school. Instead, he was privately tutored. After a couple of years at The Bancroft School, he began attending St. John's High School at the age of nine and graduated when he was 13. Ella Fallon was none too pleased to see her 13-year-old boy coming home from the senior banquet smoking a cigar.

He went on to attend Holy Cross, walking to school every day from the Fallon home at 9 Portland Street in downtown Worcester. In spite of his heavy course load, his father insisted that he be in bed every night by 8 p.m. Graduating from Holy Cross College in 1919 at the age of 17, Dr. Fallon went on to Harvard Medical School and then to the Mayo Foundation, where he served as a fellow from 1927 to 1929. While at the Mayo Clinic, Dr. McCann introduced him to his sister, Kathleen, and they were later married. Kathleen Fallon died giving birth to her second son, John Fallon, Jr. John Fallon's first son was Michael F. Fallon II.

When his father needed his help to build the operation of Fallon Clinic, "Dr. John," as he was frequently called, cut short his fellowship and returned to Worcester. Serving as a surgeon and director of the new Fallon Clinic while also performing surgery at St. Vincent Hospital, he sometimes operated side-by-side with his father.

Like his father, too, John Fallon was a prolific writer. "When I was a student, there was only one doctor from Worcester who was consistently in the *New England Journal of Medicine,*" Dr. Blute said. "That was Dr. John Fallon. His reputation was outstanding. He was well known outside of Worcester."

His essay on surgery as a career became especially well known. It is a memorable essay, not only for what it reveals about the occupation, but for what it reveals about Dr. Fallon. In the essay, he notes that "the romantic picture of the surgeon is about as close to life as that of the detective. Surgery overflows with romance. And the surgeon you would want for your own operation is no flashing figure, cutting boldly, saving you by prestidigitation just before you 'die on the table.' In some 20,000 operations I remember seeing only two patients 'die on the table.' Sometimes the patient dies later unless the operation is bold, swift, maybe inventive. But operating is more precision and caution than courage."

About the attraction of surgery, he writes, "There is something snobbish about distinguishing between professions and jobs. The surgeon shares with the machinist, the sculptor and other skilled tool-handlers a pride unknown to the executive, the confidence man and similar wit-workers. This is the third greatest reward of surgery and to the intellectual it may seem adolescent. But to the fellows who use the tools it brings a solid, masculine satisfaction. A mechanical imagination is desirable for surgery: the gadgeteering cast of mind helps solve the unprecedented at the operating table. But this is mental, not digital, and fingers which are all thumbs at your stage, after practice and Demosthenic tricks such as blind-folded (no, not on patients) or at the bottom of a bucket may make the best surgical hands.

"The second reward of surgery comes from working in a rapidly advancing field. Journals, meetings, clinical trips and the generous comradeship of surgeons bring new windfalls of knowledge to save today the patient who yesterday was hopeless.

"For that is the surgeon's first reward: saving life and stopping pain." He ends his essay concluding that "of the ordinary ways of life open to ordinary folks, only one other than surgery, I believe in my prejudice, offers such demonstrable results in this world. And that, one, motherhood, is closed to you and me."

Reflecting his own "mechanical imagination," Dr. Fallon also was an innovator and a "gadgeteer." It was not unusual for some surgeons to adapt instruments to suit their needs, but Dr. Fallon was particularly inventive, developing, for example, facile strippers for use in oral surgery. Once, when he had a cold that he did not want to spread to his patients, he carried out his work while wearing a breathing apparatus from his volunteer fire department.

While many of his attributes came from his father, his interest in fires and fire fighting came from his mother, who, when he was a baby, took him out in the middle of the night whenever there was a fire. John Fallon became a member of the Shrewsbury volunteer fire brigade, an honorary member of the Worcester fire department, and, according to *Mayovox,* a publication of the Mayo Clinic, he was "the proud possessor of a badge which let him get within scorching distance of any blaze." He owned a Model T fire engine, which he used to drive children around in during hospital picnics. The fire engine featured a "S.K.F.D." insignia across the hood, for "Shoozelberry Kids Fire Department," Shoozelberry apparently being a frivolous variation of Shrewsbury, where he had converted an old inn for his home.

Dr. Fallon had many other interests, as well. He was interested in mountain climbing, skiing, sailing, swimming and photography. He was a pioneer in the use of photography in teaching medical and surgical techniques. When he died, he was editing a book called "Handbook of Medical Photography."

Dr. Fallon also was active with the Salerno Club, a group of Mayo staff and fellows interested in medical history. He kept his father's collection of medical books and added to it, later donating many of the most valuable books to the Mayo Clinic library. He was somewhat discriminating in his book collecting, explaining that "medical books are not evergreen — but deciduous, and there are many brown leaves." Among Dr. Fallon's medical books was a collection of poems written by physicians, reflecting his own interest in writing poetry when he was a student at Holy Cross. In one of his college poems, he wrote:

Emotion is a churning main,
Why leave the rock-bound shores of brain?
  A footless periwinkle be,
  When God let me swim the sea!

But science is a firm, safe ground,
And you would sail the moon around!
  I would soar, if soar I may,
  A mile above our earthly clay!

But you may fall, and falling die,
  What matters that, if once I fly.

In 1931, Dr. Michael Fallon suffered from "a shock," according to a newspaper account, and stopped operating. He did not retire, even though he was slightly paralyzed, but he left more of the control of the clinic to his son. Dr. Michael Fallon "kept on until he was weaker than the patients he saw," according to Dr. Olier Baril, staying on as president of the medical staff until his death in 1939, just short of his seventy-third birthday. Dr. John Fallon later confided to Dr. Baril that his father suffered from cancer for the last 15 years of his life.

By the time his father died, "Dr. John" was a powerful man at St. Vincent Hospital. He had replaced his father at the top of the St. Vincent hierarchy and maintained a great deal of control over the hospital's surgical procedures.

His leadership role was not entirely inherited. He is remembered as a highly skilled surgeon with a commanding personality. As a surgeon, his distinguished career led to his appointment as a fellow of the International Society of Surgeons. He was a diplomat of the American Board of Surgery, fellow of the American College of Surgeons, president of the New England Obstetrical and Gynecological Society, and president of the Mayo Foundation Alumni Association.

He was shy and soft-spoken, but he had a way of getting people to follow his direction. According to Dr. John A. Duggan, a pediatrician and former president of Fallon Community Health Plan, Dr. Fallon "could talk a dog off a meat wagon. He would invite people to his home and they'd end up weeding his garden for him."

With his father's death, Dr. John became increasingly busy. Having taken over sole leadership of The Fallon Clinic, he oversaw the clinic's move from the Slater Building in downtown Worcester to 10 Institute Road in 1946 and its continuing growth for five years after the move. An old Tudor home that previously belonged to Ella Reed Lawton, the new Fallon Clinic office was renovated and adapted for diagnostic work.

At one point, Dr. Fallon became so busy, he had green tags placed on the charts and on the doors of his patients so he could keep track of which patients were his.

The idea caught on, and the senior members of the medical staff soon adopted their own colors. The colored tags became a sign of status. Fallon Clinic doctors Brosnan, Meyers and John J. Manning were put on "the green service," while Dr. Charles Whelan had yellow tags and Dr. McCann had purple tags to identify his patients. Dr. Joseph Hurley, the medical doctor who replaced Dr. Dumphy, had blue tags and allowed his friend Dr. Ware to share the color.

Mother Mary Loreto, who became the superintendent of St. Vincent Hospital in 1937, achieved a level of prominence at least equal to that of anyone on the medical staff.

Practically anyone who worked at St. Vincent Hospital between 1937 and 1963 has been in the office of Sister Mary Loreto. Her door was always open, and anyone who had a problem was invited to share it with her. The odds were good that she would solve it.

When Dr. Blute first came to Worcester, he saw the need for a new cystoscope, a piece of equipment for examining the bladder. Cystoscopes cost about $900 each then and would cost several thousand dollars today. He went to see Sister Loreto and told her what he needed and why.

"I expected a long session and figured it would have to be discussed by a committee," he recalled. "But when I was through talking, she said, 'Fine.' She called the purchasing agent, who called the company that manufactured cystoscopes and two days later it was there."

Another time, Dr. Kocot was with her when she heard a nurse screaming in the admitting area and stopped her work to see what had happened. The nurse panicked because a small child had vomited on the floor. Sister Loreto took off her apron, wiped up the mess and said, "Sister, that's all it takes."

The matter-of-fact demeanor with which she cleaned up the mess was a trademark of Sister Loreto, whether the mess was big or small. At the apex of her career, during the building of a new hospital in 1954, Sister Loreto showed such calm control that *The Catholic Free Press* wrote, "No one would have guessed from her unwearying smile and quiet patience that Sister Mary Loreto, hospital superintendent, has certainly been under more pressure and been responsible for more decisions during these last several months than any woman in Massachusetts, no matter what her post."

Those who knew her say that an administrator like Sister Loreto could not exist today. When someone asked her opinion, or asked for something for the hospital, she weighed the facts, made a decision and was done with it. In today's regulatory environment, she would be an anachronism.

"I don't think we have anything comparable today," Dr. Blute said. "She didn't have a lot of committees to do things. When something had to be done, she just did it."

The nurses say she was supportive of the nurses, the doctors say she was supportive of the doctors, and the nuns say she was supportive of the nuns. She also saw to it that, for the first time, interns had a place to live and were paid for their work. She is remembered as being fair, open and intelligent. And, while time has a way of building a legend, it is generally acknowledged that nothing ever happened at St. Vincent Hospital without Sister Loreto finding out about it.

Born in Pittsfield, Massachusetts, in 1893, she began her nurse's training at St. Luke's Hospital, which was operated by the Sisters of Providence in her home town. In 1920, during her training, she joined the order. After her two-year novitiate, she completed her nurse's training at Mercy Hospital in Springfield. While she is remembered as having served as a scrub nurse to Dr. Michael Fallon, her initial service at St. Vincent was brief. She worked as an anesthetist then as a nursing supervisor, and in 1930 she became the administrator of Farren Memorial Hospital in Montague City, the smallest of five hospitals then operated by the Sisters of Providence. A couple of years later, she served at Providence Hospital, then in 1937 she was appointed superintendent of St. Vincent Hospital.

She served as superintendent for a quarter of a century — longer than anyone else in the hospital's history. Sister Mary O'Leary, one of two sisters still at St. Vincent, believes Sister Loreto "never, never had an unhappy day at St. Vincent. She hated leaving here. This was her home."

When she did leave in 1963, it was to become Mother Loreto as the major superior of her order, a position she held until 1969, when she became coordinator of planning and development for Mercy Hospital. Among her many honors, she received a fellowship from the American College of Hospital Administrators in 1951, and was named Outstanding Catholic Woman of the Year for the Worcester Diocese in 1954 by the Diocesan League of Catholic Women. When she was named Woman of the Year, *The Catholic Free Press* commented that "she has borne the title for many years, but until now without public recognition." A past winner of the honor, Elise A. Rocheleau, characterized Mother Loreto as having the three qualities necessary for leadership and a religious life: "Sister has first, that unremitting perseverance which is the root of an administrator's genius; secondly, detachment, which is the heart of religious life; and third, faith, the leveler of mountains."

Mother Loreto was awarded an Honorary Doctorate of Laws Degree from Our Lady of the Elms College in Chicopee before her retirement in 1973. In 1983, the Loreto Shelter in Holyoke, a shelter for homeless women and children, was named in her honor.

Mrs. Darcy, who served as both her director of public relations and secretary in 1960, remembers Mother Loreto as someone who "took to heart any sadness in peoples' lives." When her mother was in the hospital dying of cancer, Sister Loreto sat with her at her mother's bedside after her mother died. "It was a comfort to have her there," Mrs. Darcy said. "It meant a lot to me."

Another time, during general conversation, she mentioned that her husband had a serious chest condition. Sister Loreto went to Dr. Ware, the hospital's noted chest surgeon, and made certain he was the physician to perform a bronchoscopy on her husband.

"She was never one to go against anyone. If you complained about someone else, she'd hear both sides of the story," Mrs. Darcy said. "She had an awe about her. I can't think of anybody in the hospital who didn't love and respect her. She was a real presence in the hospital. She was a role model for all of the other sisters. The medical staff thought that there was nobody else like her."

Joseph M. Monroe, the chauffeur for the nuns from 1937 to 1976, remembers that a few years before she left St. Vincent, Sister Loreto asked him to give her a driving lesson while they were visiting the Mother House in Holyoke. At the time, it was unheard of for nuns to drive.

"She wanted to see what it was like," he said. "I let her drive around the grounds. She was very careful, but she did all right. She was good at anything she tried."

Mother Loreto made such an impression on those she met, she is still remembered today. Typical of her impact is a story told by Dr. Kocot, who, as chairman of the fund-raising committee for St. Vincent Hospital's new amphitheater in 1983, approached each member of the medical staff and asked for a donation. Although his fellow doctors were mostly generous, one long-time physician was reluctant to give.

"I'm through donating," he told Dr. Kocot, and it was clear he meant it.

But Dr. Kocot kept asking and eventually, to rid himself of Dr. Kocot, the physician agreed to tour the site, a former convent that was being converted to an amphitheater and library. Dr. Kocot no sooner guided him into the lobby, when he realized that the physician was no longer by his side. In the lobby was a portrait of Mother Mary Loreto Donovan. When Dr. Kocot turned around, he found his missing companion standing in front of the portrait. "There were tears in his eyes, and he said, 'Why didn't you tell me her portrait was here?'" He immediately made a generous donation.

CHAPTER EIGHT

World War II and Beyond

"World War II was a bad war, but for medicine is was good. A lot was learned from the tragedy of war."
Elizabeth White, 1948 graduate of the School of Nursing

*D*uring Sister Loreto's early years, before World War II, the practice of medicine was still primitive by today's standards.

"It was brutal," according to Dr. Robert Abodeely, a Boston University graduate who served an externship at St. Vincent in 1938 and an internship in 1939. When he began his medical career, doctors were treating tuberculosis by placing maggots on patients' joints. Some of the younger doctors, who were pushing for changes, encountered resistance from some of the old-time members of the medical staff. When, for example, Dr. Oscar Feinsilver warned that an overabundance of oxygen in oxygen tents could push a patient into oxydosis, many old-time doctors were reluctant to accept the use of meters to measure oxygen levels.

While some in the medical profession were slow to accept change, a new era in medical care was thrust upon them almost overnight by the bombing of Pearl Harbor in 1941.

Out of necessity, medical care changed dramatically during and after the war. For the first time, the federal government provided major subsidies for private medical research, with tremendously successful results. Great advances were made in brain surgery, cardiac surgery and even maternity care. American researchers learned how to mass-produce penicillin. They developed atabrine, a synthetic substitute for quinine in the treatment of malaria, and they developed various useful blood derivatives.

Diseases like yellow fever, dysentery, typhoid fever, pneumonia, tetanus, malaria and meningitis were no longer fearful killing diseases. American doctors advanced their medical knowledge through research that was necessitated by the war. In some cases, they even learned from captured German soldiers. Through X-rays and examinations, they learned how Germany was treating its soldiers. Where World War I's advances were primarily in surgical techniques and the organization of multispecialty medical practices, World War II's breakthroughs were medical. By one estimate, more than half of the drugs in use in 1947 were discovered in the preceding decade.

Unlike in past wars, disease was not the greatest enemy. During World War I, the disease-related mortality rate was 14.1 for every 1,000 soldiers. During World War II, it was 0.6 percent. In other words, the likelihood of a soldier dying from disease was more than 23 times as high during World War I as it was during World War II.

The most dramatic change was the widespread use of penicillin. In 1942, after the discovery of penicillin, there was only enough available to treat a single case. By the end of the war in 1945, there was enough penicillin for virtually all medical needs. While St. Vincent Hospital's cautious procedures prevented infection from being widespread before the war, the use of penicillin further protected the patient and ensured a rapid recovery.

"We used penicillin for everything," Mrs. Couillard recalled. "All we did all day long was give shots of penicillin. The speed of the healing process improved and people were cured faster."

The result was shorter hospital stays. While before the war it was typical for a patient to spend two or three weeks in the hospital, after the war, it was not unusual for a patient to be home in a week. The one disadvantage to the shorter hospital stays, according to Mrs. Couillard, is that when patients stayed in the hospital longer, "you got to know your patients better."

✣ ✣ ✣

Many of St. Vincent's doctors and nurses responded to the war effort, leaving the hospital even shorter than usual on staffing and supplies. It was left to the leaders of the medical staff to decide which doctors served in the military and which doctors were indispensable to the continued operation of the hospital. Dr. Lynch appointed a board of doctors to determine which of their fellow doctors should have their names referred to the draft board.

While the draft left the hospital short on doctors, the war spurred an increasing interest in nursing, and the School of Nursing grew. A Golden Jubilee history of the school from 1950 says: "The School answered the nation's need by educating more nurses and cooperated with the United States Cadet Nurse Corps, the first class of Cadets entering in June 1944. During the war, the Alumnae corresponded with and sent gifts to their fellow nurses in the armed forces."

The war had little effect on the older, established doctors, but many of the house officers and younger doctors were called to serve. Dr. Meyers was drafted in 1942, six weeks after his daughter was born. He wasn't assigned to combat duty, though he might have preferred it to the assignment he was given — testing pilots. That meant flying with "gung ho 18-year-olds" to find how well they flew, according to Arlene Lian, his daughter. Some of them didn't fly all that well.

"It was nothing for them to let the plane straight down," Mrs. Lian said.

It didn't help that, even before his assignment, Dr. Meyers had a fear of flying and a fear of heights that he developed while painting fire escapes for his father as a boy in Brooklyn.

After five years in Texas at Maxwell Field and Ellington Air Force Base, Dr. Meyers was ready to stay on in Texas, even after the War ended. But "Dr. (John) Fallon got wind of it and went down physically to bring him back," Mrs. Lian said. Because of his fondness for New England and Dr. Fallon, he was persuaded.

Dr. Daniel Kaplan spent three years as an Army doctor in the South Pacific, and found that "it was terrible being a medical doctor during the War. There was so little to work with." He treated his patients with aspirin and not much else. He became a patient himself after developing malaria in Guam and had to spend six weeks recuperating in Hawaii.

Dr. Morrison interned at Memorial, then became a resident at St. Vincent Hospital in 1945, shortly before the end of World War II, and was soon called into the U.S. Navy.

"Doctors were being taken out of civilian life for the war, so there was a great need for house doctors," he said. There were none at St. Vincent and hadn't been any for a couple of years. St. Vincent was using residents who were moonlighting from other hospitals, and independents in private practice.

"There was really a shortage of manpower," according to Dr. Morrison. "Everybody in medical school wondered whether they would be taken out. It was a really upsetting period." Finally, the military took over the medical schools, and, "there was such a shortage of doctors that emergencies were not being properly handled."

After the war, Dr. Morrison had to go back into the Navy for duty with the Fleet Marines in China. He had a six-month-old baby, and his wife had active tuberculosis and was being treated at Belmont Hospital, a hospital in Worcester for the treatment of infectious diseases. Because of his wife's illness, he was able to get his orders changed to the Naval Hospital in Portsmouth, New Hampshire. Soon after, his wife was discharged and they lived in Portsmouth for two years.

"I like to say I fought in the Battle of Hampton Beach," he quipped.

During the war, those doctors who stayed behind had plenty of work and their practices prospered. But many of the doctors who served had to begin anew. Some found difficulty locating office space; others found it difficult to build up a base of patients. Those doctors who served in World War II banded together to form the Maddox Society, named in honor of an American ship that was sunk during the war. A Worcester doctor, Dr. James Dunn, was among those who went down with the ship.

"When we came back," Dr. Kaplan said, "you couldn't get a car, you couldn't get office space. The doctors who didn't go into the service had an unfair advantage, and it took a while to get started up again."

During and after World War II, Dr. John Fallon continued to be the most active surgeon at St. Vincent Hospital. Dr. Fallon was a surgeon with the U.S. Public Health Service during World War II.

Dr. Fallon's career at St. Vincent Hospital and The Fallon Clinic proved to be as illustrious as that of his father, but not nearly as long. It ended abruptly on a warm summer day in 1951. Dr. Fallon was at a hospital picnic at Knowles Park driving the children around in his antique fire engine on the day he died. Dr. Morrison remembers, "He drove the kids around at the picnic and had his coronary that night. He made his own diagnosis. He said he had chest pain and had given himself a shot of Demerol® and he called Dr. (John) Meyers."

When he died, Dr. Fallon was just 49, but he lived his brief life fully. Like his father, according to *Mayovox,* he had a "deeply religious spirit." And like his father, he held the title of president of the St. Vincent medical staff when he died.

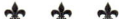

In the 1940s and 1950s, hospitals, like other business organizations, were very hierarchical, and, as president of the medical staff, Dr. Fallon was at the top of the hierarchy.

The structure of St. Vincent's surgical staff changed with Dr. Fallon's death, but remained very hierarchical. Six senior surgeons controlled the department — Drs. McCann, Richmond,

Gadbois, Butts, John J. Manning and Charles Whelan. New senior surgeons were appointed only when an existing senior surgeon retired or died.

Senior surgeons were assigned for two months at a time in the emergency room, which was then an important source of patient referrals. During the 1950s, each senior surgeon had a resident and an intern assigned on a rotating basis to help him with his work. As new surgeons were added to the St. Vincent staff, they were assigned to work with the senior surgeons. Dr. James McCann, Jr., for example, was assigned to his father; Dr. John T. Howard, now president of the medical staff, was assigned to Dr. Gadbois, and Dr. Robert A. Johnson, a neurosurgeon, was assigned to Dr. Manning. The senior surgeons had a great deal of authority over the other surgeons.

Senior surgeons also had control over the operating rooms. Operating rooms were assigned to specific senior surgeons on specified days, and junior surgeons could not operate until the senior surgeons they were assigned to completed their work.

This hierarchical system was not confined to the surgeons. Medical doctors and specialists also followed a distinctive pecking order. While some doctors helped junior staff members to establish their practices, others required complete obedience. One senior physician, for example, did not allow his junior staff member to enter a room before him.

Conversely, the structure of Fallon Clinic changed dramatically after Dr. Fallon died. When Dr. Fallon was alive, he was the sole owner of the Fallon Clinic. His staff worked not just with him, but for him. With Dr. Fallon's death, the remaining Fallon Clinic doctors, Drs. Brosnan, Meyers, Manning and M. Elizabeth Fletcher, resolved to keep the clinic running and reorganized the group practice into a partnership. They also resolved to run the clinic in as democratic a fashion as possible. Each of the four doctors purchased an equal share in the clinic from Dr. Fallon's widow, Frances Fallon.

"Democracy was practically an obsession with them," according to Dr. Robert Phaneuf, who joined the Fallon Clinic as a urologist in 1963. "Everybody came in as an equal partner."

Dr. Brosnan, whose parents emigrated from Ireland to Lowell, joined the Fallon and St. Vincent staffs after completing his residency at St. Vincent in 1934. He became president of the medical staff at St. Vincent and director of Fallon Clinic when Dr. Fallon died in 1951 and he replaced Dr. Dumphy, who also died in 1951, as chief of the department of medicine. An internist, Dr. Brosnan specialized in both gastroenterology and cardiology, and he headed St. Vincent's cardiology department from 1951 to 1968.

Dr. Brosnan is remembered as a father figure by Dr. Massarelli. He was "a nice guy who couldn't say 'No'," according to Dr. Massarelli, who remembers Dr. Brosnan calling someone into his office who had been fired. She came out smiling. He ended up giving her a raise.

He may have been good natured, but he also did not hesitate to make an unpopular decision if it was in the best interest of the hospital, according to Dr. John F. Stapleton, the hospital's first director of medical education.

For example, he changed the "apprentice" system to benefit interns, even though the change was unpopular with St. Vincent's medical staff. Under the apprentice system, the intern was matched up with a doctor and stayed with him from case to case for the duration of his stay at St. Vincent. The doctors liked the system, because they had a "personal escort" to do their bidding, Dr. Stapleton said, but "there was too much variation between the way the doctors treated them. To be assigned to a bad teacher was the kiss of death." Dr. Brosnan instead developed a system where each intern was assigned to a group of beds, so that the intern worked with several attending physicians.

Dr. Brosnan also was instrumental in organizing St. Vincent's medical training program and in hiring specialists in fields that previously were not represented on the medical staff.

Dr. Brosnan "knew we needed to have some of these specialists," according to Dr. Stapleton. "It was a concept a lot of the medical staff didn't like, but he had the bigger picture in mind."

Dr. Brosnan was a 49-year veteran of St. Vincent and Fallon Clinic and was still practicing in 1979 when he fell down a flight of stairs while attending a communion breakfast at Boston College, his undergraduate alma mater. He died as a result of his injuries. Eulogizing Dr. Brosnan in the *Worcester Medical News,* Dr. Meyers writes: "I came here in 1936, as Jim had, a stranger to Worcester, and a fellow alumnus of Boston University Medical School. From the first day, he offered his friendship and support, and was my first real personal mentor. He literally paved the way for me for a career in this community. His friendship, once given, was steady and secure, as it was for everyone upon whom he lavishly gave it."

Continuing, he writes that Dr. Brosnan "was ever mindful of the great privilege conferred on him as a member of an honored and exalted profession. He never ceased to strive to deserve this reputation as a physician."

Unlike Dr. Brosnan, Dr. Manning was pretty tough, according to Dr. Massarelli. One day when the lights went out during surgery and Dr. Ware had to finish an operation with the help of a flashlight, one of the nurses was heard to say, "Thank God it wasn't Dr. Manning." His tremendous technical facilities, especially in performing abdominal or gynecological surgery, made him an equal of Dr. McCann, according to Dr. Massarelli, but "he was a really old-fashioned surgeon. He was supremely self-confident and not tolerant of fools."

Dr. Manning, a resident of Spencer, served as director of Fallon Clinic from 1953 to 1968, overseeing much of the clinic's expansion during that period, and he succeeded Dr. Fallon as chief of surgery at the clinic. A native of Sioux City, Iowa, Dr. Manning graduated from the University of Notre Dame and received his medical degree at the University of Pennsylvania Medical School. He served as an intern at Milwaukee County General Hospital, and like so many other Fallon and St. Vincent doctors, he received his surgical training at the Mayo Clinic.

He served as president of the Worcester District Medical Society in 1973.

Dr. Fletcher, who also was trained at the Mayo Clinic, succeeded Dr. O'Connell as the Fallon radiologist in 1947. An avid deep-sea fisher, Mrs. Fletcher caught more than two dozen tuna 500 lbs. or larger and, during the 1970s, she held the record for the largest tuna ever caught by a woman.

The Fallon doctor who is best remembered, though, is Dr. Meyers, who, in addition to serving as president of the medical staff at St. Vincent Hospital, is the most influential person in the history of the Fallon Clinic next to the Fallons.

Dr. Meyers was such a fast learner, he skipped several grades growing up as a child in Brooklyn. In high school, he often was called on to teach math and science classes — when he wasn't skipping school to sneak into an opera at the Metropolitan Opera House. He attended Boston University Medical School and left six months early, in 1937, to accept an internship at St. Vincent Hospital, because he needed the $25 a month internships were paying at the time.

As an intern, he caught the attention of Dr. John Fallon when he disagreed with the diagnosis of a patient made by several other doctors. Dr. Fallon realized that Dr. Meyers, not the more experienced practitioners, had made the proper diagnosis.

Dr. Meyers was "a tremendous role model for all of us," according to Dr. Joseph A. Podbielski, president of Fallon Clinic and The Fallon Foundation, Inc. "He had an incredible relationship with his patients, a great bedside manner. He didn't miss anything. His practice was so huge, he built the practice of many young doctors," including Dr. Podbielski.

Because of his heavy patient load, Dr. Meyers began his day at the hospital by 6 a.m. One reason for his early start, according to his daughter, Mrs. Lian, is that he knew that if he approached his patients early in the morning when they were still groggy, he could make his rounds more quickly. Despite his early morning start, Dr. Meyers often worked late at night as well. He often relaxed on a recliner, listening to music. After a 15-minute nap, he returned to work, as refreshed as if he had a full night's sleep.

Dr. Meyers also was a devoted family man, according to Mrs. Lian, who remembers accompanying her father during his rounds or when he made house calls. Depending on how sick the patient was, she often waited in the car while her father tended to patients.

As busy as he was, Dr. Meyers maintained an uncanny ability to stay current with the medical literature, according to Dr. Podbielski, but where he really excelled was as "a visionary. With the idea of prepaid health care vs. fee-for-service, he was ahead of his time."

"Visionary" is a strong word. But Dr. Blute goes even further, calling him a "medical prophet," while Dr. Kocot remembers him as "a monumental individual as a medical philosopher."

Dr. Meyers' first great insight was to convince the Fallons, shortly after World War II, to look past their love for surgery and to expand Fallon's practice into a comprehensive care clinic. They followed his advice and the clinic grew.

Much of the widespread praise for Dr. Meyers comes from his development of the concept of a health maintenance organization, or HMO, in the mid-1960s. The idea of prepaid health care had been tried on a very small scale before. Worcester's St. Elizabeth Hospital was just one 19th-century example. But Dr. Meyers' ideas were much more sophisticated and included the concept of managed care.

"A physician-directed system can make the best judgment about the kind of care the patient receives," Dr. Podbielski said. "Managed care allows us to place the patient in a quality fashion, in a proper setting, from acute care through home health care. It's a seamless delivery system. The primary care physician is the quarterback. He directs the patient's care, determines where the patient goes, who he sees."

In the mid-'60s, the idea of a prepaid managed-care plan seemed fantastic. At the time, others in the medical community thought that traditional indemnity health-care coverage would be the standard form of medical insurance for many, many years. But it also was a time of great change in medical care. Medicare was created in 1964, and the health-care industry became more heavily regulated than ever before, on both a state and national level. Medical technology advanced dramatically and people began to live longer. Under Dr. Meyers' guidance, Fallon Community Health Plan was established to begin studying the idea of an HMO in 1970, in cooperation with Massachusetts Blue Cross and, initially, St. Vincent Hospital.

Congress passed the Health Maintenance Organization Act in 1973, attempting to develop and standardize HMOs. Fallon received several grants to study and then to establish an HMO with Blue Cross. The Fallon Community Health Plan finally was established in 1977. It proved to be tremendously successful.

"When we began," Dr. Podbielski said, "we figured Fallon Community Health Plan would be 5 to 10 percent of our business. It's now 90 percent," and Massachusetts has passed every state but California in its frequency of use of HMOs. Today Fallon Community Health Plan has 170,000 subscribers, and 230 doctors working at 22 sites, and continues to grow.

Dr. Meyers' bedside manner is almost as legendary as his medical philosophy. A calm man who never lost his temper, his combination of intellectual skills and people skills made him a natural leader. According to Dr. Kocot, "There was almost something ethereal about his relationships with his patients."

According to Sister Adrianella, "He gave you a sense of security just walking through the building."

He also had other skills and talents, and was an accomplished sculptor, shaping wooden busts of Christ, tiny animal figurines and other objects. He took up sculpting when, as an intern between patients, someone handed him a bar of soap that he shaped into a figurine. Today many of his sculptures can be found in Fallon Clinic's offices, and in churches and synagogues.

"Sculpture became almost a form of prayer for him," according to Mrs. Lian. "If he was under a lot of stress, or if one of us was particularly ill, he'd do a piece of religious art and give it to the church."

A religious man, Dr. Meyers converted to Catholicism with his friend, Dr. Rudolf J. Utzschneider, but later attended not only Catholic services at Our Lady of Good Counsel in West Boylston, but Jewish services at Temple Emanuel in Worcester.

He also became an accomplished violinist — at the age of 75. Although he studied the violin as a child, he disliked it and gave it up at an early age. Having later developed a great appreciation for music, he decided to take violin lessons after the death of his first wife, Anna. He approached Nelia Hopkins, a teacher of concert violin.

Amazed at the prospect of teaching a 75-year-old man to play the violin, she asked him, "What do you hope to accomplish?"

"Within a year, I hope to be first violinist for the Boston Symphony Orchestra," Dr. Meyers replied, completely serious.

"Then we'd better get started," she said.

Although he lacked the stretch and nimbleness in his fingers necessary to attain professional status, Dr. Meyers did become very proficient within a year. In 1992, he was preparing to give a recital when he became ill with liver cancer and died.

In the post-War years, Vernon Hill was poised for dramatic change. St. Vincent Hospital and its neighboring Mariemont mansion symbolized the change that was taking place.

Mariemont had stood in glory, a resplendent monument to the Industrial Revolution, when the House of Providence was still too humble, too in need of care to be called a hospital. But as kind as time was to one institution, it was unfriendly to the other. The busy healing in one contrasted, as the twentieth century progressed, with the stillness in the other.

"After the death of George Crompton," Behrman, the playwright, wrote, "his sisters lived in the house, but no one ever saw them. The place was still; no sound ever came from it. But walking back home, brushing the wall as we passed it, stopping at the gates to look through the grill at the tree-lined walk that led to the great, many-windowed house, we could populate it at will from the story books we had been reading in and out of school."

Through the 1920s and 1930s, Mariemont increasingly showed its neglect. The five Crompton sisters died, one by one, and the house deteriorated rapidly as the family dwindled. George Crompton, in a book about his boyhood home, wrote: "A house is a living thing, and changes as human beings change." Indeed, by 1946, Mariemont had entered a less-than-graceful old age, a crumbling reminder of its former greatness. The once-beautiful gardens were overgrown with brush, the only living thing that remained at once-fair Mariemont.

At the same time, St. Vincent Hospital continued to grow and was soon so crowded, patients were being treated in the corridors. In 1952, 12,938 patients were treated. In 1953, 13,505 patients were treated, stretching the resources of the aging hospital to the limit.

But the fate of these two monuments that were neighbors for so many years was about to intersect. A newspaper account of April 30, 1940 announced Bishop O'Leary's purchase of the 12-acre estate for a price "in the neighborhood of $35,000 and transfer included the 37-room mansion, the powerhouse, laundry, greenhouse and stables." In 1947, Curtin and Riley of Boston was hired as the architectural firm to design a new St. Vincent Hospital.

With the razing of Mariemont and the construction of a new hospital on the land, the rise of one institution and the fall of the other was complete. Dr. Stuart R. Jaffee, who grew up in a three-decker a block away from Mariemont, said, "I never thought when I was a kid that I would ever go through those hallowed stone walls. Now I have a parking place there. And the stone wall is the only relic left."

Despite the purchase of the land, plans to build the hospital were temporarily put on hold. From 1947 to 1950, work was at a standstill, and there were rumors that plans for the new hospital had been abandoned. But the diocese had other business to tend to that proved to have perhaps an even more dramatic impact on the future of the hospital and of Worcester — creation of a new diocese and the appointment of a bishop.

CHAPTER NINE

Ambassadors of Good Will

"The task that I have appointed you is to go out and
bear fruit — fruit which will endure."
John 15.16

Francis P. Murphy, managing editor of the *Worcester Telegram,* usually left his office by 10:30 p.m., but, acting on a tip, stuck around past midnight on the evening of January 31, 1950. He was rewarded with what turned out to be a tremendously important story for the city — important enough for Murphy to play it ahead of President Truman's decision to approve development of the hydrogen bomb.

Following episcopalian tradition, news was released at midnight that a new diocese would be created in Worcester, and that Auxiliary Bishop John J. Wright would be consecrated as the first bishop of the new diocese. Murphy's staff scrambled, scooping *The Evening Gazette,* Worcester's afternoon newspaper, and on the morning of February 1, 1950, Worcester County residents woke up to read about their first bishop. Not everything in the late-breaking, first-day coverage was accurate. Reporter Jack Deedy, who had been a stringer for *The Boston Globe* when he was a student at Trinity College in Dublin, just happened to have covered a visit from Auxiliary Bishop Wright to Ireland and recalled his interest in baseball. Twenty-five years later, when Deedy had gotten to know the bishop better, he wrote that then Cardinal Wright "wouldn't know a baseball from a Hubbard squash." But other characterizations, including Deedy's description of the new bishop's informal, approachable style, captured the essence of the new bishop quite accurately.

✤ ✤ ✤

Despite having one of the largest Catholic populations in the northeast, with more than 100 churches and missions, Worcester remained without its own diocese throughout the first half of the century, a secondary presence in the eyes of the church to the smaller city of Springfield.

All of that changed quite completely with the consecration of Bishop Wright as the first bishop of the Diocese of Worcester on March 7, 1950. Just 40 years old, he was the youngest bishop in the United States. And quite likely, the most gifted.

Recalling the huge outpouring of people who turned out to celebrate his installation and the creation of the diocese, Cardinal Wright later wrote, "In no small part it was sheer friendliness on the part of our neighbors, as well as an outpouring of the faith of our own people, the faith and openness of a people who will take everyone who is sent in the name of the Lord." Out of local pride, Cardinal Wright wrote, Worcester residents welcomed their new bishop and even presented him with a bell and siren for his car, "so that I could get all over the place in no time for anything and everything."

By tradition, Bishop Wright did not visit Worcester before his installation, so when he came to the city, he had "no hook on which to hang cope and miter," according to Deedy's account. Because the new diocese did not have a bishop's residence yet, Bishop Wright moved into the three-room bishop's suite at St. Vincent Hospital that had been used by Bishop O'Leary. Even though it took the new bishop just a month to find a separate residence, it was not uncommon to find him in his suite at St. Vincent throughout his nine-year tenure as bishop.

It is difficult to overstate the effect Bishop John Joseph Wright had on St. Vincent Hospital — and on the city of Worcester.

He brought people of all faiths together and made the city a community. As reporter Jack Tubert wrote in the *Worcester Telegram* at the bishop's death: "Until Bishop Wright came here in 1950 to create the diocese of Worcester . . . it was a city of West Siders and East Siders; the Village and Greendale. Old Yankees and cut-glass Irish. Protestant, Catholic and Jew. Each worshipping in pious houses of worship — but never together. Never as one. Break bread together? Throw mental stones instead."

Bishop Wright galvanized the community, transforming Worcester into "a community united in God," according to the Reverend John T. Murray, a radiologist at St. Vincent Hospital in the 1950s, who gave up his medical practice to join the Jesuits while Bishop Wright served in Worcester. According to Father Murray, Bishop Wright attracted a lot of young people to the priesthood.

From its inception, St. Vincent Hospital accepted everyone, regardless of faith or ethnic origin. Bishop Wright went even further. He reached out to everyone. Saul Seder, the first Jew to sit on the Board of Trustees of St. Vincent, said Bishop Wright showed respect for all religions. "Being Jewish didn't matter to him," Seder said. "He always required that kosher foods be served to patients who were orthodox. He always gave Jews the option of having the cross taken out of their room."

He considered himself to be bishop of every soul in his diocese. While Worcester County had a sizable Catholic population of 300,000 at the time, Bishop Wright later wrote, "I worked on the principle that I had been sent to the more than 500,000 persons in Worcester County (the entire civil population) and that each of them had some claim on me as the Catholic bishop. . . . The future was left to God with open minds and no hand was turned against us and every ethnic and religious group helped us become a pulsating part of the Heart of the Commonwealth."

Bishop Wright is remembered as a man of extraordinary intellect and nearly superhuman energy. One newspaper recounts that "parish priests who worked under him were astounded at his ability to recall whatever he read or saw. He could skim through a letter dropped on his desk in a glance, and then ask that the author correct a grammatical error halfway down the page."

He typically slept only a few hours a night and he used virtually all of his waking hours productively. It was not unusual for Bishop Wright to walk the corridors of St. Vincent through the early morning hours, visiting the patients. Many a priest was called at 3 a.m. with an idea or sudden inspiration that struck the bishop.

A poem, written for the laying of the cornerstone to the new hospital, includes the following verse about Bishop Wright:

> We worry about him quite a lot,
> He does so much, never seems to stop,
> A heavy schedule he does keep.
> When — oh when — does our Bishop sleep?

Despite his intellectual gifts, or perhaps because of them, Bishop Wright could communicate with anyone on any level. At a time when patients with contagious diseases were shunned even by many hospital employees, Bishop Wright was often found playing cards with patients who were stricken with polio or tuberculosis. He also took a special interest in the unwed mothers and mothers-to-be at Marillac Manor, which he helped to establish across the street from St. Vincent Hospital. Marillac Manor was a favorite project of Bishop Wright. Much to the despair of their doctors, Bishop Wright frequently brought the young pregnant women lasagna dinners and boxes of chocolates.

Bishop Wright was both cordial and unassuming. "He was a bishop, but didn't want to be treated like a bishop," according to Mrs. Healey. He was so down-to-earth, in fact, that those who did not know him would hardly mistake him for a bishop. Two days after starting his internship, Dr. Kocot was with another intern who stopped by a water bubbler to take a drink. A person in front of him who was dressed in a T-shirt turned and said, "Hello, doctors." Dr. Kocot responded with a "Hello, Mac," and the man chuckled. He later found out that "Mac" was the bishop, and that he was wearing a T-shirt because he was staying in the bishop's suite.

"He'd sit down with interns and residents and have a cup of coffee," Dr. Kocot said. "He didn't ask why you needed something, but, 'What do you need to make this a better hospital?'"

His sister, Margaret Wright Haverty, described Bishop Wright as being "a normal boy," but his fascination with St. Joan of Arc, which began when he was in sixth grade, hints at intellectual accomplishments to come.

"When the soldiers were coming home from World War I, they stopped near his school and his teacher released his class to see them," she said. "They sang something about Joan of Arc, and he asked his teacher who Joan of Arc was. She told him, and the next day she brought him in a book about Joan of Arc. He took it home and read it that night. He was fascinated. From then on, he collected books, music and memorabilia about Joan of Arc everywhere he went, all over the world."

Collecting Joan of Arc memorabilia, he said, was his "substitute for cigarettes." Judging from his collection, he might have become a chain smoker. His 6,000-volume collection, which was donated to the Boston Public Library in 1976, is believed to be the world's largest collection outside France of memorabilia about St. Joan of Arc.

"Sometimes," he said in an interview published by the Pittsburgh Bibliophiles, "I am asked the reason for this strange veneration on the part of a bishop for someone who died at the hands of a bishop — condemned as a witch, a heretic and a sorceress. My reply is now automatic: what saint could be more appropriate as a reminder to a bishop to be very careful when passing judgment, particularly where conscience is involved and where the alleged heretic is appealing over his head to the Pope?"

His quick wit and active mind are legendary and can only be hinted at in a few of his comments, which are gleaned from his speeches and interviews.

On criticism of the church by sociologists using computerized statistical information: "No computer is so omnicompetent that a baby crawling on all fours can't pull out the plug." He said he hoped to live long enough "to see the last sociologist fed into the last computer, which will then self-destruct in five seconds."

On a crisis in priestly identity, in a speech before a congress of priests: "I am almost afraid to declare what I often suspect it is: a preoccupation with the kingdom of this world and a forgetfulness of the life to come . . . It may well be that the faith of our fathers is burning still — but that does not explain most of the healthy tans we see among us."

On professionalism in the hierarchy of the church: "There are those of us who believe that professionalism, despite all its virtues, can ruin religion more quickly than sin — at least if the sinners have contrite and humble hearts."

On the use of expensive cars by the clergy: "I never learned how to drive and the only cars I owned when in America were ostentatiously inexpensive, except for a year's fling with a Jaguar in which I was nearly killed. It had desks, lights and a telephone so one could work on the road. On what might be called 'state occasions,' local undertakers always proved kind."

Dr. Robert Blute remembers Bishop Wright for his wit and humor as much as for his intellect and accomplishments. During one committee meeting, after hearing one doctor deliver a report on increasing incidents of patients falling out of bed and another delivering a report on the need to reduce the length of hospital stays, Bishop Wright responded, "You have two committees going in opposite directions. One committee is trying to get patients back in bed and the other is trying to get patients out of bed. These two committees need to get together."

He also placed great importance on education and on doing whatever was needed for the hospital. When the doctors went to him with the idea of establishing an educational program for residents — a program that cost $100,000 to implement — Bishop Wright looked up and said, "I think it's a great idea and we ought to do it." His presence was so powerful that anyone who had a negative thought about it kept silent.

Bishop Wright is also remembered as an accomplished speaker, having polished his rhetorical skills as a member of the

Boston Latin School debate team from 1924 to 1927 — years in which the team won every debate. "He could talk about doors for two hours and keep you spellbound," according to Dr. John Howard.

Bishop Wright remained in Worcester for nine years, until he was appointed bishop of Pittsburgh. He later served as a cardinal, and as Prefect of the Congregation for the Clergy, a position that put him at the head of 350,000 priests around the world. He became the first American to serve as head of a congregation of the Roman Curia. Many believe that, if his health had not failed him in 1979 at the age of 70, he may have become the first American Pope.

And yet he never forgot Worcester.

During the 25th anniversary of the diocese, Bishop Wright was asked by *The Catholic Free Press* to write about his days in the new diocese. Responding with "a love letter," he wrote, "What does the silver jubilee of the diocese mean to me? The beginning of a joyful love adventure unforgettable in a life that has been blessed with love, activity and adventure beyond my (or almost anyone else's) possible hopes."

Bishop Wright was a much-sought-after speaker, and, as Mrs. Haverty remembers, he accepted speaking engagements everywhere. "After he left Worcester, he traveled all over the world. Whenever anyone asked him to speak, wherever it was, he went. He never said 'No' to anyone. That was partly his downfall. He never really took care of himself. I miss him terribly."

Betty Lilyestrom, a reporter for the *Worcester Telegram* who covered Bishop Wright as part of her beat for four years, remembers his return to Worcester to deliver a speech: "I caught up with the bishop at St. Vincent Hospital and asked for an advance text of his speech — a pointless request, I was sure, since he seldom prepared speeches in advance. True to form, he had no text. But he accommodated the press by composing and dictating one to me as he paced the sunny courtyard of the hospital building. When he was done, I had a text that went 10 typewritten pages, which he delivered nearly word for word from memory that night as I followed along, amazed."

Bishop Wright acted quickly and decisively, as if making up for the long years that the Worcester area was without a bishop. Just two months after his consecration, he created the Guild of Our Lady of Providence and, almost immediately, he resurrected plans for the new hospital.

Just as Ella Fallon, Dr. Michael Fallon's wife, had served as the first president of the St. Vincent Hospital Aid Association, Frances Fallon, John Fallon's second wife, was named the first president of the Guild of Our Lady of Providence. Like the Aid Association and the Society of Patrons, the guild was made up of a mix of doctor's wives, women who lived near the hospital, women who were active in the church and people who were merely interested in volunteering their time for a worthy cause. Unlike the first two organizations, though, the guild had the added benefit of Bishop Wright's support. Filomena DiTomaso, a member since the guild began, credits the bishop with drawing people into the guild. "He took Worcester by storm," she said.

At a tea held on May 7, 1950, at the School of Nursing, Bishop Wright and Sister Loreto detailed the group's mission and gave the 230 interested women the opportunity to choose between two names — the Guild of St. Elizabeth of Hungary and the Guild of Our Lady of Providence. Providence, quite naturally, was the chosen name. With the bishop as a catalyst, membership reached 842 by October 1950 and 1,060 a month later. By 1951, the guild had 1,300 members.

In November of its first year, the guild sponsored a concert by the Little Symphony with Harry Levinson conducting, raising more than $5,000 for a portable respirator. The fund raiser began a tradition of holding an annual assembly to raise funds for an item that was needed by the hospital. The guild has held annual assemblies every year since, except 1968, when the administration was already soliciting pledges for a building project, and

1977. The guild has brought Arthur Fiedler and the Boston Pops, Mantovani, Henry Mancini and other popular names to Worcester. It sponsored "The Sound of Music," "Camelot," "The Prisoner of Zenda" and other plays that brought stars such as Tyrone Power, Anne Baxter, Stewart Granger, Deborah Kerr and Raymond Massey to Worcester.

Each year, the funds raised from the assembly paid for something different. The proceeds paid for furnishing the pediatric unit, renovating the maternity department, and purchasing equipment such as a deep-therapy X-ray machine for cancer treatment, an image intensifier for the heart catheterization laboratory, a scanner for use in nuclear medicine and, more recently, equipment for the critical care unit. In 1963, to celebrate Sister Loreto's 25th year as superintendent, the guild saved up for a scintillating spectrometer and put a bronze plaque on the machine in her honor. The guild also commissioned the oil painting of Mother Loreto that hangs in the amphitheater lobby. One year, at Bishop Wright's request, the guild raised $10,000 for the statue of St. Vincent that is currently in the hospital lobby.

Mrs. DiTomaso, who has been dedicated to St. Vincent Hospital since being hospitalized there for 30 days in 1946 and 1947, received a pin in 1987 for 15,000 hours of volunteer service. If she were paid a wage of just $5 an hour, her volunteer work would be equivalent to a $75,000 donation. And there are many others on the guild who have donated as much time, or nearly as much time. A 1990 proclamation signed by Mayor Jordan Levy in honor of the guild's 40th anniversary says that from 1950 to 1990, the guild accumulated more than 1,225,000 volunteer hours, awarded more than 1,600 scholarships totaling $108,800 to student nurses, donated $50,000 for a diagnostic building and more than $167,000 for St. Vincent's amphitheater and library. The proclamation estimates that the guild raised $1,847,000 for the hospital. By 1992, donations passed the $2 million mark.

The guild has held art auctions, gold sales, dances and mini-fairs, and has sponsored movies. It has sold cookbooks and remembrance cards. It sponsors an annual fall fashion show, two rummage sales a year and a concession stand at the Pleasant Valley Golf Tournament.

From 1952 to 1969, the guild sponsored a consignment shop at 195 Pleasant Street. "They'll sell anything for you — from a set of golf clubs to an outgrown jacket — and at a small commission, too," according to a newspaper article written shortly after the opening. "We heard about one guild member who asked the exchange to sell a dress on which she had splurged last year. She had brought it home from downtown, worn it once, and ever after disliked it, because she had suddenly decided that it made her look fat. It was sold within two weeks."

One regular customer, according to the article, came in looking for an oversized coffee cup that she wanted because her coffee-loving son was coming to visit. The store didn't have an oversized cup in stock, but Mrs. Francis J. Steele, the shop treasurer, had one at home and gave it to the customer as a gift.

In November 1950, the guild started a coffee shop in a renovated waiting room, selling brownies, cakes and other food baked or donated by the volunteers. It proved to be so popular, a kitchen was added, but it later closed because the hospital needed the space.

The guild's activities include much more than just fund raising.

"We're ambassadors of good will," Mrs. DiTomaso said. "Our concession at Pleasant Valley Country Club, for example, didn't make much money, but there was a huge sign with 'St. Vincent Hospital' on it. We'd wear our smocks. It was public relations, to project the image of St. Vincent Hospital."

During its first couple of years, the guild held birthday parties on the hospital lawn for patients. Each year, the guild holds a Mass to honor the dead. A junior guild was created for 15- to 20-year-old girls, who worked in the record room, took care of patient flowers and mail, and made surgical dressings. Adult guild members also made dressings and sewed. In the 1951–1952 fiscal year alone, 86 volunteers made 147,568 dressings. In 1959–1960, volunteers made 260,763 dressings. In 1992, the guild added a book cart to the intensive care area, and in 1990 it began a care program for the elderly. The guild has made holders for cards, knit hats for babies and taken pictures of newborns.

Mrs. DiTomaso particularly enjoyed taking the baby photos. "It was one of the happiest places I've been in," she said. "No matter what the baby picture looked like, the mother was happy with it."

One year, guild member Margaret Bonner went to a national convention for hospital guilds and came back with Guildy the Puppet, which was dressed in a volunteer's smock. "Every child, when they left the hospital, got a puppet after that."

The most successful and steadiest form of funding comes from the guild gift shop. While it has been in the lobby of the current hospital for many years, it was started under a staircase in the old hospital with just two china closets and a bureau. The gift shop was turned over to the guild to manage in 1954. Mrs. Philip Sheridan, chairman of the gift shop that year, wrote, "In addition to the regular lines carried in the past, we have added magazines, cigars, which were being repeatedly asked for, jellies from the Trappist Monastery, and lastly, African violet plants, which were a sellout on the first day we received them."

Monsignor John F. Reilly, pastor of St. Stephen's Church, was named the spiritual director of the guild, and showed a constant dedication to its members, according to Mrs. DiTomaso. "Msgr. Reilly came to every meeting and he would sit in a corner and, God love him, how he stood 50 to 60 women conducting a meeting. He never said anything unless he was asked to." One year the guild bought a Christmas crèche for the hospital, and Msgr. Reilly walked up Vernon Hill during a snowstorm for the dedication ceremony.

In the mid-'50s the guild had its first volunteer dinner, inviting anyone who volunteered at least five hours during the year. "We had so many people, we didn't know what to do," Mrs. DiTomaso recalled.

Later, Sister Miriam Regina, then superintendent of St. Vincent Hospital, described the work of the guild as she saw it: "The pathway of the work of the Guild of Our Lady of Providence is somewhat like a mountain road. At times it seems to double back and cover the same ground as if to see how great has been its accomplishments."

Establishing the guild was only one of many accomplishments that took place at St. Vincent Hospital during Bishop Wright's tenure. Certainly the most visible and most important advance that took place was the construction of a new hospital. Plans for the hospital were revived in 1951, and the project was put out to bid. On July 5, after a review of a dozen bids, the contract was awarded to Granger-Loranger, a Worcester firm. Mariemont was demolished, ending one era and signaling the beginning of another. All that remained was the stone wall that still outlines the hospital's perimeter today. On July 11, 1951, ground was broken for a $7 million, 400-bed hospital. The plans called for the continuing use of the existing hospital for maternity patients and for patients with chronic illnesses.

"Daily experience of the dangerously overcrowded condition of the hospital and immediate admiration for the work of the Sisters of Providence, even under such hampering conditions as confronted them in the old building, prompted the bishop to call for early consideration of the plans already drawn by the architects," according to the *Worcester Telegram.*

With a third of the $7 million set aside already by the Sisters of Providence, Bishop Wright decided there was no need for an organized fund drive. Instead, he made quiet personal appeals to individuals and groups in the community for assistance in raising $700,000 for hospital equipment. The *Worcester Telegram* noted that the bishop's method of fund raising reflected his confidence in the loyalty of Worcester's Catholics, but added that it also showed his confidence that the non-Catholics in the community would support the hospital and "show their appreciation for what St. Vincent Hospital has come to mean in this area."

Construction of the new hospital proceeded on schedule, in spite of a nationwide steel strike and a local work stoppage. The new hospital combined with the old hospital building gave St. Vincent nearly 600 beds, making it one of the largest hospitals in New England.

Another special project of Bishop Wright's during his tenure as bishop of the Worcester diocese was Marillac Manor, a home for unwed, pregnant girls that was named for St. Louise de Marillac. A companion of St. Vincent de Paul, she dedicated most of her life to helping the sick and the poor, and she was especially sympathetic to the needs of unwed mothers and mothers-to-be.

Marillac Manor was opened in 1956 at 36 Winthrop Street, across the street from St. Vincent Hospital, in a home previously occupied by the Xaverian Brothers. The home was located next to St. Vincent so that pregnant girls could be examined easily by St. Vincent doctors and deliver their babies discreetly when the time came. Marillac Manor's medical staff was headed by Dr. Philippe W. Ouellette of St. Vincent and other St. Vincent doctors assisted.

Bishop Wright opened the home, according to Irish writer Alice Curtayne, who wrote about her visits there in *The Catholic Free Press,* because he was troubled by the double standard by which unwed mothers were judged. The boys who were equal partners in the pregnancy were not treated as social outcasts and considered immoral. The girls were. Bishop Wright wanted Marillac Manor to be a home for the girls, where they could be treated with care in a home-like setting. With its crucifixes and pictures of bishops on the walls, Marillac Manor has been described as looking like a cross between a sorority house and a convent.

Because being pregnant and unmarried still created a difficult social stigma when Marillac Manor opened, precautions were taken to ensure the privacy of the girls in the home. A stockade fence discouraged the curious, and few visitors were allowed. The girls were never addressed by their surnames. Even when they crossed the street to deliver their babies at St. Vincent Hospital, their identities remained secret. They were signed into the hospital under assumed names and even the nursing staff didn't know who was being treated.

Outside the house, the girls usually wore fake wedding rings. They were discouraged from going out between 2:30 and 3:30 p.m. to avoid insults from boys getting out of school.

Being pregnant out of wedlock and "having a keen desire to be rehabilitated morally and socially" was the only common bond between the residents, according to Ms. Curtayne's article. The only requirement for admission, other than pregnancy out of wedlock, was a psychiatric screening to determine whether the mother-to-be could adjust to the community living of Marillac Manor.

The home served girls as young as 13 and women as old as 42. Many were from Worcester, but others came from as far away as St. Louis, Atlanta and Indianapolis. Although priests were available daily for confessions and Mass, the home was open to girls of all religions. Many could afford to pay for their stay. Others paid nothing. By 1972, the top price was nearly $20 a day, but the cost of operating the facility was nearly $35 a day per patient. The remaining costs were paid for by contributions through Catholic Charities of the Diocese of Worcester, which operated the home.

The pregnant girls who lived at the Manor spent their days cooking, sewing, reading and singing. They made many of their own meals, attended ceramics classes, watched soap operas and split up the housekeeping duties. They also received regular medical care and counseling. Girls enrolled in the program were cared for according to a philosophy called PAD, for protection and shelter, affection and direction. Through counseling, they decided whether to keep their babies or give them up for adoption. When the home opened, most of the babies were given up to adoption. In later years, as social values changed, most mothers kept their babies.

As abortion began to become increasingly available as an option, and the Catholic Church became increasingly vocal in opposition to abortion, Marillac Manor provided an outlet for counseling pregnant girls about alternatives to abortion.

As pregnancy out of wedlock became less of a stigma, and as the use of birth control pills and other contraceptives increased, the number of girls using Marillac Manor's residential program decreased. When Marillac Manor opened, the residential program had the capacity to serve up to 20 girls at a time. When it closed in 1988, only eight beds remained and most of the time fewer than half of them were in use. Today Marillac Manor continues to operate its obstetrics clinic, and to provide individual and group counseling, pregnancy testing and parenting education.

Reflecting on the closing of Marillac Manor's residential program, Msgr. Edmond T. Tinsley, director of Catholic Charities, talked about the decreasing demand for the home's services and said, "If it reflects a more compassionate society, that would be great. If it reflects a lessening of the sacredness of human sexuality, that would be negative. I think it's a blend of both."

Bishop Wright's efforts extended well beyond St. Vincent Hospital. In addition to overseeing the building of the new hospital and the establishment of Marillac Manor, he also oversaw the opening of 30 new parishes and the organization of a number of Catholic organizations, including the Holy Family League of Charity, the Diocesan League of Catholic Women, the Diocesan Council of Catholic Men, the Society for the Propagation of the Faith, and various Catholic organizations for trade groups, from taxi drivers to lawyers.

Before entering the priesthood, he worked briefly as a reporter for *The Boston Post,* ending his journalistic career when he refused to interview the mother of a girl who had just killed herself by jumping off a bridge. He renewed his journalistic interests after coming to Worcester by founding a widely respected diocesan newspaper, *The Catholic Free Press.*

In addition, of course, he also established the administrative structure of the diocese. When he became the bishop of Pittsburgh in 1959, he left behind "a fully functioning ecclesiastical organization, as well as a tremendous good will toward the Church that before his arrival was still seen as 'something foreign and for immigrants,'" according to *The Catholic Free Press.*

Bishop Wright also was an able leader during times of crisis. When the Greendale campus of Assumption College was leveled by a tornado in 1953, Bishop Wright supervised the construction of a new campus on Salisbury Street.

In a personal letter written on behalf of Bishop Wright, Archbishop Richard J. Cushing of Boston urged the members of his archdiocese to contribute to Bishop Wright on his behalf.

"My dearly beloved in Christ, please help," he wrote. "I appeal not for ourselves but for a good neighbor, a brother in Christ, one of our own, and his afflicted spiritual children who are dependent upon him.

"The need is so urgent that, if you are contemplating a gift for one of my charities, please forget me and my projects and give to this collection for the Bishop of Worcester."

Archbishop Cushing made a personal donation of $5,000 and his letter resulted in the collection of $250,000.

Bishop Wright's accomplishments at St. Vincent Hospital were, of course, not his alone. Sister Loreto was an equal partner, in as much as Bishop Wright had an equal. She played an important role in the construction of the new hospital — a more day-to-day, hands-on role than the bishop — and she supported the hospital completely.

She had to deal with day-to-day crises, like a couple of fires set by an arsonist in 1952. And after the tornado ripped through Worcester, while Bishop Wright tended to those in need throughout the city, Sister Loreto tended to the hospital.

The two fires, which were set in the kitchen section of the hospital in a frame building adjacent to the main building, caused a total of $5,500 in damage to the hospital and resulted in the hospitalization of five people. Four firefighters were hospitalized in addition to Joe Monroe, who fought the fire with hand extinguishers until the firefighters arrived. An orderly at the hospital was later arrested and charged with the arsons. During the fires, Sister Loreto tended to the patients, making certain they didn't panic.

Sister Loreto's efforts after the tornado are chronicled in an article she wrote for *The Modern Hospital*. The article not only highlights her efforts, but provides insight into life in the early 1950s. She explains that St. Vincent Hospital fared well after the tornado, because it had a plan in place for dealing with disasters — although the plan was written for use in case the city was hit by an atomic bomb.

"About the time of the onset of the Korean affair, the nation in general and Worcester in particular again began to plan for trouble," Sister Loreto wrote. "Worcester, being a highly industrialized community of 205,000, was felt to be a possible primary and surely a secondary target in the event of an all-out atomic war."

Still, the plan, which was organized by a hospital civil defense committee working with government officials, was effective after "the big blow," even though the blow was not man made. Of the city's five hospitals, St. Vincent was the farthest away from the tornado's path, so it had more time to prepare for casualties.

The tornado hit at 4:40 p.m. on June 9, 1953, crossing the city in about 15 minutes. Miss Weeks, a scrub nurse at the time, was in the operating room when it struck. Cyclopropane, an explosive gas, was being used as a general anesthesia for the operation, so the results could have been deadly if the tornado had struck closer. "We knew there were terrible thunder storms, but we didn't know there was a tornado," she said. The surgical team completed the operation, and she completed her shift. She went home, still not knowing that a tornado had struck. But, like many others, she heard an appeal for blood on the radio and knew that a catastrophe had struck. She returned to the hospital and worked for 24 hours without relief.

"We still didn't know what had happened; what catastrophe had struck," she said. In those pre-television days, such news traveled slowly. And in this case, she said, city officials deliberately kept quiet. They did not want anyone to panic.

Like Miss Weeks, scores of other hospital personnel began reporting for duty. They may not have known what happened, but no one had to tell them they were needed.

Sister Loreto wrote, "The response to a radio appeal to donors was dramatic. By 6:30 p.m. they began to appear, and by 7 p.m. there was a line of 200 donors formed and blood was being drawn." Charity presented its own problems, however, as the crowd of donors clogged the corridor on the ground floor until it was detoured outside the building. By 10 p.m., 190 pints of blood were drawn by six teams, and the blood was typed and Rh factored.

Members of an order of nuns from Assumption College were the first patients to arrive at St. Vincent, according to Sister Mary John Bosco, and "one woman, Mrs. Jackson, had her baby blown our of her arms and killed." Sister Loreto reported that the first casualty arrived at St. Vincent at 6:35 p.m. By 11 p.m., when the flow of incoming patients had slowed down, 68 people were treated for minor injuries and an additional 27 were admitted. Memorial Hospital, which was closer to the path of the tornado, saw about 300 patients.

St. Vincent was able to handle its heavy rush of patients by using the nurses' dining room, which was 40 feet from the ambulance entrance, as a sorting station. Medical personnel at the sorting station assessed incoming patients, treating those with minor injuries, and dispatching those with serious injuries for emergency surgery or admission into hospital wards.

"The hospital switchboard was flooded with calls and frequently it was easier to go after things than to call for them," according to Sister Loreto. "Too many people used the telephone unnecessarily." A separate telephone line independent of the switchboard was set up in Sister Loreto's office, which was used to coordinate information with other hospitals. Because of the separate line, it was easy to reach suppliers for needed items. For example, because of a shortage of large-gauge needles for drawing blood, a call was made, and, within a half hour, 100 needles were delivered.

Dr. Morrison was among the medical staff that worked through the night to collect blood. He and Sister Mary Trinita collected 72 pints of whole blood. Even with the delivery of extra needles, there were insufficient needles to draw enough blood, so they sterilized and reused the needles they had. Because that violated the requirements of the American Red Cross, the blood had to be discarded. Overall, however, the hospital's response to the disaster proceeded smoothly.

"We have now had a small experience — when one thinks in terms of the atom bomb — but it is better than no experience at all," Sister Loreto concluded. "Now we must enlarge on our plans and improve them in the minor details, at the same time praying to God that we'll never have to use them."

CHAPTER TEN

Our Hospital

"More than one person remarked on the wholesome spirit of 'proprietorship' which permeated the thousands of area citizens whose steady stream gave vitality to the hospital building Sunday afternoon. Observers suddenly realized that the popular sense of 'owning' St. Vincent's was an accurate reflection of the realities. These were the people who ultimately build hospitals like St. Vincent's, who love them with a family attachment no other institutions can claim, and who take a pride in the monuments of the Church comparable to that which others take in their narrow personal possessions." **The Catholic Free Press**

The postwar years were a time for building hospitals. Projects stalled by the war were resumed with a new urgency and a heightened awareness of the value of life. World War II created a tremendous number of medical breakthroughs, and physicians made great strides in their ability to save lives and to cure disease. So hospitals finally were built with a confidence that hospital-based medical and surgical treatment indeed held the central position in the future of health care.

The availability of federal funds for hospital construction further accelerated hospital expansion. The 1946 Hospital Survey and Construction Act, commonly known as the Hill-Burton program, was approved by Congress and provided $75 million a year for five years to finance hospital construction projects. There was little federal discretion for disbursement of the funds and hospitals expanded with little attention paid to health-care needs. A commission organized by the American Hospital Association, not surprisingly, concluded that the number of hos-pital beds nationwide should be increased by 40 percent. The results of the survey were used to rationalize funding of Hill-Burton financed projects across the country.

Hospitals throughout the Worcester area expanded. The Memorial Hospital completed a 75-bed addition in 1948, a two-story maternity wing in 1951 and a new emergency ward in 1953, giving the hospital a total capacity of 269 beds. Hahnemann Hospital, which had 125 beds, moved and by 1954 was building a million-dollar addition. Fairlawn Hospital com-pleted an addition, and City Hospital, which had 480 beds and was the largest hospital in Worcester, was planning a moderniza-tion program. Belmont Hospital grew into a 250-bed hospital. Outside of Worcester, Holden Hospital expanded, a new wing was added to Clinton Hospital and a new $850,000 hospital was built to serve the Webster area.

But the most ambitious plans were carried out by St. Vincent Hospital. The new 400-bed hospital building, which gave St. Vincent a total of nearly 600 beds, used enough concrete to build a road six feet wide connecting Worcester to Boston, enough wire to wrap around the equator five-and-a-half times, and enough bricks to build an outdoor barbecue for every family in Worcester. Some people, in fact, thought the plans for the new hospital were too ambitious.

Owen Murphy, former editor of *The Catholic Free Press,* believes Bishop Wright took great pleasure in having a huge white hospital built on top of a hill, where it could be highly vis-ible from many points in the city. Bishop Wright loved symbol-ism, according to Murphy, and must have been delighted with the huge white structure. He once suggested to the bishop that St. Vincent reminded him of Sacré Coeur, the famous Church overlooking Paris. Bishop Wright only smiled at the suggestion.

The hospital was so big, many in the community called the white-brick building "the white elephant" and said it would never be filled. Mother Loreto, though, was confident that the hospital would fill quickly. "When she built the new hospital, Mother Loreto was a very daring woman," according to Sister Adrianella. "She had a lot of vision." Her vision, in fact, proved to be 20/20. In a short time, the hospital was so full, the solariums at the end of each corridor were converted into extra rooms.

After the hospital was completed, a three-day dedication ceremony was scheduled, beginning on March 26, 1954. Nurses and students volunteered their time to clean and polish the new hospital for the grand opening, according to Mrs. Healey, because "we were so proud of our new hospital. We were so very proud and knew it was going to be the greatest."

On the opening day of the dedication, the 50-mile-an-hour wind was so blustery, it toppled chairs, whistled into the microphones and prompted Archbishop Richard J. Cushing, the keynote speaker, to say, "I thought you had the tornado last year." One reporter wondered why the small hats of some of the women blew off their heads, while the wing-like habits of one order of nuns seemed unaffected. Bishop Wright told the crowd he had asked the Sisters of Providence to pray for wind to blow away the previous day's rain clouds, and implied that their prayers had been too effective. Despite the cold weather, 2,000 people attended the dedication ceremony. In all, 23,800 attended the three-day celebration. Most of the crowd, about 15,000 people, came on Sunday afternoon, the last day of the dedication, for an opportunity to tour St. Vincent Hospital. They waited for nearly two hours in a line snaking around the hospital.

Even though the wait was long and cold, the atmosphere was festive. Bishop Wright signed souvenir booklets for autograph seekers. Families posed for photos at the shrine for St. Vincent. One of the 25 police officers on duty for the event "regaled visitors with the competence of a Gilbert and Sullivan counterpart," according to a newspaper account. And Mrs. Bonner sold commemorative plates with an enthusiasm that led one reporter to admire her ability to make plate sales appear to be the main event.

Once inside, the spectators saw a seven-story, ultramodern hospital with medical technology and patient amenities that almost no other hospital could match. The hospital featured a third-floor suite of 16 operating rooms, more than five times the number in the old hospital. The operating rooms included eight major surgeries, four equipped with X-ray controls and all with X-ray viewers. Two operating rooms had spectator galleries.

The new St. Vincent Hospital was among the first hospitals in the country to have a separate wing solely for the treatment of psychiatric cases and alcoholism. The hospital included a groundbreaking new medical training center with lecture halls and libraries. An affiliation with Georgetown University Hospital and Medical School in Washington, D.C., though considered to be second in importance only to the building of the new hospital, was not announced until the dedication ceremony. The new hospital was fully equipped to treat polio, and had an iron lung, hot-pack units and a rocking bed. It also included facilities for the treatment of tuberculosis and diabetes, as well as a fully equipped X-ray department, a pediatric department, a cystoscopic section and more.

The chapel in a Catholic hospital like St. Vincent was as important as the surgical center. The new St. Vincent chapel, which was built in a service wing that also included maintenance shops, dining rooms, storerooms and a cafeteria, had a seating capacity of more than 400, with provisions for wheelchair patients and the ability to broadcast special services throughout the hospital on loudspeakers located in every room. The new hospital also included a convent for the Sisters of Providence, which by then numbered more than 200.

Guild members and their aides guided the visitors through the corridors to view the building, and later, under the direction of Mrs. Hanrahan, wielded mops, vacuum cleaners and waxers, and cleaned the entire seven-floor hospital.

Despite the crowds, *The Catholic Free Press* noted, "With scores of nurses on hand to help, the most modern equipment in the world for handling accidents, and doctors available a dime a dozen, the three days of crowds passing through the hospital yielded nary a call for first aid — not even an aspirin, a band-aid or a smelling salt."

The first operation in the new hospital was an appendectomy performed on Robert Benoit by Dr. McCann.

"Our Hospital," a history of St. Vincent Hospital published to commemorate the building of the new hospital, notes that "'futurity' is a very stern judge, and today it looks on the year 1899 in the hospital's history with the same detachment as it does 1918, when a 60-bed addition was built onto the building, and 1922, when a residence for Sisters and student nurses was constructed at the rear of the property on Providence Street. And as the year 1954 may be looked upon by our generation as 'the most memorable' in the hospital's history, a succeeding generation may regard it as just another year of continued growth in the evolution of a great Medical Center."

Yet futurity, in this case, was not stern, and 1954 was not "just another year." The year 1954, and the years immediately following it, were years of greatness for St. Vincent Hospital.

By the time the new hospital opened, the admitting office of the old hospital had become chaotic, to say the least. There were too many patients and too few rooms. But Sister Loreto told Sister Devota to be patient, because working conditions would be better in the new hospital. So she was patient.

Instead of transferring patients to the new hospital, Sister Loreto planned to leave them in the old hospital until it was time for them to be discharged. Keeping them where they were, she reasoned, allowed the hospital to operate more efficiently. But that was before the city volunteered to make the transfers with its ambulances at no charge. Not being one to pass up a free donation to the hospital, Sister Loreto accepted the offer, much to the dismay of Sister Devota. For a short time, her task of admitting, billing, running the switchboard and handling mail was extremely difficult, and the transfer of patients from the old hospital made it even worse. She did not even have a chance to learn the layout of the hospital, but somehow she managed.

✤ ✤ ✤

With the addition of the new building, St. Vincent Hospital had a complete hospital campus. While the new hospital and its adjoining convent were the center of attention, the first two versions of St. Vincent Hospital continued to be widely used.

A chapel attached behind the old hospital was razed in 1954 and a $250,000 renovation program was begun. The wing that was added to the hospital in 1919 was converted into a 40-bed maternity unit, while the rest of the hospital housed 110 beds for chronic patients. The exterior of the building remained unchanged, except for the addition of a one-story refrigeration and storage area. The interior was refinished in 18 different colors.

When the old hospital was built, most mothers-to-be were still having their babies at home because they could not afford hospital care. By the time the new hospital was built, health insurance was fairly widespread, and almost all births were taking place in hospitals. Reflecting advances in health care, the renovated maternity unit featured three delivery rooms, including one for Cesarean deliveries, three labor rooms, and six nurseries, including a nursery for premature deliveries. The maternity section included facilities that allowed new mothers to have their babies "rooming in" with them during their entire hospital stay, if they desired. There also was a special room for Rh factor babies, where blood transfusions could take place immediately after birth.

During the 1950s, St. Vincent Hospital was a progressive hospital, willing to carry out new ideas. It was one of the first hospitals to offer free training classes for new mothers to teach them to prepare for the responsibilities of motherhood. In an article reviewing the ongoing renovations, *The Catholic Free Press* wrote, "A unique feature of the new maternity center will be a demonstration room where the new mothers will be taught in organized classes how to care for their babies. It will be the first such organized class in this area, it is believed. Mothers will attend only during the period of their hospitalization.

"For expectant fathers, on the other hand, there will be a waiting room with television."

The chronic care section was a nursing home for people with an average age of 80 or more, according to *The Outlook,* a St. Vincent Hospital publication. Patients there had illnesses requiring constant care, including arteriosclerosis, hypertension, strokes, heart and kidney diseases, anemia, diabetes, brittle bones, severe arthritis and other diseases.

In honor of the Sisters of Providence, the remodeled hospital was renamed Providence House in October 1955, though it was still commonly referred to as the "1898" hospital.

The first St. Vincent Hospital, which had been known for many years as the St. Vincent Home, underwent major renovations in 1956 and was renamed St. Mary's Hall during a dedication ceremony in the basement cafeteria on August 12. The renovated building continued to be a home for the aged, accommodating 71 women. Msgr. Griffin would have approved.

At times, history can be serendipitous. Through a magical combination of events, a person or an institution may be elevated to a new, heightened stature. Such was the case with St. Vincent Hospital in 1954.

The size of the old hospital and the inadequacy of the facilities held back the hospital's growth. But with the new hospital in place, the restraints on growth were removed, and the hospital filled rapidly. At the hospital's December 9, 1955 annual meeting, the Sisters of Providence reported: "The effectiveness of a new physical plant, modern equipment and added facilities was shown by the result of the past year's work. A 46 percent increase in admissions and patient days over the same period last year, together with an increase of from 35 to 50 percent in the use of the various services . . . indicates that the hospital is now running at a constant high rate."

Admissions for the year totaled 21,077, including 13,856 in-patients staying for 139,361 hospital days. Charitable care for the year was worth $119,227, and enrollment in the School of Nursing reached 214, its highest level up to that date.

When the new St. Vincent Hospital opened, it was perhaps the first major hospital built in Massachusetts in the post-World War II years, and it remained the only new hospital in the Commonwealth for many years. This alone would have put St. Vincent at the center of the community. But it was the people behind the brick and mortar that gave the hospital a sense of greatness.

Valerie T. Mancini, who emigrated with her family from Italy in 1956, still remembers her uncle pointing out the new hospital and saying, "This is the finest hospital in Worcester." She was so impressed, she was determined to work there one day. "From that moment, I told my parents I wanted to be a nurse. I used to drive them crazy. I never thought of doing anything else." She later became the vice president of nursing.

The greatness of St. Vincent came from the combined talents and dedication of many people, from the administration to the nursing students, from the medical staff to the maintenance staff. It was not just Bishop Wright, who remained intimately involved with the new hospital and spent many nights there, and it was not just Sister Loreto. People took pride in their new hospital, and treated it as if it were their own special place. The hospital emanated a positive attitude.

"We were a dominant force in the area and had earned a reputation for the manner of delivery of medical care," Dr. Kocot said. "There was a sacred attitude about what the hospital promised and what it delivered."

For all of its innovations, St. Vincent Hospital remained a community hospital. The hospital staff and the community truly viewed the new hospital on the hill as "our hospital" and took great pride in it. Together in their hospital, the entire staff, doctors and nurses, sisters and patients, all seemed part of an intimate community, perhaps even a family.

✠ ✠ ✠

Ask anyone who worked at the hospital at the time, no matter what position the person held, to describe the relationship among the people who worked there, and the chances are good that the word "family" will work its way into the conversation. The nursing students, who spent so much time together in close quarters, talk frequently about being part of a family. House officers lived together like members of the same family. Chauffeur Joe Monroe said the sisters treated him as part of a family, cooking him a meal when he worked late and showing concern about his health.

In many cases, the word "family" can be taken literally. It is a tradition for sons to follow their fathers into practice at St. Vincent. Dr. John Fallon followed Dr. Michael Fallon; Dr. Denis J. FitzGerald, current president and chief executive officer, followed his father, Dr. Arthur FitzGerald, who served as president of the medical staff. Dr. McCann, chief of surgery for many years, relinquished the post and it was shared by his son, James McCann, Jr., and Dr. Howard. The younger Dr. McCann, who joined his father's private practice when he began his medical career, represented the third generation of McCanns to be elected to the American College of Surgeons. Dr. Robert D. Blute, Jr. is a urologist with his father, Dr. Robert D. Blute, Sr. Dr. Paul F. Bergin, an obstetrician, and his brother, Joseph, a urologist, followed their father, Dr. Stephen A. Bergin, who was an obstetrician at St. Vincent from 1903 to 1945.

Many of the doctors had large families and their children played an important role in their lives. Dr. Blute had 11 children. Dr. Whelan and Dr. Utzschneider each had 10. Dr. Ware had eight, the senior Dr. McCann had seven and Dr. John Fallon had six. Despite their large families, the doctors cared for their patients and did not expect special treatment. They were doctors, and they recognized that they were unable to spend much time with their families, so they didn't complain about their long hours. "If you had five kids," according to Dr. Gerald J. Carroll, co-director of thoracic surgery, "you didn't open your mouth."

In addition to raising large families, many of the doctors' wives were active at the hospital through the Guild of Our Lady of Providence. Vera Massarelli, wife of Dr. Massarelli, has been especially active in the operation of the hospital gift shop. Rita Scanlon, whose husband, Dr. Joseph C. Scanlon, Sr., was on the St. Vincent staff for 46 years, was in charge of the Junior Guild and worked in the guild coffee shop when she wasn't raising her six children.

"Fathers participate more in bringing up kids today," Mrs. Scanlon said. "When the children were growing up, you had to hire good help. They didn't see much of their fathers."

Given the doctors' busy schedules, the hospital itself played an important social role.

"The hospital was viewed differently," according to Dr. Denis FitzGerald. "It was part of the social fabric of the medical community. They used to congregate and exchange ideas at the hospital. They would come here whether they had patients in the hospital or not. Every aspect of a doctor's life rotated around the hospital."

He spent so much time with his father at St. Vincent, he said, "I made more rounds than most doctors do today."

The doctors usually made Sunday a family day, even when they came to the hospital. It was a tradition for many of the doctors to attend 8:30 a.m. Mass at the chapel, and to leave their children with Sister Devota. She especially remembers babysitting for the children of Dr. FitzGerald and Dr. McCann. She was strict with them, but occasionally indulged them with ice cream. One day, young Jimmy McCann got his head stuck in the round window in the wall that separated the telephone switchboard from the admitting office. His father, although not very pleased about having to perform the operation, put his surgical skills to work, and separated his son from the window.

Many times, the sense of "family" went beyond blood ties. In a life-and-death business, the word "family" takes on a higher and broader meaning. Working together, the people of St. Vincent Hospital sometimes touched each other's lives as intimately as if they were members of one big family.

One night, Sister Mary Francis found Dr. Paul Bergin pacing quietly outside the emergency room. He looked troubled. She knew he was waiting for a room to perform a Cesarean section, and she asked him if the unavailability of a room was bothering him.

"It isn't that, sister," he replied solemnly. "My brother Joe was killed."

He had just been told that his brother had died in an automobile accident. Another doctor volunteered to take over the Cesarean operation, but Dr. Bergin insisted on proceeding. He completed the operation silently, but faultlessly.

Soon after, Dr. Blute arrived at St. Vincent. Dr. Blute began his medical career in Boston and at first expected to stay there. But after a few months of private practice, he began to grow weary of Boston traffic. His office was on Commonwealth Avenue, and he often finished work at the same time as the Boston Red Sox, so he routinely was caught in traffic jams. At the persistent urging of Dr. Frank Sheddan, his chief of staff during his residency, he came to Worcester for an interview.

The new hospital had just opened, and it was attractive to Dr. Blute. But he was even more attracted by the people he met. During his interview, he met with the hospital's senior surgical staff; Dr. Frank Steele, the chief of urology; Sister Loreto; and Bishop Wright, who was chairman of the Board of Trustees.

"All of these people convinced me my future was not in Boston, but in this new, dynamic place," Dr. Blute recalled. "I look back and I have no regrets."

He arrived in Worcester on December 10, 1954 ready to work. Three days later, his wife, Ann Marie, who was seven-and-a-half months pregnant, went into labor prematurely.

"We had not met any of the obstetrical staff," Dr. Blute said. "When I called the hospital, Dr. Paul Bergin answered and told me to come right in." Dr. Blute brought his wife to the obstetrical unit, which was still in the old hospital. It appeared deserted when Dr. Blute arrived. A sister found the young couple and showed them to the obstetrical unit, where Dr. Bergin delivered twins. The twins were a surprise to the Blutes, who had no indication in those days before ultrasound that they would be adding their sixth child as well as their fifth.

Dr. Blute was both impressed by and appreciative of the attentive care his wife and newborn children were given. When he encountered Bishop Wright the day after the twins were delivered and told the bishop about the premature delivery, Bishop Wright saw to it that the twins were confirmed (they already had been baptized). With this extra measure of spiritual grace, and the attentive and professional care of the hospital staff, the twins, Carol and Mary, survived. Today Carol Ryan heads the science department at St. Peter-Marian High School while Mary manages the food service department at the College of the Holy Cross.

Dr. Bergin worked to save the twins' lives just months after he had lost his brother Joseph. His brother was a urologist. And Dr. Blute was his replacement on the St. Vincent staff.

The feeling of family also extended to the house staff. The house doctors were literally house doctors and lived on a corridor of the hospital. "It was a different camaraderie then," Dr. Howard said. "Not being married, the guys used to hang around together. We'd work together and live together."

Sometimes the shifts were long and uneventful. Working shifts from Friday morning until Monday afternoon, the surgical staff sometimes played cards. One day, when the junior Dr. McCann was losing at cards, he asked his father for an advance on his salary.

Dr. McCann, Sr. had not realized that the house officers were playing cards, let alone gambling, so he determined to punish them. Dr. Howard, who was seen as a ringleader, and another doctor were told that they had to take a week off and would not be allowed to perform surgery. To Dr. McCann, whose whole world was surgery, this was a serious punishment.

"We grinned, and finally he realized he had given us the whole week off," Dr. Howard said. Dr. McCann instead told the doctors they had to continue to work their shifts, and, within a day or two, he allowed them to perform surgery again.

The relationships between doctors and patients also reinforced the "family" atmosphere at St. Vincent. This was especially true of Dr. FitzGerald. Described as "a Norman Rockwell kind of doctor," he was the Dr. Delahanty of his day — the beloved general practitioner who worked hard and long, and cared for two or three generations of his patients' families, delivering their babies, removing their tonsils, and treating their coughs and sore throats. Shirley Fornier, whose family was cared for by Dr. FitzGerald for more than 20 years, remembers when she was giving birth to her second son and complications occurred.

"I was told that he left an office full of patients, and he came across town and never even stopped for a light to get here," she said. "He saved my life."

There were no appointments in Dr. FitzGerald's office. When a patient needed to be seen, "you just got there and sat," Mrs. Fornier said. "It was on a 'first come' basis. There were people in his office afternoon and evening."

She remembers him coming to her home in the middle of the night to treat a daughter with a temperature of 105°F. Her husband didn't own a car at the time, so Dr. FitzGerald drove her husband to his father's home so he could borrow the car and get a prescription filled.

"He was part of the family," she said.

Dr. Denis FitzGerald also remembers his father treating his patients as an extended family.

"He was a tremendous role model," according to Dr. FitzGerald. "The beauty of what my father did is that, if you were his patient, he knew you and where you came from. He knew your roots. He knew your problems. He talked to all of his patients in terms they could understand."

Dr. FitzGerald is also remembered for his sense of humor.

"I worked with Fitzy on maternity," Mrs. Hanrahan said. "He was always playing tricks on people. My boyfriend was coming home from the service, and I was told that I had a long-distance phone call, that he was on the phone. It was Fitzy. He strung me along."

"We all loved him. He was a terrific guy," Sister Devota said, recalling that his one bad habit, not counting cigar smoking, is that he used to swear. "I told him he was going to give me a nickel every time he swore. By the end of the week, I had $5."

The money went into a kitty the sisters had that was used to pay cab fare for the poorer patients who had no way of getting home from the hospital.

During the post-World War II era when the hospital was being built, staffing needs changed. The Sisters of Providence no longer could fill all of the nursing slots with nuns and students, so they broke with tradition and began hiring lay nurses, including many who graduated from the School of Nursing and were working as private duty nurses. Some had left nursing to raise a family and were ready to return. As the hospital grew, there simply were not enough nuns to fill every slot. Mrs. Hanrahan, for example, said that in 1951, "I was asked to return for three months, and I stayed for 27 years." Mrs. Healey finished her nursing training shortly before the new hospital opened, and was invited to stay on as a nurse.

The need for adding to the nursing staff increased with the opening of the new hospital, which was more than twice the size of the old one, and the old hospital still had to be staffed, too.

"We came at night," said Miss White. "We made the beds, washed the dishes . . . we thought we should. St. Vincent Hospital was a part of our lives." The facilities at the new hospital were a big attraction to many of the nurses. "We thought we were in heaven," she said. "There was a bathroom in every room, big utility rooms, nice sterilizing equipment."

Mrs. Swift also was asked to return to her alma mater, and, she said, "it was the best thing that I ever did."

The nuns at St. Vincent also increased at all levels with the opening of the new hospital. In 1955, the all-encompassing position of superintendent was split into the positions of local superior and administrator. Sister Loreto continued as the administrator, performing her usual hospital management duties, but Sister Mary Madelina was appointed local superior, relieving Sister Loreto of many of the duties relating more directly to the order.

Among the new arrivals who were part of the order were Sisters Mary Denise, who supervised medical nursing, and Mary Adrianella. As they had for the first 70 years of the hospital's existence, the Sisters of Providence continued to move personnel from position to position, at times without consideration for the person's training. Sister Adrianella had no knowledge of accounting when she was transferred to St. Vincent's accounting department in 1955. But having contracted tuberculosis as a laboratory technician, an office job was considered more appropriate for her.

"I was brand new to the field and learned on the job," she said. "I started in payroll when we were still handwriting payroll checks."

Fortunately, she readily took to accounting. Her first challenge was keeping the books in order at a time when the hospital had assumed a large financial burden with the building of the new hospital. Soon after the new hospital opened, the entire front of the hospital had to be rebuilt, because water was seeping in behind the bricks whenever it rained. Even though the hospital was going to be reimbursed, it had to come up with money for the repairs right away. Given that practically every penny the sisters saved already went into the new hospital, it was difficult to keep the hospital's accounts in balance.

In addition, accounts receivable often were difficult to collect. Until Medicare and Medicaid were established in 1964, many people were still uninsured and often lacked the money to pay their bills. Even if they had the money, they didn't always pay up.

"A lot of people figured, 'the sisters are taking care of you.' A lot of people took advantage of it," according to Sister

Adrianella. "They were astounded that we asked them to pay their bills."

But, knowing that other people legitimately could not afford to pay, "I hated to ask people for money. I designed the cashier's office so people could sit down to talk about their bills."

Sister Adrianella, the accountant who had never taken a course in accounting, became the treasurer of St. Vincent Hospital and a board member from 1968 to 1977.

The medical staff also increased significantly after World War II, and especially after construction of the new hospital. Many of the key doctors who built the reputation of St. Vincent Hospital were winding down their careers. But they were being replaced by a new generation of physicians and surgeons — doctors like Dr. Frederick J. McCready and Dr. Robert A. Johnson.

Dr. McCready's surgical skills were on par with those of Dr. McCann and Dr. Fallon. The busiest of surgeons, he was particularly well known for his neck dissections of parathyroid tumors, a tricky operation in which the slightest mistake could kill the patient.

"He would start his rounds at 6:30 or 7 a.m., turn out a dozen operations and work until 10 or 11 p.m. every day," according to Dr. Massarelli. "Clearly, he performed the most surgery of anyone on the staff when he was at St. Vincent. He was very intense. He lived for this. It was all he did, all he thought about continually."

"He was an artist," Dr. Howard said of Dr. McCready. "He was an excellent surgeon. It was not unusual for him to do five or six majors in a day, then he'd have office hours until 11 or midnight and be back in at 5 a.m. In two-and-a-half years with him I saw a lot of good surgery. He was a performer. His stage was the operating room."

Joining the St. Vincent staff in 1949 after earning his master's degree in surgery from the Mayo Clinic, Dr. McCready performed more than 1,000 operations a year during most of his 39 years on the St. Vincent staff. His record is all the more incredible, considering that he was never appointed to be a senior surgeon, a position that provided other top surgeons at St. Vincent with an important source of referrals. Dr. McCready performed the first vascular transplant at St. Vincent in 1954, and performed more than 20 new procedures during his career. Working with Dr. McCready, one doctor joked that he was so busy, he had to schedule his haircuts in the operating room.

Dr. McCready served as chief of the St. Vincent medical staff in 1975 and 1976, and served on the Fallon Clinic staff and the clinic's Board of Directors for many years. He later became an associate professor of surgery at the University of Massachusetts Medical Center, where he was named professor of the year.

As he aged, Dr. McCready's lifestyle changed and he developed other interests. He became especially interested in golf and became a fairly good golfer, but, like anyone who learns the sport late in life, never an exceptional one. Still, he showed the same intense devotion to the game that he earlier showed to surgery. A fierce competitor, he started every game negotiating handicaps to his advantage. He even assembled a series of reference notebooks on subjects such as putting, driving, uphill lies and downhill lies.

Another distinguished surgeon at St. Vincent during the 1940s and 1950s was Dr. Johnson, a neurosurgeon who served as president of the Worcester District Medical Society.

"When I first came here, the three intellects that were respected the most were Dr. Ware, Dr. Johnson and Dr. Meyers," said Dr. Kocot, who began his career at St. Vincent in July 1957. "It is unusual to see three such people in one period of time. They each could talk about anything. At a meeting, when any of the three got up and spoke, there was absolute silence. They had a great influence on my future."

Dr. Johnson was especially well known for his sharp wit. Dr. Kocot recalled operating with Dr. Johnson on a sailor who had been hit on the head. As Dr. Kocot suctioned "debris" from the sailor's brain cavity into a jar in preparation for surgery, Dr. Johnson cautioned him and said, "Careful. Before you know it, that mason jar will be smarter than the patient."

Although the doctors, sisters and nurses receive most of the credit for the success of the new hospital, there are others, according to Sister Adrianella, who deserve recognition for "holding us together."

Chauffeur Joe Monroe was "a real brother to us," she said. "He knew the sisters inside out." During meetings of the Rate Setting Commission in Boston, "he would bring us to a nice place and park the car, then he would leave the car while we had lunch" because the sisters were not allowed to eat in public. He often stood behind the car and ate the sandwiches the sisters brought him. After the Second Vatican Council in 1963, many of the restrictions on nuns were relaxed, and they were allowed to eat in public for the first time. Shortly after Vatican II, Monroe took them into Boston on a rainy day. As usual, he picked up his lunch and began heading toward the back of the car when the sisters stopped him and explained that he could finally join them for lunch.

Pop Logan also was a familiar face to the sisters, and probably spent more time with them than any other member of the laity. He is, according to Sister Adrianella, "part of our history."

It was common in the early days of the Brightside orphanage for babies to be left on the doorstep, and that's how Pop Logan came to the Sisters of Providence. He was just a few days old, and he wore handsome hand-embroidered baby clothes that suggested he came from a prosperous family. Most orphans stayed with the sisters only until they reached high school age. Pop Logan stayed on and soon became a father figure to the other orphans. He became a fixture in Holyoke, raising funds for the orphans wherever he went.

When the old Brightside orphanage was razed, he moved to Worcester to help the sisters at St. Vincent Hospital. "He became a messenger, delivering things between the old and new hospital," Sister Adrianella said. "The employees always bought their stamps off of him. He stayed there at the hospital all day, doing odd jobs. He loved to be of service to people. There were no hours for Pop. We were his to take care of."

He worked for the sisters until a few years ago, when he suffered a stroke and died. He is buried in the cemetery at the Mother House, along with his "sisters."

Soon after the new hospital was built, it faced its first medical challenge.

Throughout its history, St. Vincent Hospital has been ready to respond to medical crises in the community. From the early typhoid fever and flu epidemics to the constant battles against tuberculosis, pneumonia and other diseases, St. Vincent always played an important role, as did other hospitals in and around Worcester. But when an epidemic of polio struck Worcester in 1955, no other hospital in the area was as well equipped to fight it as the new St. Vincent Hospital.

A viral disease that spread quickly and easily, poliomyelitis strikes the nerve cells in the spinal cord, causing the muscles to waste away. Striking mostly children, polio often resulted in paralysis, deformity and even death. It was perhaps the most feared disease of the day. The crippling disease was so dreaded, Bishop Wright ordered perpetual adoration in the hospital chapel and left the Blessed Sacrament exposed for prayer for six weeks during the epidemic.

From August 12 to early September, St. Vincent admitted 45 polio patients from all over the county, and during the entire epidemic the hospital treated 83 polio cases — more than all of the other Worcester hospitals combined. Although polio is often referred to as infantile paralysis, the 45 patients ranged in age from two to 40 and included 10 adults. In November, at the tail end of the epidemic, a mother and her four-year-old son were both stricken with polio. The mother was treated on a separate floor to keep the boy from finding out that she was sick.

To prevent the disease from spreading, during the epidemic all patients were treated on the west wing of the sixth floor, which was turned into an isolation ward with its own kitchen, utility room, sterilizers, gown and cloak room, nursing station and incinerator. Iron lungs from other hospitals were added to St. Vincent's existing machine, giving the hospital a total of five iron lungs. Under the direction of Dr. Brosnan, the medical staff agreed to set policies for treating polio patients. All suspected cases of polio were kept in private rooms until diagnosis was verified. Three wards adjacent to the isolation ward were used for patients when they were no longer infectious. Patients were limited to one 15-minute visit a day from either a father, a mother, a husband or a wife. The visitor had to wear a sterile gown and mask and stand in a corridor facing into the room. Visitors were not allowed into the isolation ward.

Children, separated from their parents and suffering from a crippling disease, were treated with hot dry-steam packs and placed in iron lungs during their first 72 hours of treatment. They were required to remain absolutely flat and were spoon-fed and given intravenous injections. The Sisters of Providence hung rosary beads from the mirrors on the iron lungs, a spiritual medication that brought hope to afflicted patients. As patients were weaned off the iron lung, they were placed on a rocking bed, which restored rhythm to their breathing and helped them breathe naturally.

According to a newspaper account of the epidemic quoting Sister Loreto, "Nurses who had been trained for polio nursing were scarce, and we had little success in recruiting any outside our own nursing staff. In this crisis, however, our nursing staff, both religious and lay, graduate and student, responded heroically, and under the tutelage of the few trained persons we had, soon acquired a more than adequate working knowledge for the task. They labored tirelessly and unselfishly, often 15 and 18 hours a day."

Miss White, who was working as a private duty nurse, said even some nurses were reluctant to treat polio victims. "A lot of people didn't want to do it," she said. "They were afraid of it.

One of my cousins had been stricken and we were exposed to it." The doctors and nurses took precautions, changing their clothes to go to lunch, and changing between patients. They received gamma globulin shots and wore isolation gowns, according to Mrs. Healey, but, "when I walked down the hall, everyone parted, the fear was so great."

The treatment of the polio patients was painstakingly long and difficult. "If we could get a patient to move a big toe that they couldn't move before," she said, "we felt like celebrating." She recalled one patient in particular, a young boy who was stricken with both cerebral palsy and polio. "On December 8th, he received his First Communion, and we lined the hallway."

Some of the sisters and nurses who worked in the isolation ward look back on the epidemic as one of the most important times of their lives, because it gave them an opportunity to apply their training in a way that could relieve the suffering of children and save their young lives. According to Mrs. Healey, "It was just fantastic nursing."

Medical Pioneers

"High on the hilltop, against the sky,
A beautiful picture meets the eye,
The new St. Vincent, 'Healing Fount,'
Preaching a 'Sermon on the Mount.'

"A friendly home for the sick and weak,
What e're their race; what tongue they speak,
Christ the Healer's here to welcome all,
He knows their needs; He'll heed their call.

"The gleaming cross, shining bright,
Makes safe the path like a beacon light,
Flashing a message constantly,
Sweet and consoling, 'Come unto Me!' "

"A Sermon on the Mount," from **Old Timer**

The idea of a wing dedicated to psychiatric care would have been groundbreaking for any hospital in 1954, but it was especially progressive for a Catholic hospital.

Psychiatry at the time was associated with Sigmund Freud and Carl Jung. And Freud and Jung agreed with Karl Marx that religion is the opiate of the masses. In fact, according to Dr. George E. Deering, one of the first psychiatrists to work in the wing, psychoanalysis in those days was practically a religion in and of itself.

"You didn't sing hymns, but you would quote Freud," said Dr. Deering, who was not a Freudian psychiatrist. "Freud was always there. And talking was the answer to everything."

In the 1950s, all of psychiatric treatment was perceived as being antireligion, Dr. Deering said, but "Bishop Wright just said that was a lot of nonsense." With the support of Bishop Wright and Sister Loreto, as well as Dr. Jesse Arnold, the psychiatry unit was added to the new hospital, but it was not always easy to get Catholic patients to submit to treatment.

"I had a terrible time with the Catholic patients, because they thought you would try to get them to do something against their religion," said Dr. Deering. "They'd tell me, 'I can't say too much, because I'm going to have to go to confession and tell the priest what we talk about.'" Dr. Deering had a couch in his office, he said, but because of the perception his patients had of psychoanalysis, "I was the only one who used it."

Dr. Deering trained under Dr. William Malamud, president of the American Psychiatric Association, who trained with both Freud and Jung. "He lasted three weeks with Freud, two with Jung, and he concluded, 'This doesn't make any sense at all.'" While the Freudian and Jungian psychiatrists were opposed to religion, Dr. Deering said, "My attitude always was that you use the Church and faith as a power to help the patient."

When the psychiatric unit opened, the only medical treatment available was shock therapy and Thorazine®, two forms of treatment that are still in use. About 49 out of 50 patients received shock treatment, he estimated, and it usually was very effective and helpful. Unfortunately, he said, some doctors abused shock treatment because of its potential as a money maker, and the abuse gave it an undeservedly bad reputation.

"There were two doctors in Boston doing eight to 10 treatments a day on each patient," he said. "With 90 seconds per treatment, they were getting $75 to $100 each back in the '50s. That adds up to a lot of money."

As medication has improved, shock treatment has become almost unnecessary, though it is still used occasionally.

Even though the psychiatric unit's work was controversial, Dr. Deering said neither the nuns nor Bishop Wright ever tried to influence what he did. And, like other hospital services, the psychiatric unit remained open to all types of people with all types of mental disorders. Many of his early patients were veterans of World War II or Korea, including a Marine with over 200 notches on his rifle who was a paranoid schizophrenic.

"Occasionally they begin to like to kill," Dr. Deering said. "He told me he could run through the woods of New England on dry leaves in the fall and not make a sound. During deer hunting season, he said, he used to line up the sights of his rifle on hunters' hearts and pull the trigger halfway. Killing was a normal thing for him."

Another patient, who served as a commando during World War II, "was pretty normal until he was assigned on his 16th birthday to pick up the pieces of bodies on Normandy Beach." He lied about his age to join the military, and he became involved in clandestine operations. His partner was captured, and he killed six or seven people with his bare hands to rescue him.

"He was in my office and said, 'Do you have a knife?' I handed him a jackknife, and he said, 'See that fly on the wall?' He threw the knife and cut the fly in two, and he buried the blade an inch deep in the oak paneling."

But unlike the paranoid schizophrenic patient, Dr. Deering said, "He hated the killing. At some point, he had witnessed some kid being shot with a bow and arrow, and he fell apart. He saw how senseless and unnecessary it was."

In June 1954, Francis Holmes, director of the Worcester County Council on Alcoholism, worked with Dr. Morrison and Dr. Deering to obtain a $20,000 state grant to add a clinic to the psychiatric wing to provide treatment for alcoholism.

"There was a lot of argument about whether alcoholism was an appropriate psychiatric disease. We were probably the first hospital in the area to admit chronic alcoholics on the same priority as other patients," Dr. Morrison said. "As a general hospital, we treated the whole person. I treated the medical problems, and Dr. Deering treated the psychiatric problems. Our batting average was pretty good."

In November 1956, the House of Delegates of the American Medical Association approved a resolution recommending that general hospitals admit without prejudice those alcoholic patients who seek hospital admission, "rather than following the punitive and prejudicial rule that no alcoholic patient be admitted to the hospital."

St. Vincent Hospital's alcoholic clinic was already well ahead of the rest of the country. In "The Chronic Alcoholic in the General Hospital," a paper on starting up clinics for alcoholics, Dr. Morrison wrote, "The physician, whose training and experience should qualify him in such matters, recognizes alcoholism as a disease. He recognizes it as a disease clinically and pathologically, and he views it as a rather complex illness with physical, emotional and spiritual aspects." The St. Vincent clinic's approach reflected a belief in Dr. Morrison's statement. Early on, it developed corporate programs, treating alcoholics in the workplace with Antabuse®, a drug that made them ill if it was in their system when they drank alcohol. The clinic was an early prescriber of Librium®, which is still recommended by the National Council on Alcoholism. And, from its inception, it held group therapy sessions for alcoholics, treating both the physical and psychological consequences of the disease. The alcohol clinic had more than 300 admissions in its first year and 3,000 in its first six years.

In 1956, the clinic received national attention on the television series *Medical Horizons,* which was sponsored by Ciba Pharmaceutical and produced by its advertising agency, J. Walter Thompson. The program, which was called "The Hidden Disease," showcased the St. Vincent clinic as a model for the rest of the country. The program was broadcast on a Sunday afternoon on 86 ABC stations.

Television, like hospital treatment of alcoholism, was also in its early days. In 1956, American families had begun their love affair with television and were buying millions of televisions a year, but still had few programs to choose from, so a program like *Medical Horizons* was widely seen. Dr. Deering was not nervous about the show until the cameraman told him it was going to be viewed by 10 million people.

Unlike most of today's documentary programs, "The Hidden Disease" worked with dialogue that was scripted in advance and developed to fit the half-hour program perfectly. The St. Vincent doctors, patients and staff had to memorize and rehearse their lines.

"We sat in a room rehearsing for nine hours the day before the show and nine hours the day of the show," Dr. Deering said. "We sat for so long we got sunburned under the incandescent lights. Finally, the cameraman said, 'Do it now, or everyone's going to have to have makeup.' My nose was getting red."

Although Dr. Deering had some experience acting for theater, Dr. Morrison was the official director of the clinic, so he was the focus of the program's interviews. He had so many lines to memorize, he found it difficult to sound spontaneous. To this day, he regrets having gone along with the script.

While Dr. Morrison remains self-conscious about his performance, it was good enough to draw attention to the St. Vincent program. The national exposure brought to St. Vincent by the program enhanced the hospital's image and created a great deal of pride among the hospital staff. "We got a lot of telephone calls," Dr. Morrison said.

One of the stars of "The Hidden Disease" was Sister Mary Joseph, the Sisters of Providence supervisor in the psychiatric wing. Sister Mary Joseph, looking professional yet welcoming, describes alcoholism as "a non-sectarian disease," and she says her alcoholic patients are "a very likable group of people."

Both Dr. Deering and Dr. Morrison have high praise for her work in the wing. "At night, she would do the history and physical of the patient for me, whatever she felt capable of doing, and let me sleep," Dr. Morrison said. "She was never wrong. She had a special knowledge of the patients."

"She was great with alcoholics," according to Dr. Deering. "She simply understood what it was like. She could talk to a patient for two or three minutes and make decisions that were valid. She was a wonderful observer." Being a nun gave her an advantage, because alcoholics knew that certain behavior was unacceptable in front of her. "An alcoholic with the DTs might be cursing and swearing," Dr. Deering said, "and she'd come into the room and they'd stop."

Even volunteer workers who did not have a great deal of training seemed to have a tremendous sensitivity and intuition on how to deal with the psychiatric and alcoholic patients. Dr. Deering remembers a frail and elderly ward aid who was spoon-feeding a patient when another patient, who was very hostile and aggressive, held a heavy oak chair over her head and said, "I'm going to kill you." Still feeding her patient, she calmly asked, "Why?" The patient put down the chair.

Despite the seriousness of treating alcoholism and mental illness, the wing had its occasional light moments. Once, a good friend of Dr. Deering was admitted to St. Vincent Hospital with prostate trouble. Because of a lack of space, after surgery he was given a room on the sixth floor.

"I went to see him," Dr. Deering said, "and, after I left, they moved his bed away from the window and put him on 24-hour watch." Because Dr. Deering had been to see the man, it was assumed that his illness was mental, not physical.

Another time, Dr. Deering was confined to a wheelchair after striking his foot with an ax. The door to the psychiatric wing was locked, and he was one of the few people with a key. Because he was in a wheelchair, no one on the other side of the door could see him when he unlocked and opened it. An alcoholic patient saw the door seemingly open by itself. The seeming hallucination caused the patient a bit of anxiety, according to Dr. Deering.

As psychiatric treatment expanded, and there was no longer any room for the alcoholic clinic in the same wing, the clinic moved into the basement, then into the convent building and then into the nurses' home.

Over time, increasing governmental regulation made it difficult to sustain the clinic, according to Dr. Deering. In the 1980s, some alcoholic treatment clinics became very profitable, and there was a lot of abuse and even fraud in the way some of the clinics were managed. The abuse led to increasing regulation.

"Until seven or eight years ago," he said, "if a patient came in, you saw them. Now there's a four-week wait. You have to have three one-hour sessions and fill out a 16-page patient history. It's all totally irrelevant. Alcoholics don't tell the truth anyhow. You ask questions like, 'How often do you go to Church and why?' You don't see too many good Church-going people coming in. You have to ask questions like, 'If you're 57 years old, and you started drinking when you were 12, how many beers did you drink every day?' The people who were most likely to get better don't come in any more. We mostly get the people who are mandated to come or go back to jail."

While government regulations have made treatment difficult today, Dr. Morrison feels good about looking back at all of the people the clinic has helped over the years.

"There are a lot of people who came to the clinic and put their lives in order," he said. "It's a beautiful feeling when I get Christmas cards from some of these people and they say, 'You had confidence in me when no one else did.' . . . I'm not sure doctors do much for them except provide encouragement, but I'm glad I was able to help."

One person who saw "The Hidden Disease" on television was Dr. Massarelli, who was finishing his training at the Mayo Clinic in Rochester, Minnesota, and trying to determine where to begin his career.

He found out that the Fallon Clinic had an opening for an internist, and that members of Fallon's medical staff routinely practiced at St. Vincent. He wrote to Dr. John F. Stapleton, St. Vincent Hospital's first director of medical training, because "I knew that if he was at St. Vincent, it was a good place." An interview followed, and he's been at St. Vincent and Fallon Clinic ever since.

Like many of St. Vincent's innovations, the idea for the medical training center is believed to have originated with Bishop Wright, whose brother, Dr. Richard Wright, served as the director of the diagnostic clinic at Georgetown before he returned to Boston to practice at Holy Ghost Hospital. Dr. McCann, a graduate of Georgetown who helped develop an earlier affiliation between St. Vincent and Tufts Medical School, also may have initiated the affiliation with Georgetown.

In the fall of 1953, when the idea of a medical training center was under consideration, five of St. Vincent's top doctors visited Georgetown to check it out — Dr. Brosnan, who was chief of medicine; Dr. McCann, who was chief of surgery; Dr. Meyers; Dr. Steele; and Dr. Richmond. The medical training center and the appointment of Dr. Stapleton were strongly influenced by Dr. Meyers, who believed a well-educated medical staff was essential to the future of the hospital. But Dr. Meyers himself, writing a eulogy, gives credit to Dr. Brosnan for establishing the training center at St. Vincent.

The concept, though, of establishing a training center in a Catholic community hospital clearly came from Dr. Harold J. Jeghers, who was chairman of medicine at Georgetown. Dr. Jeghers was a medical education innovator whose two great contributions were the concept of a community teaching hospital and the creation of a uniquely classified index of medical articles.

Dr. Jeghers, who later figured even more directly in St. Vincent's medical education program as the hospital's first medical director, envisioned community hospitals as playing an increasing role in medical education. Dr. Jeghers already had helped to establish education centers at two other community hospitals when he approached Dr. Stapleton, who was then a part-time instructor at Georgetown, and persuaded him to become St. Vincent's director of medical education.

"He told me St. Vincent was a much better hospital than the other two, with a brand-new, shining physical plant, and a progressive young bishop whose brother was Dick Wright," Dr. Stapleton said. "Harold was impressed by the medical staff. He thought the credentials of the leaders of the medical staff were stronger than those of most hospitals. He was impressed that there were lots of graduates of Boston colleges. He thought that Boston was the Athens of America."

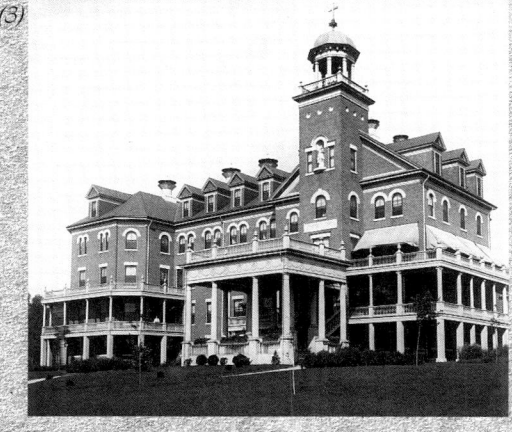

(1) The Bartlett farmhouse, known as "House of Providence Hospital," 1893

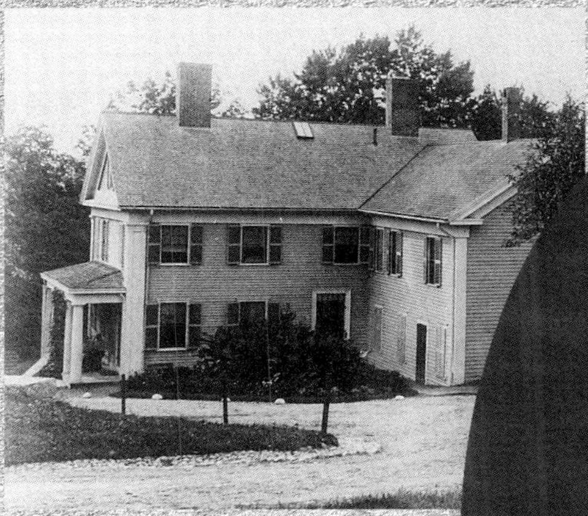

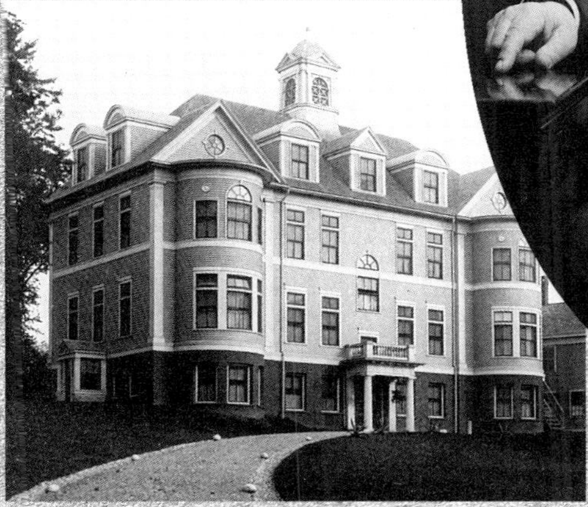

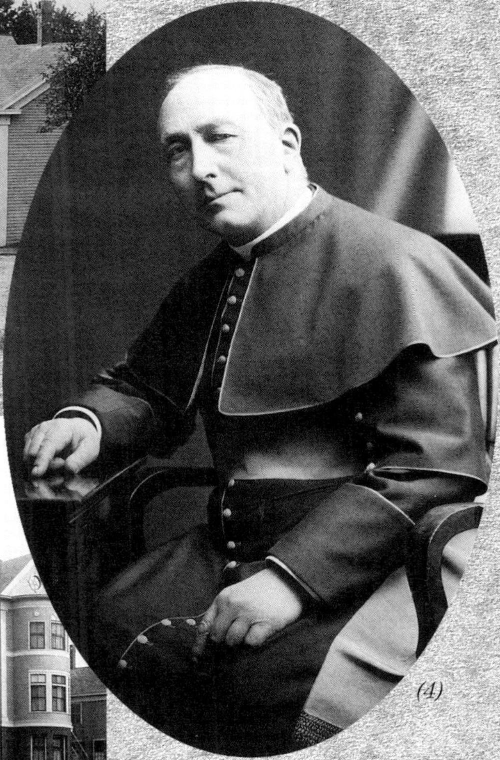

(2) The 1895 expansion, called "Saint Vincent Hospital"

(3) Saint Vincent Hospital, 1808

(4) Msgr. Thomas Griffin, hospital founder, 1893

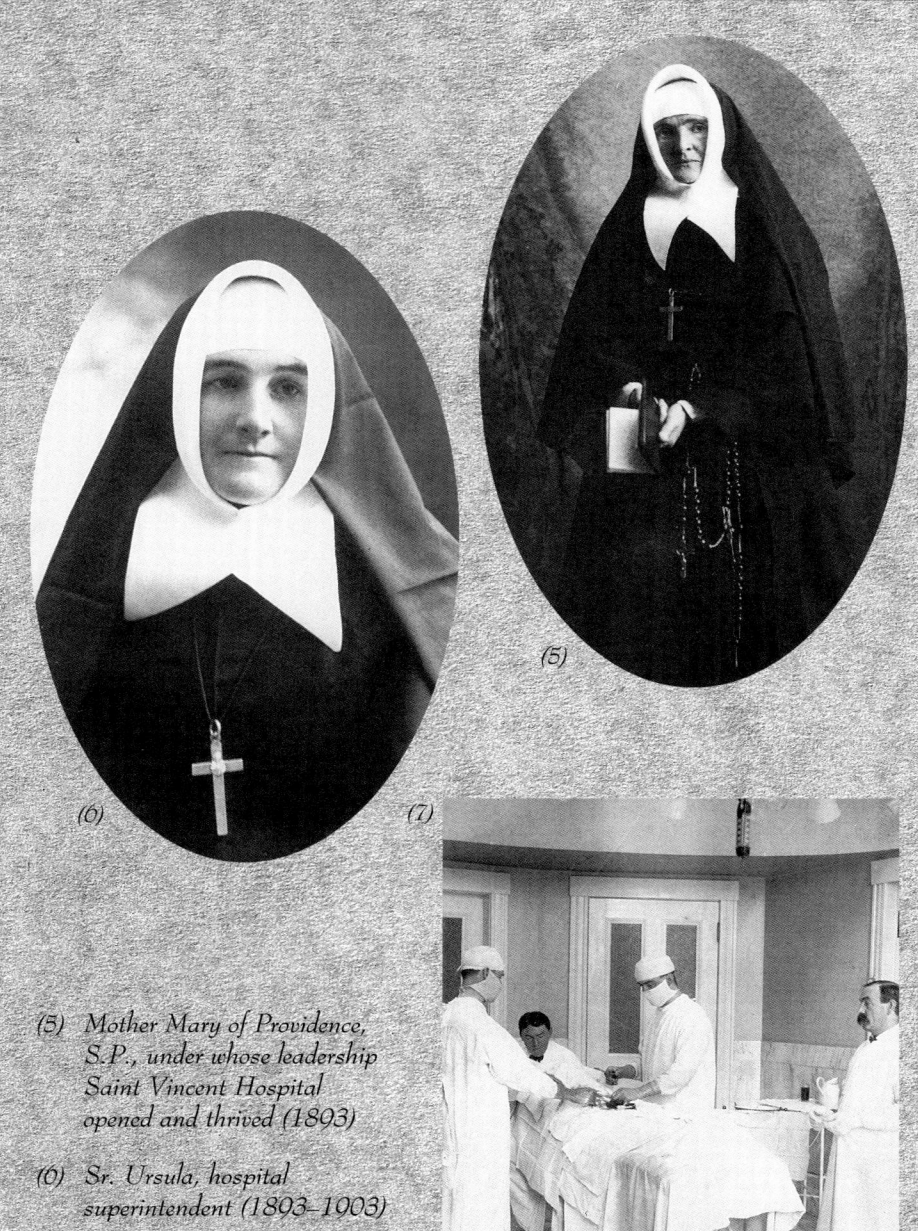

(5) Mother Mary of Providence, S.P., under whose leadership Saint Vincent Hospital opened and thrived (1893)

(6) Sr. Ursula, hospital superintendent (1893–1903)

(7) Dr. Michael Fallon (second from right) performing surgery (1901)

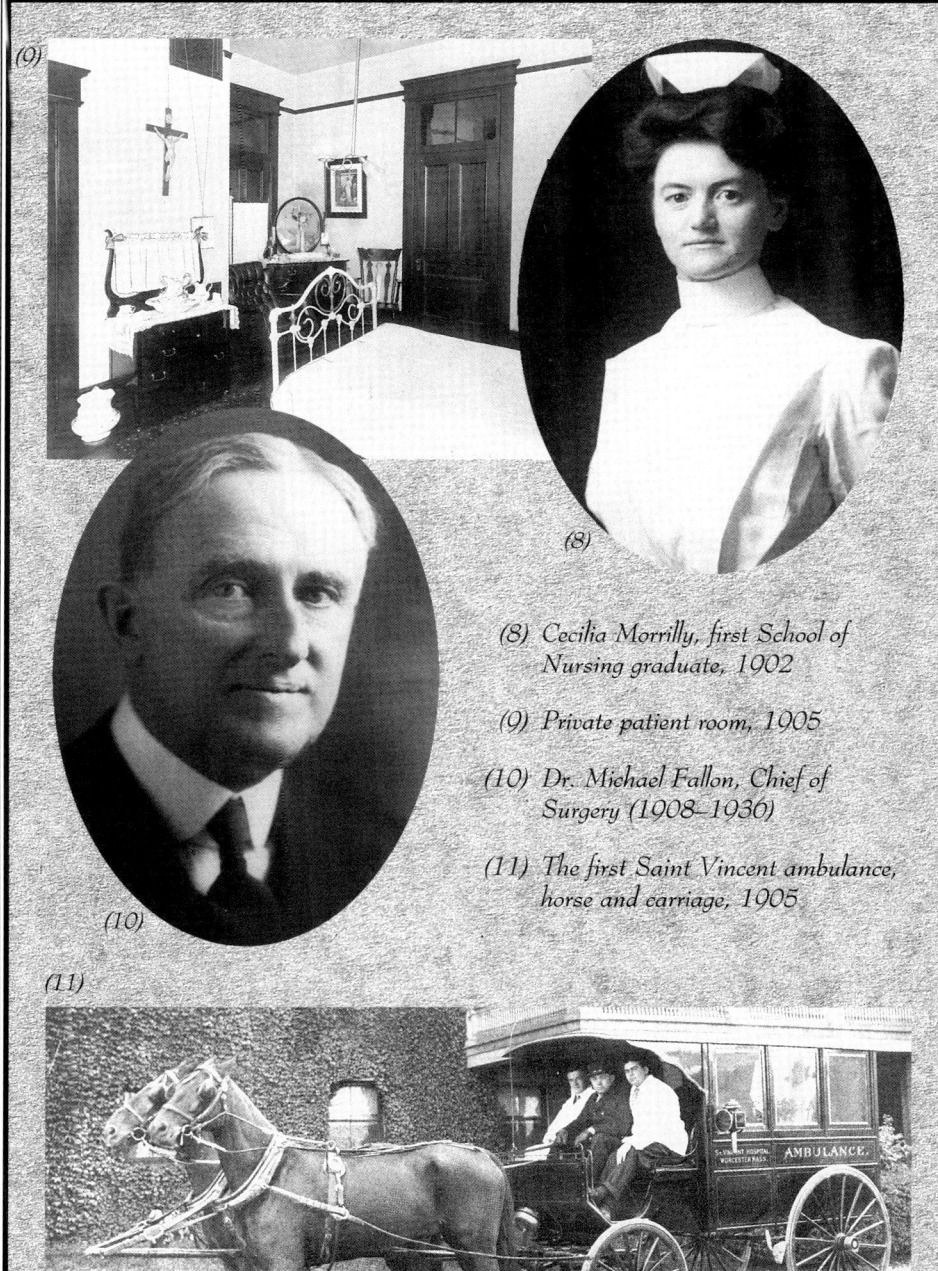

(8) Cecilia Morrilly, first School of
Nursing graduate, 1902

(9) Private patient room, 1905

(10) Dr. Michael Fallon, Chief of
Surgery (1908–1936)

(11) The first Saint Vincent ambulance,
horse and carriage, 1905

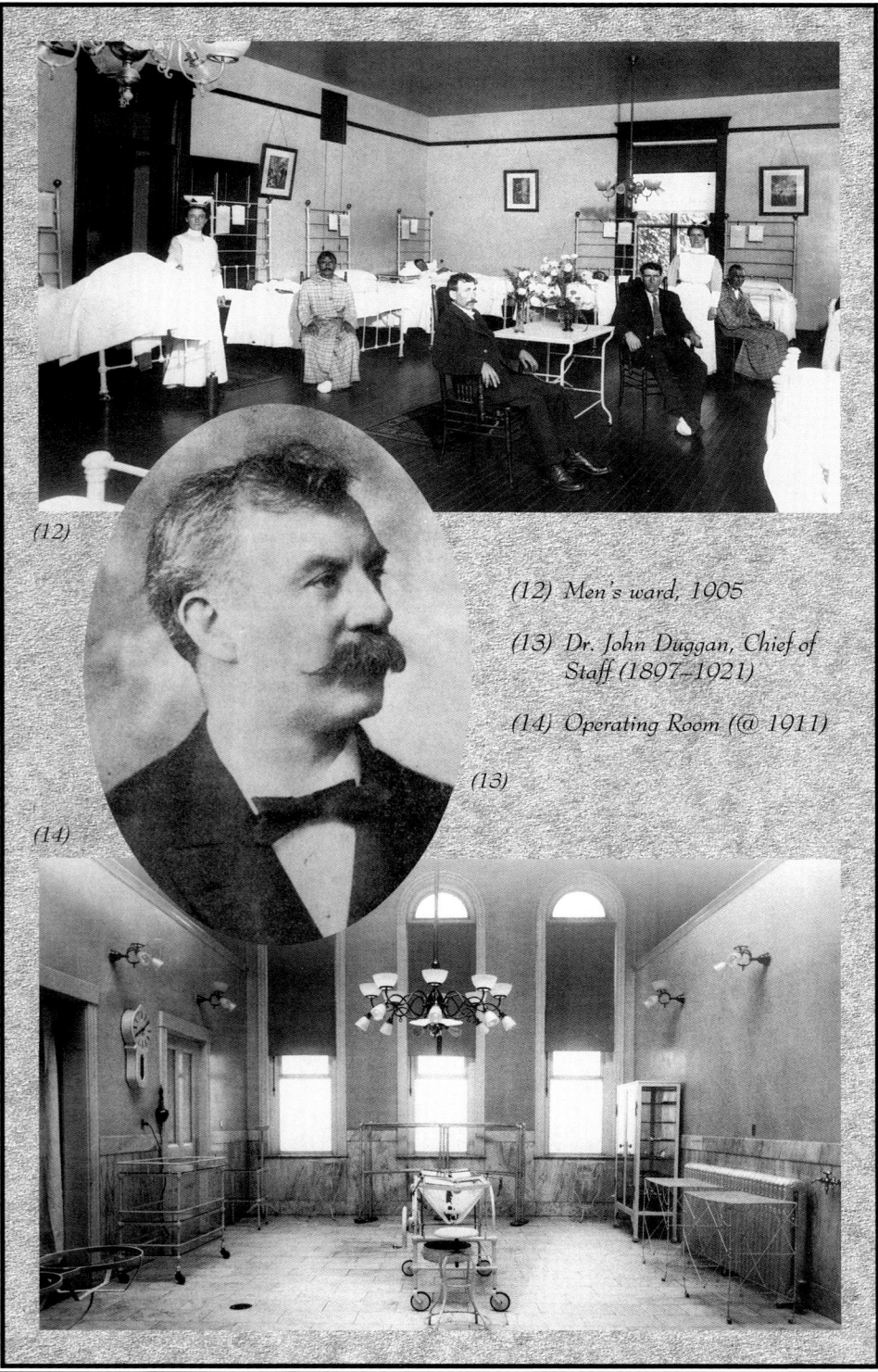

(12) Men's ward, 1905

(13) Dr. John Duggan, Chief of Staff (1897–1921)

(14) Operating Room (@ 1911)

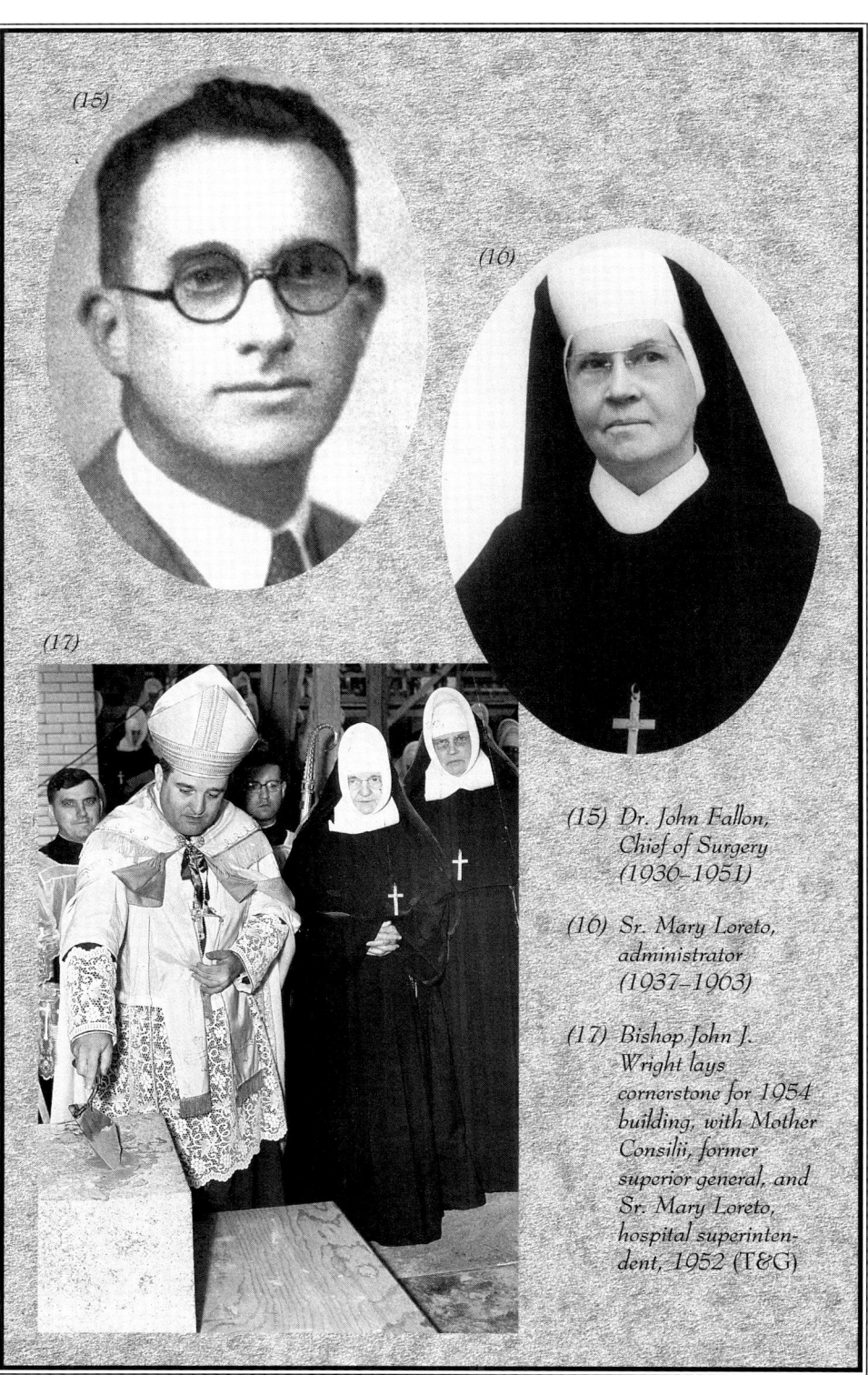

(15) Dr. John Fallon,
Chief of Surgery
(1936–1951)

(16) Sr. Mary Loreto,
administrator
(1937–1963)

(17) Bishop John J.
Wright lays
cornerstone for 1954
building, with Mother
Consilii, former
superior general, and
Sr. Mary Loreto,
hospital superinten-
dent, 1952 (T&G)

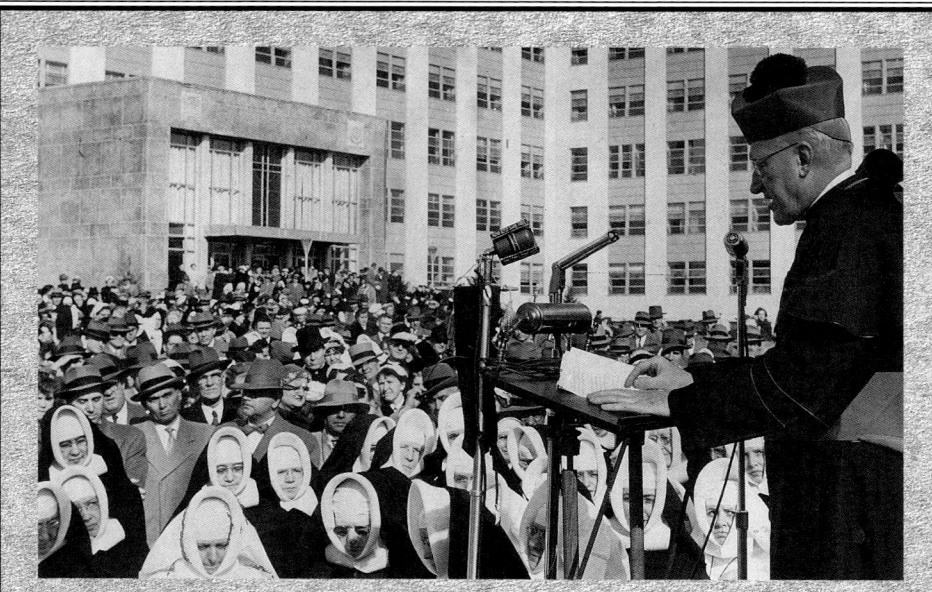

(18)

(18) Archbishop Richard J. Cushing speaks at the dedication of the current Saint Vincent Hospital, 1954 (T&G)

(19) Sr. Mary Dolorum attends to a polio patient in an iron lung, August 1955 (CFP)

(19)

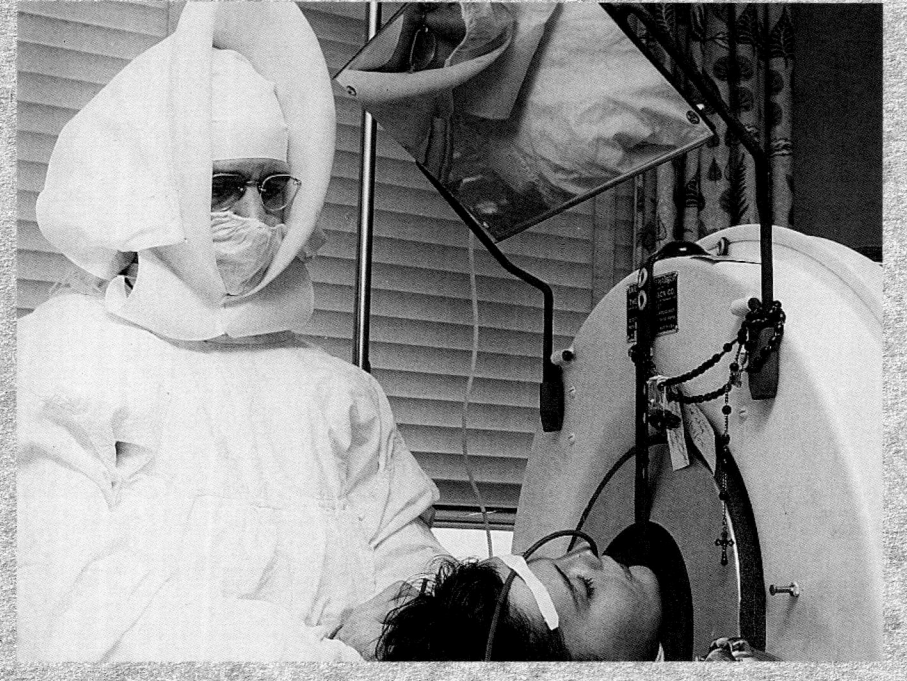

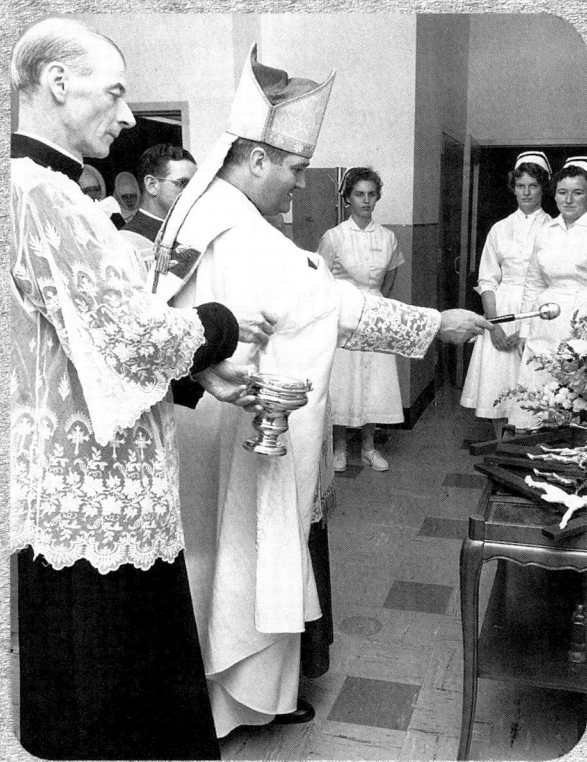

(20)

(20) Blessing of nurses'
residence, with
(L to R)
Fr. Hendran,
Bishop Wright,
Anne Houle,
Patricia Ronan,
Jane Healey,
August 29, 1957

(21) Rose Marie Picard,
first open-heart
patient, with
(L to R) Jean
McLaughlin, R.N.,
Dr. Paul Ware,
Mrs. Agnes Picard,
and Sr. Mary
Parquelette,
October 1959

(21)

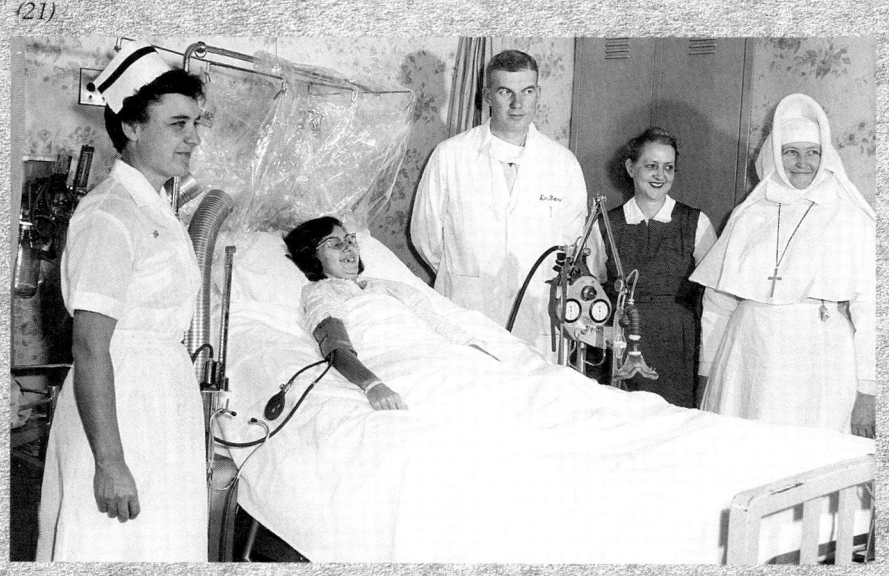

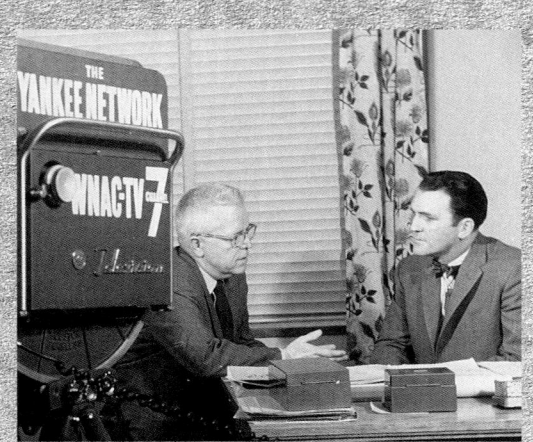

(22)

(22) Dr. James Morrison
being interviewed by
WNAC-TV 7,
December 27, 1957 (CFP)

(23) Mrs. F. Joseph Donohue,
Mrs. James C. Donnelly,
Mrs. John E. Butts,
Mrs. Frank R. Bowler and
Miss Gertrude E. Mullaney
(L to R) of the Guild of
Our Lady of Providence
members compile a report
on the Fall Assembly,
December 11, 1953 (CFP)

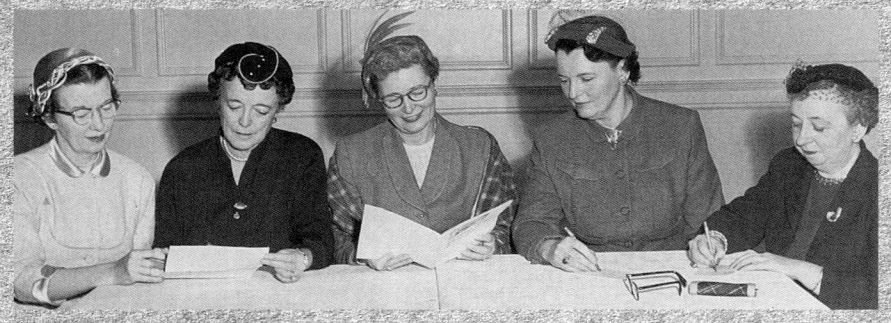

(23)

(24)

(24) Dr. Stanley
Kocot with
Rosemary
Hallinan
Foley, R.N.,
in Outpatient
Pediatric
Clinic, 1958

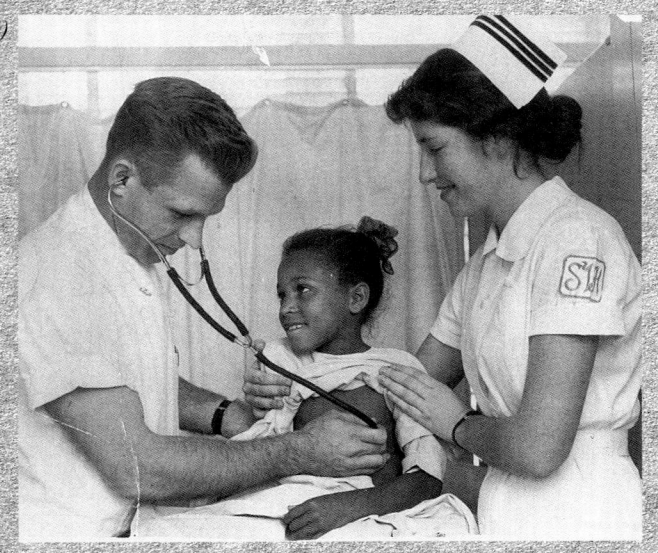

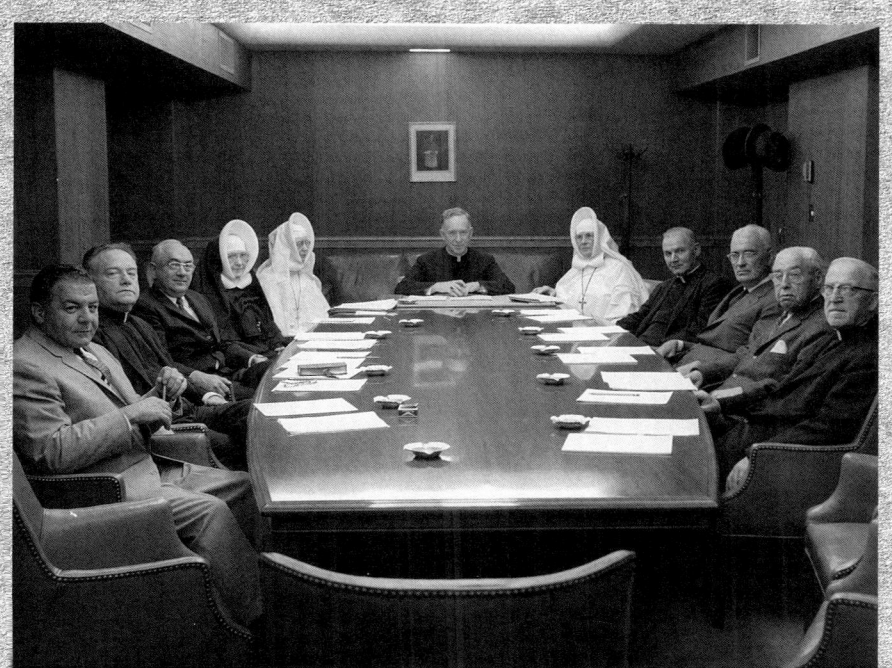

(25)

(25) Meeting of Executive Committee, Board of Trustees (1965):
(L to R) Cosmo Mingolla, Msgr. Timothy O'Connell, Saul Seder,
Sr. DeLasalle, S.P., Sr. Agnes Marie, S.P., Bishop Bernard
Flanagan, Mother Mary Loreto, S.P., Rt. Rev. John F. Gannon,
Ray Heffernan, James Crotty, Msgr. John G. Reilly

(20) Dr. Arthur FitzGerald (left) with his son, Dr. Denis FitzGerald

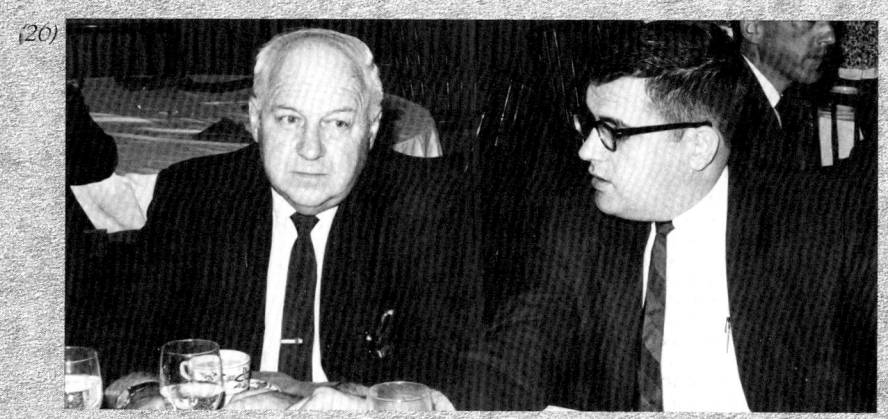

(20)

(27) Sr. Helen Smith
(right) with
Sr. Adrianella,
1905

(27)

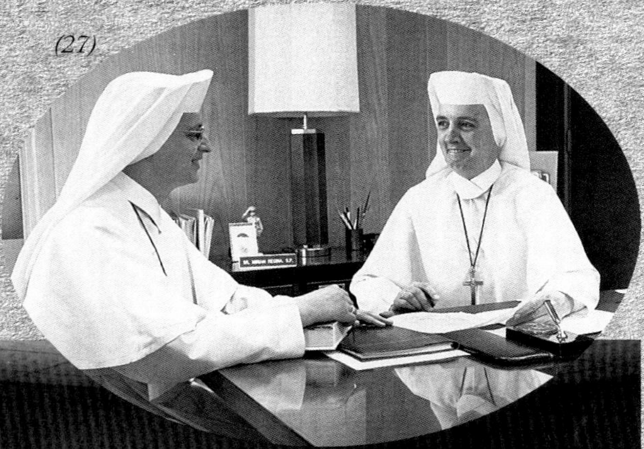

(28)

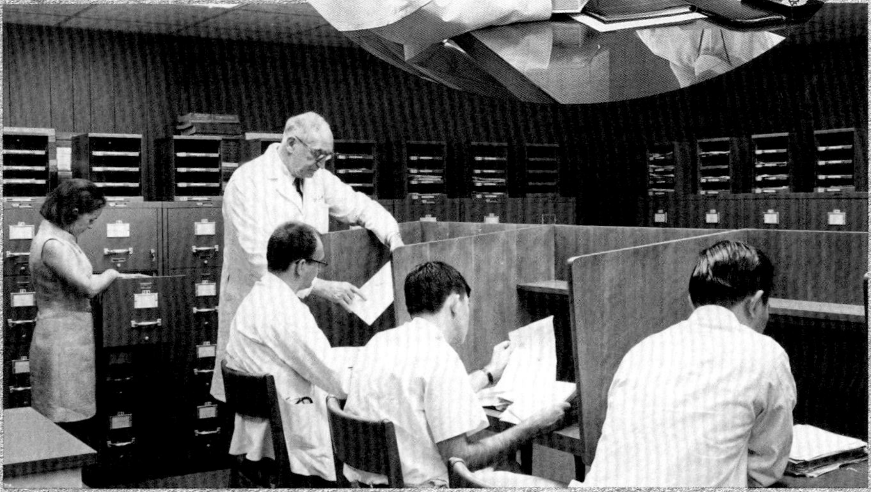

(28) Dr. Harold J.
Jeghers working
on his Medical
Index System,
with secretary
Anne Carter and
medical residents,
1968

(29) Mr. & Mrs.
Philip Rose at
dedication of the
Diagnostic &
Research Center
in their name,
1972 (T&G)

(29)

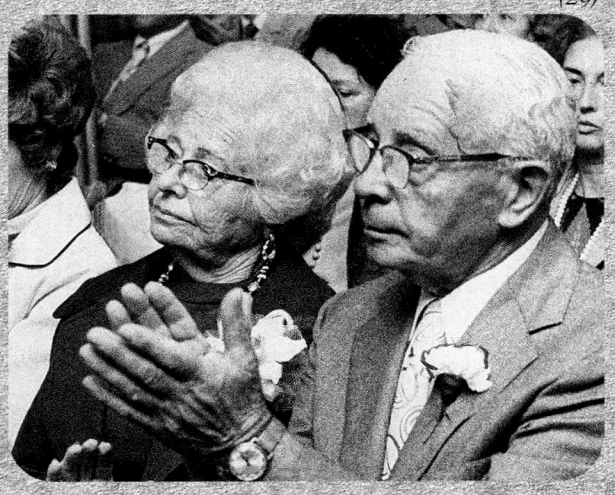

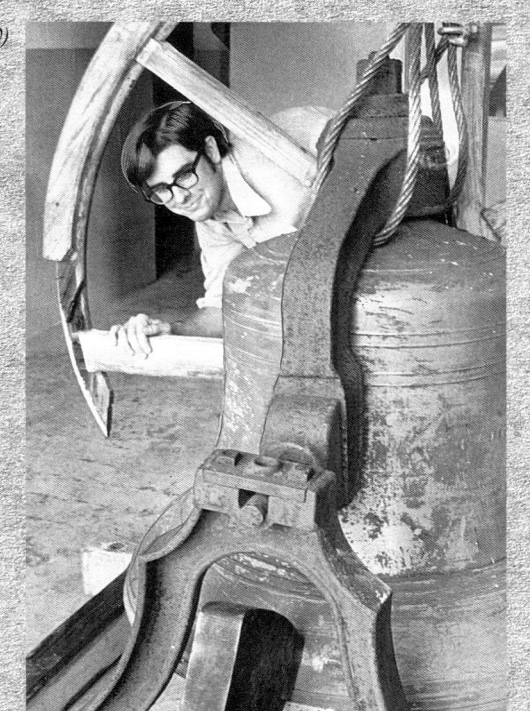

(30)

(30) Bruce Frieswick
assists with moving the
bell, donated in 1899 by
Mr. & Mrs. Peter Baker,
when the 1898 hospital
building was razed, 1973
(T&G)

(31) Groundbreaking for
amphitheater: (L to R)
Helen M. Smith,
Dr. Stanley Kocot,
Msgr. O'Connell,
Ethel Noonan,
William Fox and
Sr. Catherine Laboure,
1982

(31)

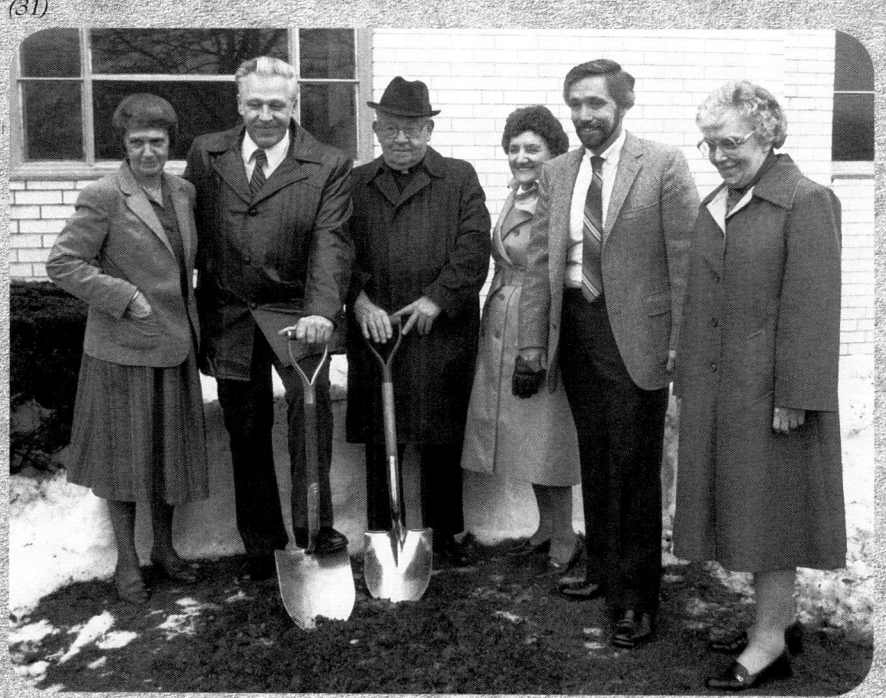

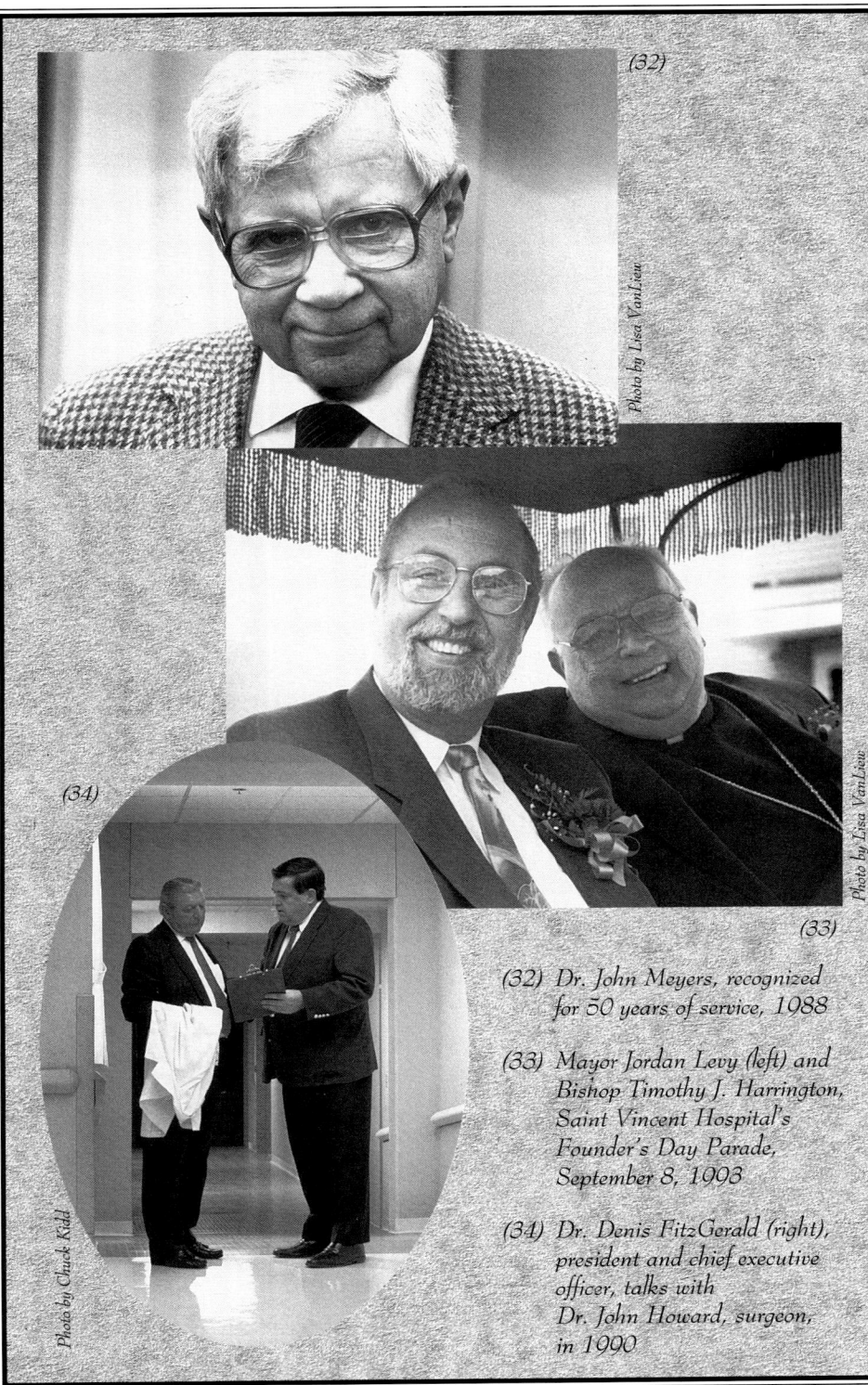

(32)

Photo by Lisa VanLiew

(34)

Photo by Chuck Kidd

(33)

Photo by Lisa VanLiew

(32) Dr. John Meyers, recognized
for 30 years of service, 1988

(33) Mayor Jordan Levy (left) and
Bishop Timothy J. Harrington,
Saint Vincent Hospital's
Founder's Day Parade,
September 8, 1993

(34) Dr. Denis FitzGerald (right),
president and chief executive
officer, talks with
Dr. John Howard, surgeon,
in 1990

Dr. Jeghers had reason to be fond of Boston, the city that launched his career. In 1932, he had been one of the first interns at the new Fifth Medical Service, which was formed by Boston University at Boston City Hospital. In 1936, after serving a research fellowship at the Evans Memorial Institute in Boston, he was appointed to the BU faculty. At the time, Boston City Hospital was affiliated not just with BU, but with the Harvard and Tufts medical schools. Dr. Jeghers was the only full-time paid teacher at the hospital.

While at BU, Dr. Jeghers developed a 10-page form house officers could use to ensure that their patients were receiving a thorough examination. A patient who was subjected to the lengthy questioning and examination necessary to complete the form was said to have been "Jegherized," according to Dr. Gilbert E. Levinson, who was recruited to St. Vincent by Dr. Jeghers.

In addition to being impressed by the Boston roots of the St. Vincent staff, Dr. Jeghers found the active role of the bishop and the abilities of the nuns to be unlike anything he had seen at other Catholic hospitals. At the time, the nuns who operated many of the other Catholic hospitals throughout the country "had little interest or understanding of how to run a hospital," Dr. Stapleton said. "They thought that the only thing important was keeping the hospital clean. When we arrived at St. Vincent, we found that the nuns were, for the most part, quite the opposite of what we had expected."

Dr. Stapleton understands why Dr. Jeghers found the St. Vincent Hospital affiliation attractive, but he is less than certain why he was chosen to manage the program — although, having served as a "reading resident," helping to research and catalogue articles for Dr. Jeghers' medical index, he must have understood that he was well thought of by Dr. Jeghers.

"I don't know why Dr. Jeghers picked me," he said. "Maybe he thought that I was in tune with bedside teaching. As a cardiologist, you listen and have a feel for things that others don't usually have."

With a medical training center in place and Dr. Stapleton at its helm, St. Vincent Hospital was able to attract a better quality of intern. Many of the hospital's physicians and interns, like Dr. Massarelli, came from other parts of the country, attracted by St. Vincent's newly enhanced reputation. Many came directly from Georgetown.

"Georgetown University students all knew about St. Vincent Hospital," according to Dr. Robert J. Phaneuf, a Georgetown graduate who came to St. Vincent as an intern in 1958. "There were 15 slots in St. Vincent's matching program, and in 1958, 10 were filled by Georgetown University students, and Georgetown graduated only 100 students a year."

Dr. Jeghers worked with Dr. Stapleton to get the St. Vincent program started. As part of the agreement with Georgetown, many of the physicians from the Georgetown staff lectured at St. Vincent.

Dr. Stapleton served at St. Vincent for nearly a dozen years before returning to serve as the medical director of Georgetown University Hospital. A student of Dr. Proctor Harvey, Dr. Stapleton is remembered as being second only to his teacher in his ability to use a stethoscope.

"He could do with a stethoscope what one needs the most sophisticated equipment to do today," according to Dr. Kocot. Dr. Massarelli also noted Dr. Stapleton's agility with a stetho-scope. "He was an excellent electrocardiologist — one of the best in the world with a stethoscope. Listening to a heart, he could tell 'that sounds like the opening snap of mitrostenosis' because the second snap was 0.006 seconds after the first."

According to Dr. Massarelli, with the creation of the medical teaching center and the opening of the new hospital, "St. Vincent was on the cutting edge."

The new St. Vincent Hospital offered some of the most advanced and innovative services of any community hospital in the country. Its new medical training center and its dedicated wing for psychiatric treatment marked the hospital as an innovator. So did its clinic for the treatment of alcoholism.

In 1956, St. Vincent also became the first hospital in New England to open a muscular dystrophy clinic. The clinic, under the direction of Dr. Philip Lahey, was only the 30th muscular dystrophy clinic in the United States. It was established under the sponsorship of the Worcester County Chapter of the Muscular Dystrophy Association of America to provide physical therapy, and recreational and entertainment programs.

St. Vincent also established a Social Service Department in 1956. The hospital's social services and clinics for the poor were, if not necessarily groundbreaking, well in advance of what might be expected at most community hospitals.

St. Vincent Hospital was among the first community hospitals to establish an intensive care unit for cardiac patients, one of the first Catholic hospitals to establish a research foundation, and one of the first to establish full-time positions for many members of its medical staff.

But what really set St. Vincent apart most, and enhanced the hospital's reputation nationally, was that it was one of the first community hospitals to establish an open-heart surgery program.

Until World War II, when doctors had to operate on a large number of chest wounds, cardiac surgery did not exist. Heart surgery was so new in the 1950s, that when Cecilia Benoit gave birth to a baby girl at St. Vincent in 1959, it was announced that she and her husband, Richard, were perhaps the first parents in the world to have both survived heart surgery. Heart surgery's greatest advance came in 1954 with the invention and successful use of a heart-lung pump. The pump made open-heart surgery possible by functioning during surgery as the patient's heart and lungs, oxygenating the blood and keeping it flowing through the patient's body. The first patient for open-heart surgery, in which the heart muscle is actually cut open to expose the heart's inner tissue, was a cat.

By the end of the decade, many of the largest and most sophisticated city hospitals were using open-heart surgery on humans. So was St. Vincent Hospital.

A brand new hospital with spiritual leaders like Bishop Wright and Sister Loreto, with innovative medical programs and some of the best physicians anywhere, St. Vincent's open-heart surgery program enhanced the hospital's reputation perhaps more than any other factor.

That a community hospital offered open-heart surgery at the time was highly unusual. But so was the surgeon who started the program, Dr. Paul F. Ware.

A ruggedly handsome man who stood 6'4", Dr. Ware left an impression on everyone he met. "Dr. Paul Ware was the most commanding person I have ever encountered," Dr. Jaffee said. "He was a guy who you wanted to be your commander. He would say, 'In my opinion . . .' and everyone would agree with him."

But his commanding presence masked his vulnerabilities. He suffered from both asthma and a bleeding ulcer — conditions that individually would discourage a lesser man from pursuing a career in thoracic surgery. Yet Dr. Ware refused to give in to his frailties. When his bleeding ulcer weakened him, it was not unusual for Dr. Ware to give himself a blood transfusion and return to work the next day.

Growing up in Clinton, he was inspired by a neighbor who was a doctor, and at an early age, he began to bandage up other children in the neighborhood. As a student at Holy Cross College, he met his future wife, Louise, who was a student at Wellesley College. He attended Harvard Medical School, losing a year of schooling because of his bleeding ulcer. After graduating, he was a resident at Boston Children's Hospital with Dr. Robert E. Gross, who wrote a classic textbook about pediatric care. In the foreword to his textbook, he praises a resident who he says helped him achieve dramatic advances in postoperative care, particularly in the treatment of peritonitis. That resident was Dr. Ware.

After his stay at Boston Children's Hospital, Dr. Ware became one of the first thoracic surgeons, or chest surgeons, trained at Boston City Hospital. At the time, the inside of the heart was still unexplored territory for surgeons, and thoracic surgery itself was still a brand-new field. Dr. Ware was one of only about 50 certified thoracic surgeons in the country. Working under Dr. John Streeter, he learned how to perform chest surgery on tuberculosis patients, removing the infected tissue in their lungs, and he learned "closed" cardiac surgery, primarily how to crack valves, or what is called a mitroaocommurotomy.

After completing his residency, Dr. Ware began his practice in Boston, but by 1953, he was performing chest surgery one day a week at Memorial Hospital in Worcester. Enlisting in the U.S. Army in 1953, Dr. Ware served as commander of a mobile medical unit in Korea, then as chief of thoracic surgery at Fitzsimmons Army Hospital in Denver, Colorado, and as an Army advisor to Chinese nationalists in Formosa on the treatment of tuberculosis, the number-one cause of death in the world at the time. Dr. Ware completed his military service in 1955.

A native of Clinton and a deeply religious man, it is not surprising that this man who could have had his choice of hospitals at which to practice chose to base so much of his practice at St. Vincent Hospital. He soon moved his practice to Worcester permanently, and was in great demand at hospitals throughout the county, according to Clare Weeks, his full-time scrub nurse. Because of his skills, he became "a celebrity" throughout the county and regularly performed surgery from Milford to Rutland. While other hospitals sought out his skills, St. Vincent was always a special place to him.

"He was a man ahead of his time," according to Miss Weeks. "He had a great love for St. Vincent and he wanted to see it succeed — to see it become the best it could be."

By 1957, Dr. Ware had determined that he wanted to bring open-heart surgery to St. Vincent. But without an endowment and with limited resources, the hospital could not afford to subsidize the program. An open-heart surgery program required not only the purchase of a heart-lung pump, but many man-hours of training. A single open-heart operation required a dozen or more trained specialists, including the surgeon in charge, two or three assistants, two anesthetists and an assistant, a cardiologist to monitor the heart, three or four nurses, and a specialist to monitor the heart-lung pump. Additional personnel were required in the laboratory, in the preparation and recovery rooms, and in the patient's sick room, where 24-hour nursing care was required for more than a week. Unlike the large, urban hospitals, St. Vincent also lacked the patient volume to warrant such large expenditures. That failed to stop Dr. Ware. Even with eight children, a thriving private practice and a demanding lecture schedule, he found time to get an open-heart surgery program up and running at St. Vincent Hospital.

To start the program, Dr. Ware first needed a heart-lung pump and a dedicated medical team willing to volunteer the thousands of hours of preparation it took to train for open-heart surgery. Dr. Ware's first step was to assemble a team of specialists that included Miss Weeks; Dr. Carroll, a junior resident in thoracic surgery at the time; Dr. William J. Martin, Jr., chief of anesthesiology; and others. Once the team was assembled, it went to the Mallory Clinic in Boston once a week to participate in its open-heart surgery operations, helping out and observing while the Boston team operated on pigs, dogs and horses. The Boston clinic was experimenting and learning to use the machine itself in preparation for operating on human patients. The work of Dr. Ware and his team continued at the Mallory Clinic for about a year.

As soon as the team was assembled, Dr. Ware set out to obtain a heart-lung pump. A desk-sized console on wheels, the heart-lung pump oxygenates the blood and performs the heart's role in the circulation system during surgery. Dr. Ware went into the community seeking to raise nearly $10,000 — a small amount by today's standards, but a great deal of money in the 1950s. Wherever he went — medical meetings, social functions and seminars included — he solicited donations. Within a few months, an anonymous philanthropist donated the money for the pump, and an order was placed with the Olson Manufacturing

Company in Ashland for an Edward A. Olson Heart-Lung Pump, the same type of pump the team used in Boston. The machine was "the Rolls-Royce of pumps," according to Dr. Carroll.

In addition to buying a pump, they had to learn how to use it, which Dr. Carroll describes as being "like learning to fly an airplane with no instructors."

In November 1958, the pump was shipped to St. Vincent. Dr. Ware and his team were ready to conduct their own animal operations. Describing the pump, *The Catholic Free Press* writes, "The heart-lung machine is an imposing fixture, replete with many dials and parts. At its center is a cylindrical-shaped unit known as the oxygenating unit, composed of 68 oxygen discs which are filled with whole blood. As the blood leaves the patient, it passes through a de-bubblizer, through the oxygenating unit where it receives oxygen, through filtering units, and then back into the patient." The pump tapped into the circulatory system through catheters inserted in the major veins leading into the heart and returned blood to the patient through an artery in the patient's leg, bypassing the heart and lungs completely. To operate, the pump required 20 pints of whole blood, donated within 24 hours of an operation.

The heart team had to find a suitable place to conduct its work. At first, Dr. Ware considered setting up shop at his barn in Southboro, but "we thought that was a little too crude," Dr. Carroll recalled. Dr. Ware succeeded in getting the cooperation of the owner of the Witt Animal Hospital in Webster Square, whose young daughter had died of a heart disease that may have been cured if open-heart surgery were available. He allowed the medical team to set up the heart pump and use the animal hospital on Saturdays.

Dr. Joseph G. Murphy, a young anesthesiologist who joined the team, rigged up an electrical system made from Heath amateur radio kits to anaesthetize the dogs during surgery. His system, which worked on the same principles as electric shock therapy, was based on an anesthetic method that was popular in the Soviet Union at the time. The pump was modified by the addition of a tape deck that allowed the surgeons to listen to music while they worked, according to Dr. Carroll. "At that time, music in the operating room was a no-no, but today everyone has it," he said.

St. Vincent Hospital endorsed Dr. Ware's efforts and encouraged him, providing him with bundles of sterilized surgical instruments and anything else he needed. The Massachusetts Heart Association provided consultants. Every Saturday, the medical team, which volunteered its time for the work, met at the hospital at about 8 a.m., gathered its instruments and headed for Witt Animal Hospital, where the team worked until mid-afternoon. Each week, Dr. Ware operated on a stray dog. The heart of a large dog is similar to that of a human. A pig heart is closer to a human heart, but there was no readily available supply of pigs to work with. Dr. Ware organized a variety of experiments to simulate conditions in an operating room. One week he might, for example, cut open a vessel on a dog's heart and operate to close it back up. Another time, he might let the dog lose a large amount of blood and then operate to save the animal.

"Part of it was he was preparing us to see how everyone would react," Miss Weeks said. "He was causing situations that might happen to a patient." Whenever possible, the dog was saved. Dr. John I. Sanders, feeling sorry for one dog, took it home and kept it as a pet. "None of us wanted to harm animals, but we realized this was the only way to learn this — that by doing this we would learn how to save lives," Miss Weeks said.

Although Dr. Ware kept a low profile, everyone in the hospital knew about the experiments, and many of the doctors and nurses came out to help or to watch, and to see how the stainless steel "wonder on wheels" worked. Although the work at all times was serious, and only qualified personnel were allowed to participate, "everybody was so interested, it became a social gathering. Everyone from the hospital would come out," Miss Weeks said. "We had a very friendly group." The core team by then included Dr. Ware, who performed most of the actual surgery; Dr. Stapleton, the supervising cardiologist, who monitored the patient's heart during the operation; Dr. Sanders, first assistant to Dr. Ware; Dr. Murphy; Dr. Carroll; and Miss Weeks, who ran the heart-lung machine. Others, including Sister Mary Clare, also participated and helped out each week.

After nearly 10 months of experiments, the team was ready for its first real case.

Fifteen-year-old Rose Marie Picard presented a relatively easy case by today's standards. She had a congenital heart — a hole in the chambers of her heart which, if left unattended, would have severely shortened her life. A hole in the heart causes the heart to pump blood faster and work harder. Today, such an operation on a 15-year-old would be rare. A congenital heart usually is detected early in life and corrected during childhood.

But on October 13, 1959, when Dr. Ware and his team first ventured inside the human heart, the operation was still risky.

"The length of time on the pump became an important factor," according to Dr. Carroll. "The blood circulating in the pump becomes traumatized. The longer it stays in the pump, the more damage it sustains." A patient could be kept on the pump for no more than 90 minutes, and ideally complete reliance on the pump lasted for only about a half hour. The blood in the pump had to be carefully monitored at all times, to ensure that the temperature, the composition and the amount of blood remained constant. Throughout the operation, blood samples had to be taken and rushed to the laboratory for analysis of oxygen saturation. Also critical was the time immediately after the operation, when it was time to transfer the patient off the heart-lung machine, according to Sister Mary Clare.

The operation initially was scheduled for October 6, but Rose Marie was scheduled to be confirmed on that day. The operation was postponed so that she could receive the sacrament with her friends. In the meantime, members of the medical team studied and restudied their roles. Everyone on the team knew, according to Miss Weeks, that if something went wrong, it would jeopardize not only the safety of the patient, but the future of the open-heart surgery program. Two years of effort would be wasted.

"Preparations were plotted with the precision of a road map," according to an account in *The Catholic Free Press.* "The operating room was made ready with equipment of all kinds. Each piece was placed in a pre-designated position, thus assuring its accessibility. The machine itself was tested and retested to ensure that each and every part was in perfect working order. Even the unforeseen was foreseen. In case of electric power failure, tests were made on the manual operating apparatus.

"Each and every person, from Dr. Ware, the surgeon, to the lab technicians who would carry the blood, were present at a series of 'dry-runs,' during which time every step of the operation was rehearsed again and again."

In addition to the core team members, staff who participated in the first operation included Dr. Utzschneider, chief surgical resident and second assistant; Sister Mary Aloysia, laboratory supervisor; Robert Hair, chief chemist; Sister Mary Clare, operating room supervisor; Rachel Robitaille and Helen Lashenski, surgical nurses; and Nivart Gumusian, Ethel Duggan and Barbara McCarthy, circulating nurses.

The operation went smoothly, taking about six-and-a-half hours to complete. During that time, the heart-lung machine took over the function of breathing for Rose Marie for about a half hour. After the operation, Rose Marie remained on 24-hour watch for 10 days. Reporters were allowed to visit and conduct interviews. Talking to a reporter about her pet bird, and her interests in roller skating and Fabian, a pop singer, she said of her operation, "I wasn't afraid at all."

During the 12th open-heart operation, a *Worcester Telegram* reporter was allowed to witness the surgery. His account makes note of the well-coordinated efforts of each member of the 13-person surgical team. "Other routine preparations common to all major surgery were accomplished with a cool efficiency," he wrote. "Each member of the team went about his own task, seemingly indifferent to the others — but under the all-encompassing coordination of the nun in charge."

While there were only a few candidates for open-heart surgery in the beginning, eventually there were one or two open-heart cases a week. As the program progressed, and the team built up confidence, the program took on more difficult, more complicated cases.

For many patients, open-heart surgery was a last resort. Because of the nature of the work, the mortality rate was higher than for other operations. The greatest difficulty was often after the surgery, when the team had to get the heart working again and the patient off the heart-lung machine. Sister Clare remembers having to tell the mother of a child that Dr. Ware could not get the child's heart working on its own again.

Dr. Ware was the kind of doctor who stayed up all night with his patients, according to those who knew him. "For a famous surgeon, he had wonderful patient relationships," according to Sister Adrianella, who was cured of her tuberculosis by Dr. Ware's operation. "When a child died, you would think it was his own child."

"If someone didn't make it, the whole team was down," Miss Weeks said. "We were always searching for something we could have done differently."

Even as the program grew, Dr. Ware always found time for his family, according to Mrs. Ware. When he could, he brought some of his children to the hospital with him, and sometimes he brought his work home with him. Dr. Ware often took the 68 discs from the heart-lung pump home with him and Mrs. Ware worked with him to coat them with silicone and bake on the silicone in their kitchen oven. The coating had to be perfect, otherwise it could result in a blood clot in the patient.

The entire medical team shared Dr. Ware's dedication to the program. One day in 1960, Dr. Martin, trying to ignore his own medical problems, excused himself from the operating room, and, without telling anyone he was feeling ill, went back to his office and died at his desk. He was 51.

"He went and had an EKG done, and he had it in his pocket and wouldn't let anyone see it," Sister Clare said. "We had an operating room practically ready. If he had spoken about it early in the day, maybe something could have been done."

Eventually, the team went on to perform other groundbreaking operations. The team was among the first anywhere to perform valve replacement operations, although the early operations proved ineffective. Neither plastic surgery to repair valves, nor synthetic valves worked well. Valves are in constant motion, and synthetic materials or patched valves eventually wear out. Only during the past 15 years has the grafting of arterial tissue proven to be an effective means of valve repair or replacement.

The team also worked to fine tune its operating procedures to maximize the patient's chances of recovery. One factor that physicians at St. Vincent and at other hospitals experimented with was body temperature. The physicians understood that cooling down the patient before the operation was helpful. An important part of the operation preparation was packing saline solution into the deep freeze. "We had to shake it a lot so it would get slushy and not turn to ice and have a lot of sharp edges," Sister Clare said. Doctors in some hospitals even experimented with "profound hypothermia," or severe freezing, Dr. Carroll said, but it proved to be deadly in some cases. Patients appeared to recover, but would drop dead weeks or even months later for no apparent reason.

"Everything in medicine, unfortunately, is trial and error," he said.

In 1965, Dr. Ware again showed his pioneering spirit, working with Dr. Johnson to establish an intensive heart care unit at St. Vincent Hospital. Some of the St. Vincent staff opposed the intensive-care unit, because they believed the hospital could not afford to give up the space. Using patience and persistence, Dr. Ware won them over. The new 13-bed unit, which was located on the fifth floor in a wing that was added to the hospital, included four beds to monitor cardiac surgery patients. Recognizing that the 72-hour period following a heart attack was most critical to a patient's survival, the special unit was created to provide heart patients with 24-hour attention. A nursing station in the unit allowed nurses to monitor patients electronically, so that any abnormalities could be readily observed.

A newspaper article announcing the opening of the unit says, "The section is in keeping with St. Vincent Hospital's reputation in the forefront of medicine's advances. At the American Medical Association meeting this June, it was reported that fewer than 20 such heart sections were operating in the country."

As the St. Vincent open-heart program advanced, the strain began to show on Dr. Ware. While he succeeded in curing medical conditions that before his time had been fatal, his own medical condition began to deteriorate.

"Toward the end, when he was not feeling well, he tried to keep up his work," Miss Weeks said. "He'd be ill for a week or two, then he'd be back. He wouldn't give in. He'd come back and act like nothing was wrong with him. He pushed himself to the very end."

Dr. Adams remembered speaking with a sickly looking Dr. Ware and being told, "I'm not long for this world." Dr. Ware died that day, on March 14, 1968, a day short of his 51st birthday.

"His myocardiopathy required a heart transplant," according to Dr. Howard, "and at the time, he was one of the only guys anywhere who could have carried it off."

"He was a unique person," according to Miss Weeks. "Walking down the corridor, he talked to the man washing the floor. The women in the kitchen he knew by name. When he died, some of the women in the kitchen collected money and gave books in his name. He was that kind of man. Whether you were president of the United States or you swept the floor, you were an individual, and he respected that."

Dr. Ware touched many people's lives, and many of them wanted to remember him. As one former patient wrote, "he could fortify even a healthy heart." After his death, St. Vincent Trustee Cosmo E. Mingolla, who had been a patient of Dr. Ware, was instrumental in organizing an annual lecture series as a living memorial to Dr. Ware. Francis D. Hart, Jr. of Holden, another grateful patient, helped to establish a memorial fund in his memory. Others remembered him in other ways. A road between West Boylston and the former Worcester County Sanatorium in Boylston, where he operated on many tuberculosis patients, was named Paul F. Ware Memorial Drive. The *Southbridge Evening News* eulogized him in an editorial, recalling that he had operated on two employees of the newspaper and had perhaps saved their lives.

"Some people are going to question the master plan that let him save so many, but pass on himself at 51," the eulogy reads. "Only men of his faith, and his strength and wisdom will not question it."

Open-heart surgery was a costly program for St. Vincent Hospital to keep up, and, soon after Dr. Ware's death, it was dropped. At the time, valve replacement operations were decreasing, and the ability of the program to succeed was uncertain. No one foresaw that, beginning in 1969, coronary artery bypass surgery would revolutionize cardiac surgery. If Dr. Ware lived a little longer, St. Vincent, no doubt, would have been on the front lines of the revolution.

Sometime later, the Olson heart-lung machine that played such an important role in Dr. Ware's success, and in the success of St. Vincent Hospital, was discarded.

The New Frontier

"Chance favors the prepared mind."
Louis Pasteur

$\mathcal{A}$mbroise Parè, a noted surgeon of the 1500s, is remembered for saying, "I dress the wound, God heals it." This modesty was appropriate for Parè. In the 1500s, God, not medicine, was the patient's best hope.

If Parè had lived in the 1960s, his attitude might have been closer to that of Dr. Robert Johnson, the prominent St. Vincent neurosurgeon. When a monk from St. Joseph's Abbey in Spencer was hit in the head with an I-beam, he was not expected to live, let alone walk and function normally. But Dr. Johnson was a gifted surgeon, and, soon after he operated, the monk was able to walk, to everyone's astonishment.

Observing the Lazarus-like recovery of the monk, one of the sisters proclaimed, "God created a miracle."

"God created the accident," Dr. Johnson countered. "I created the miracle."

By the early 1960s, the powers of the doctor must have seemed almost godlike. Killing diseases like pneumonia and tuberculosis, polio and smallpox were all but eradicated.

Much had been discovered and learned since the turn of the century, when fresh air and sunshine were still the most commonly prescribed medications. Penicillin and other miracle drugs were by then commonplace, and new diagnostic tools were making it possible to detect disease at an earlier stage. It was a time of great discovery, and, as President John F. Kennedy led the country into space with the earliest manned flights, medical scientists also were exploring a new frontier in the laboratory.

As medical treatment advanced, so did medical education. While it was typical when St. Vincent Hospital first opened for a new doctor to proceed directly from the classroom to the operating room, or to work as an apprentice for a solo practitioner, the use of house officers became widespread by the early 1900s. In 1904, a study by the American Medical Association showed that half of all doctors included hospital training as part of their education. By 1912, 75 to 80 percent were trained in medical schools.

The role of the house officer grew, not just because the house officers could benefit from intensive hospital training, but because the doctors and the hospitals could benefit from the availability of a low-cost — often no cost — labor pool.

By 1957, American medical schools were graduating only 7,000 students a year, but there was a demand for more than 12,000 interns a year, according to *The Social Transformation of American Medicine*. With the freedom to choose where they wanted to go, the best American students, quite naturally, went to the prestigious, big-city hospitals.

The need to attract high-quality house officers provided the strongest argument for St. Vincent's new medical training center, but it was nearly as important to create a program that could help the medical staff stay current with the latest medical developments.

"The ulterior motive of the program is to serve as a source of continuing education for the medical staff," according to Dr. Stapleton. "By continuing their exposure to young men and women in training, and by continuing to have to stay on top of their questions, and to prepare conferences and formal teaching sessions, it serves to improve the education of the medical staff."

While much of the teaching was done by the St. Vincent staff, the medical training center also succeeded in attracting some of the best doctors of the day, not just from Georgetown, but from Harvard, Tufts and other medical schools. Several times a month, world-class medical experts spent a day or two making rounds and teaching at St. Vincent. Dr. Arnold S. Relman, editor of the *New England Journal of Medicine,* and Dr. Stapleton's mentor, Dr. Proctor Harvey, the world's leading authority on the use of a stethoscope, were among the many renowned medical experts who came to St. Vincent Hospital.

Intrigued, perhaps, by this community hospital with big-city ideas, the guest lecturers who were asked to come to St. Vincent almost never turned down the offer.

Dr. Stapleton discussed the program in more detail in an article in the *Harvard Medical Alumni Bulletin* in April 1956: "Although at first glance, affiliation with a school five hundred miles away would appear cumbersome, the feasibility of this arrangement has been borne out by the experience of St. Mary's Hospital of Rochester, New York, and the Mercy Hospital of Buffalo, New York, who have been associated with Georgetown for five years. The affiliation provides a number of qualified teachers chosen from the medical school faculty who visit the hospital and serve as professors *pro tempore* for two- or three-day periods. During this time, the bedside physician conducts bedside rounds, presides over conferences, gives a formal lecture and usually discusses a case summary at a clinicopathological conference. He is provided quarters in the hospital and often has the opportunity to sound out interns and residents on the ups and downs of being a house officer. Many times he is entertained socially by attending physicians; fruitful exchanges of ideas often occur in the relaxing environment provided on such occasions."

And he concludes: "More important perhaps than contact with visiting instructors is the stimulus provided by teaching. It is common pedagogical experience that the teacher learns more than the pupil. One is hard put to conceive of better postgraduate education than that provided by exposure to the enthusiasm of young doctors in training. This aspect of the program may well turn out to be a more important contribution in the field of medical education than improved house officer training per se."

At first, Dr. Stapleton was in charge of the entire medical training program. As it evolved, it became more specialized. Dr. Donald Brown was appointed director of surgical education, and Dr. Stapleton limited his participation to internal medicine, though he was still responsible for recruiting for the entire program.

Although he became attached to the Worcester area and his home in Holden, Dr. Stapleton left St. Vincent in 1965 when he was offered the position of chief of cardiology at the Medical College of Pennsylvania "where I was assured I would always have a class to teach," he said. He was succeeded by Dr. Allen Shuster, a Michigan native and former house officer at Boston City Hospital. He came to St. Vincent after spending a year conducting kidney research at the Boston Veterans Administration Hospital.

While the medical education program at St. Vincent was a success by any measure, "The difficulty was that I had to recruit a class each year," Dr. Stapleton said. "At that time, it was not easy. It was a little bit like recruiting patients. You couldn't really advertise much. You had to hope the quality of the program shone through."

House officers were not the only group to be provided with new educational opportunities at St. Vincent. Responding to the ever-increasing complexity of medical care, St. Vincent established special schools for medical technology, X-ray technology and anesthesia.

The standards for a medical technologist, for example, were still very basic before the 1960s. The Registry of Medical Technologists was established in 1928 to develop criteria for certification. In 1933, the level of required training increased and medical technologists were required to complete a year of college training. In 1938, the requirement was increased to two years of college training. Requirements remained unchanged for 24 years, when they were raised in 1962 to include three years of college followed by a year of clinical work. Master's degree programs became available, and it was anticipated that doctoral programs also would soon be available. The School of Medical Technology affiliated with Merrimack College in Andover in 1960, and with Anna Maria College in Paxton and Stonehill College shortly afterward.

In 1966, St. Vincent opened a School of Inhalation Therapy. In an 18-month program, students learned how to prevent hypoxia, a lack of oxygen to the tissues and organs. When the school was accredited in 1968, the *Worcester Telegram* reported, "The treatment consists of administering medical gases (oxygen, carbon dioxide and helium-oxygen mixtures) through a variety of mechanical devices such as vapor machines, intermittent positive pressure breathing units, nasal catheters and oxygen tents.

"The intermittent positive pressure breathing unit allows a therapist to regulate the amount of oxygen entering the patient's lungs. It can vary from a gentle puff to a force great enough to fill the lung with oxygen. Drugs are also administered in aerosol form. Sometimes the drugs are coupled with one of the medical gases so that medication can be carried past obstructions in the air passageways."

St. Vincent also became affiliated with the Worcester Girls' Trade High School to provide special training for surgical technicians and licensed practical nurses. Through the affiliation, courses in "homemaking" also were offered.

At the same time, the School of Nursing continued to provide an important educational program for the hospital. By 1965, the school was graduating about 75 nursing students a year, and many of the graduates were employed by the hospital after graduating.

In the late 1950s and early 1960s, St. Vincent Hospital continued to grow, but in smaller increments than when the new hospital opened. In 1960, the hospital treated 34,092 patients, including 17,477 inpatients and 16,615 outpatients. In 1961, the hospital treated 35,832 patients, including 17,775 inpatients and 18,057 outpatients.

In 1957, a wing was added to St. Camillus House to increase the size and number of classrooms. In January 1959, St. Vincent received a $50,000 grant from the Massachusetts Chapter of the Arthritis and Rheumatism Foundation to expand the hospital's arthritis clinic. In September 1959, the hospital purchased a home on Providence Street and converted it into St. Joseph's Hall to serve as housing for unmarried interns and residents. Like the medical training program, having housing available helped St. Vincent attract higher quality house officers.

By the mid-'60s, St. Vincent was providing acute, obstetrical, pediatric and psychiatric services, and outpatient clinics were available for alcoholism; allergies; cardiac disease; dental care; dermatology; diabetic treatment; eye, ear, nose and throat conditions; gynecology; hematology; general medical care; muscular dystrophy; pre- and postnatal care; psychiatric treatment; surgery; urology; and well-baby care.

The Saint Vincent Research Foundation, established in 1963, was as important as the medical training center in advancing the reputation of St. Vincent Hospital. In December 1960, St. Vincent Hospital received a $75,000 research and development grant for the center from the National Institutes of Health, but it was soon clear that sustained funding from the community was necessary if research was to influence the future of St. Vincent Hospital.

William J. Carroll, retired president of the Rockwood Sprinkler Company, was named president of the foundation. During his eight years as president, the foundation raised $350,000, a sizable sum at the time.

Research was divided into five areas. Dr. James B. Lee was appointed director of metabolic research and endocrinology, Dr. Stapleton was named director of development and educational research, Dr. Leonard J. Morse became director of infectious disease research, Dr. George Kwass headed steroid research and Dr. Benjamin G. Covino led cardiovascular research. For a community hospital, even one as large as St. Vincent, the establishment of a research foundation was as innovative as the hospital's affiliation with Georgetown.

Dr. Lee's mother, Mary B. Lee, became the foundation secretary, and her friend, Frances G. Donahue, became treasurer. In 1970, they became the first women elected to the foundation's board of directors. In addition to keeping the foundation's finances in order, their duties ranged from taking care of the white rabbits that were kept for experiments to buying sausage for Dr. H. Brownell Wheeler, who used the sausage in his classroom projects to teach students about veins.

With the establishment of the foundation, it was not uncommon for members of the St. Vincent staff to be published in the *New England Journal of Medicine (NEJM)* and the *Journal of the American Medical Association (JAMA),* the country's two most prestigious medical journals.

"A community hospital usually doesn't do research in the true sense of the word, like a university or an institution," Dr. Stapleton said. "But at St. Vincent, Jim Lee was doing some honest-to-God, grant-supported research."

Dr. Lee's early research centered around a substance called medullin, which could be found in the kidneys. He found that medullin affected a person's blood pressure and reasoned that, in drug form, medullin could be used to control high blood pressure.

Most of the doctors at the foundation performed the type of research that might be expected at a research foundation. Dr. Lee, for example, studied hypertension and kidney disease. Dr. Joseph Baldwin researched leukemia, Dr. Covino researched the effects of lowering the body temperature during heart surgery and brain surgery, and Drs. L. Michael Snyder and William J. Reddy researched the link between blindness and glucose-6-phosphate dehydrogenase, a substance found in the blood of anemics. Their research was based on a study of an extended family in Worcester in which six of the 40 family members were either almost blind or had serious eye defects.

Drs. Leon Edelstein, Snyder, Sean Murphy and Normand Fortier researched the effects of L-Dopa on a family with Heinz body anemia, a disease that affected 10 million people world-wide, primarily blacks. During four years of research they also discovered a link between the cause of Parkinson's disease, which also was treated by L-Dopa, and Heinz body anemia. In presenting the results of their work in 1975, the doctors said they were hopeful their research would contribute to an understand-ing of the aging process, and lead to further study about the degeneration of cells caused by hydrogen peroxide buildup and enzyme system breakdown.

Dr. Morse's research was different. He might, in fact, be called a medical detective. A native of Worcester, he was attracted to St. Vincent by the hospital's medical education pro-gram and joined the medical staff in 1960. For his early work, Dr. Morse used alcoholic rabbits to study the susceptibility of alcoholics to infectious disease. After five years of working part-time in private practice and part-time at the hospital, he began working full-time at St. Vincent in 1966.

That year, he published his first major study, which traces a case of paralytic polio to the changing of a soiled diaper from an infant who received a polio vaccine.

"The patient, a 43-year-old white woman, has never received poliomyelitis immunization," he wrote. "On December 30, 1964, while under spinal anesthesia, she was delivered of a full-term living male child, who received his first dose of triva-lent oral poliomyelitis vaccine on March 20, 1965. Twenty-two days later, numbness of the lower extremities developed in the mother; this condition was followed in 48 hours by low back pain. . . . On the 5th day of the disease, the right-lower-extremity weakness had increased, making the patient totally paraplegic."

Dr. Morse said the case showed the need for adults to become immunized against polio. The polio vaccine given to an infant contains the live polio virus, which is shed in the infant's stool, but in a more virulent form. If someone who is not immunized comes in contact with the diaper, he or she runs the risk of contracting polio.

In 1967, Dr. Morse traced an outbreak of septicemia, or blood poisoning, in the St. Vincent intensive care unit to a hand lotion dispenser. In his study, which appeared in *NEJM,* Dr. Morse wrote, "Within a seventy-two-hour period (February 15 to 17, 1967) 6 patients in the medical intensive care unit had fever, shaking chills, mental confusion or transient hypotension," which he traced to *Klebsiella pneumoniae.* "The source of this outbreak was a lanolin hand-cream dispenser. With frequent meticulous hand washing between patient chores using soap containing hexachlorophene, the nurses, in an attempt to minimize severe drying of the skin, provided their own supply of lanolin hand cream. The decanter bottle had been filled repeatedly during the winter months with a variety of common skin lotions, and it is assumed to have become contaminated." The contamination was spread at the point where catheters entered the patients' tissue.

Wondering how the hand lotion became contaminated, he studied 26 brands of lotion and found that four of them were teeming with bacteria. Two of the contaminated brands were produced nationally and two were produced locally for both hospital and commercial use. Bacteria were found in both opened and unopened samples, indicating that contamination took place during production. Many hospitals continue to dispense hand lotions to patients who are at risk from infection, but Dr. Morse believes hand lotions should be kept out of hospitals.

In another case, which he investigated in 1966, Dr. Morse traced an outbreak of 167 cases of salmonella to the use of frozen, unpasteurized egg yokes in the preparation of ice cream.

Dr. Morse's most famous case was an investigation of an outbreak of hepatitis that struck 90 of the 97 members of the Holy Cross varsity football team in 1969, ending the team's season with only two games played. Mysteriously, 50 resident assistants and the entire freshman football team used the same facilities with no resulting cases of hepatitis. To crack the case, a research team was assembled that included Dr. Morse, staff members from the Worcester Department of Public Health and from Holy Cross, and Sister Mary Dolorum Leavy, Helen D. Johnson, Dr. Robert E. Bessette and Dr. Edward Hutchinson, all from St. Vincent Hospital.

"Epidemiologic investigation revealed that an infected group of children in the neighborhood, an imperfect drinking water supply, a warm August day, a football team in training, and a local fire were links in the chain which resulted in this most unusual outbreak of infectious hepatitis," Dr. Morse wrote in an article published in *JAMA* in 1972.

The research team eventually linked the source of the infection to the municipal water system that led to the team's practice field, ending at a faucet hooked up in a small building used to store equipment. The line had six subsurface faucets that were used to irrigate the field. The base of the faucet in the equipment building was the lowest point on the line, because the line also was used to drain the field during the winter.

Testing the system, the researchers found the water pressure in the line to be extremely sensitive. Opening a couple of fire hydrants in the area, for example, resulted in negative water pressure, causing surface water to siphon back into the system. The team discovered that four children and an adult who lived in a condemned building adjacent to the field had contracted hepatitis. The children used the practice field as a playground. The weather had been warm with no rainfall, and the children liked to turn on the subsurface faucets and play in the water that accumulated around them.

On August 29, 1969, a fire took place two miles from campus. Dr. Morse concluded that the demand for water to fight the fire created a large-enough drop in pressure that the line on the Holy Cross practice field siphoned off the surface water where the infected children had recently been playing. The team members then contracted hepatitis when they drank the water.

Not all of the research at St. Vincent was connected with the foundation. Dr. Richard Myler, a noted cardiologist who was recruited to St. Vincent by Dr. Ware in 1966, began working out his methodology for heart catheterization procedures while at St. Vincent. With assistance from Dr. Kocot, he set up a cardiac catheterization laboratory, so that there was no longer any need to send catheterization work to Boston. Based on research he began at St. Vincent, Dr. Myler later developed the first purcutaneous transluminal catheter angioplasty, or PTCA, an operation to "plasticize" a vessel of the heart using a catheter to reach under the skin, rather than cutting the patient open.

Dr. Michael Polanji, a researcher at American Optical Corporation in Southbridge, developed a cigar-box-like reflection oxymeter, which measures the level of oxygen in a patient's blood. Because of his friendship with Dr. Ware, he held clinical trials for the machine at St. Vincent. The machine measures oxygen saturation in blood and provides results almost instantaneously, making it unnecessary to go through the time-consuming process of sending blood to the hospital lab for testing. Because of the hospital's assistance, American Optical donated an oxymeter to St. Vincent.

Not all of the research at St. Vincent Hospital was performed by doctors. Sister Dolorum became an authority on fungus and even wrote poetry about it.

Her work in mycology — the biology of fungi — earned her state and national awards, and a listing in *Who's Who of American Women*. She also tracked down the cause of a rare fungal infection that produced fist-sized tumors over half of a woman's face. The tumors persisted for 56 years, and three operations failed to cure her before Sister Dolorum identified the fungus producing the tumors.

Sister Dolorum graduated from the Mercy Hospital School of Medical Technology in Springfield, Mass., in 1936 and became a medical technologist at St. Vincent. In the 1950s, with the support of Sister Loreto, she became a certified mycologist.

"At the time, antibiotics were just becoming widely used, and I was examining urine and sputum, and I was seeing things and I didn't know what I was looking at," she recalled. "Penicillin is an antibiotic, but it is also a fungus. I went to the Centers for Disease Control in Atlanta, and they taught me everything about it, and I taught the others."

In 1959, she assembled a fungus exhibit that took first place in a competition before the Massachusetts Association of Medical Technologists. She took the exhibit to a national competition in Atlantic City, N.J., and won there as well. The exhibit included dozens of live fungi, many of which were deadly or at least harmful. One, for example, could cause pneumonia just from touching it.

In addition to containing an impressive collection of fungus and information about its effects, Sister Dolorum's exhibit proved her abilities as a showman. A friend of hers, who was a designer of the X-15 rocket, let her use a model of the rocket in her exhibit, and a taxidermist gave her a rabbit, a guinea pig and a mouse, which she dressed as a pilot for her X-15. The stuffed animals and the rocket didn't have much to do with her project, but they attracted attention. Pretending that the mouse had dedicated its life to laboratory experiments to find cures for fungus infections, she wrote the mouse a poem for the exhibit that reads, in part:

"I'm the smallest, most used and most abused.
Serving humanity gives me the blues . . .
B. dermititides, H. capsulatum and P. erasilienses
Have no respect for my little body's defenses . . ."

She continued her education, earning her bachelor's degree from Anna Maria College in Paxton in 1966, and her master's degree in mycology and science education after receiving a two-year fellowship from C. W. Post College at Long Island University in 1972. She learned about the Post fellowship program by accident. "I was looking at a book and I saw that the government was looking for people to take lab courses and that the government would pay," she said. "I wrote without telling anyone, and two days later a doctor called and said, 'Come quick.' "

Hearing about her expertise, a nurse who was training at St. Vincent told Sister Dolorum about her mother-in-law's tumors. The woman was being treated at the University of Massachusetts Medical Center, and doctors there thought they had identified the fungus that was producing the tumors.

The doctors sent Sister Dolorum a small amount of tissue, she said, and, "when I saw the slides, I knew it wasn't what they said it was." She identified the fungus as *Loboa loboi,* a rare fungus that produced a skin infection called lobomycosis. Only 102 cases of the disease had previously been reported, all in Central America and South America.

At first the doctors refused to accept her analysis, so she wrote to the Centers for Disease Control. After CDC confirmed her analysis, the doctors accepted it.

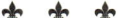

During the 1960s, three factors made St. Vincent superior to most other community hospitals, according to Dr. Stapleton. The first was the medical training center and its affiliation with Georgetown. The second was the establishment of a research foundation. And the third was the hiring of full-time specialists on the medical staff. Full-time staff members provided the hospital with consistency, stability and loyalty, and a higher level of professionalism than could be achieved through affiliations.

During the 1940s and 1950s, St. Vincent had full-time pathologists and radiologists, but everyone else on the medical staff was a "volunteer" with an independent practice. After Dr. Stapleton was hired in the new position of full-time medical director, Dr. Joseph Baldwin followed as full-time hematologist, and soon others became full-time St. Vincent doctors.

"Slowly, the development of a cadre of full-time specialists took place," Dr. Stapleton said. "I thought it was a good idea, but couldn't have persuaded them to do it all on my own. There were many good leaders among the medical staff who recognized the need for special facilities — a hematologist needed a lab, for example. The doctor with a downtown office could no longer do it alone."

With the development of a full-time staff of specialists, patients had improved access to their physicians, and St. Vincent was better prepared to keep up with the rapid advances in modern medicine. St. Vincent was also more self-reliant and independent than it otherwise could have been.

With an increasingly specialized staff, and a growing number of full-time staffers, St. Vincent was able to offer services that typically were unavailable at a community hospital, such as the cardiac catheterization laboratory.

Another area where St. Vincent was more advanced than most other hospitals was in its accounting department, which was run by Sister Agnes Marie Anderson. With the assistance of Sister Adrianella, Sister Agnes Marie oversaw the early computerization of the hospital.

The hospital bought a General Precision computer for its payroll and credit records in the early 1960s, but, after the company was sold, the hospital could no longer service the computer and it soon became defunct.

"We had to recreate all of our records," Sister Adrianella said. "We reconverted to manual records to preserve our accounts receivable." Soon after, the department computerized again, this time on IBM equipment.

In June 1963, St. Vincent also became the first hospital in the country to install teletype machines, which were used to send lab reports to nursing stations, and billing for medical tests to the business office. When St. Vincent Hospital was highlighted in Ohio Chemical's *Items & Topics* in May 1966, the publication noted how the hospital borrowed the idea of teletype machines from the newspaper industry and put them to an innovative use.

"There are two sending stations in the laboratory, two receivers in the business office and ten at various nursing stations," the publication notes. "Laboratory test results are raced to the appropriate floor, while the business office is automatically notified of the charge."

The 1960s were a time of changing attitudes in health care, as in society as a whole. The formal, regimented style of hospital management was breaking down. Nurses began to abandon the white uniform and four-cornered hat that were required dress in earlier days, and their relationships with the medical staff also became less formal.

But the Sisters of Providence still hung on to tradition. The strict discipline accorded to nursing students by the Sisters continued. For example, the nursing students continued to participate in morning Communion rounds.

"If you were on the floor where Communion rounds were taking place, you had to get on your knees with your hands folded, and you had to stay on your knees until the priest was done," according to Val Mancini, a nursing student from 1965 to 1968.

She also remembers that students were not allowed to leave the dormitory wearing shorts. Dates were not allowed into the school. And during training, she had to wear the traditional St. Vincent nurse's uniform, complete with the four-cornered hat.

"There were only two Chinese laundromats that knew how to take the hat apart, launder it and put it back together," she said. "There was a whole ritual to it."

CHAPTER THIRTEEN

The Age of the Laity

"Changing times have wrought tremendous and radical changes in the operation of hospitals. It is no longer possible for a religious community to be the exclusive agents of the hospital's many facets of responsibility in care of the sick."   Bishop Bernard J. Flanagan

*J*ust as St. Vincent Hospital was reaching its full potential, the Sisters of Providence were facing new challenges. They were, in a sense, victims of their own success. As St. Vincent Hospital grew, and as the need for professional staff became more apparent, the Sisters of Providence no longer had the personnel to fill all of the hospital's managerial positions.

In the early 1960s, the number of sisters needed to staff the hospital was growing, while the number of sisters in the order was shrinking. It was a time of great social change. On the whole, religion was playing a less prominent role in people's lives than it had when the hospital was founded. Fewer people were willing to devote themselves to the difficult life of a religious community. And there were other new and difficult challenges to deal with as well.

Two major stories, each of which, in its own way, had a major impact on the future of St. Vincent Hospital, shared space on the front page of *The Catholic Free Press* on January 30, 1959.

One story announced that Bishop Wright was being transferred to the Diocese of Pittsburgh. The other announced the decision of Pope John XXIII to convoke the Second Vatican Council.

Where previously the Catholic Church had segregated itself from other religions, ecumenism became the rallying cry of Vatican II. The Council's work, which continued under Pope John's successor, Pope Paul VI, culminated by the end of 1965 in a series of decrees that, among other things, changed the rules for the nuns. The strict barriers between the sisters and the laity were suddenly breaking down. Sisters could talk to lay people and even eat with them. They could dress like lay people, and they could use their family names. While "Mother" or "Sister" continued to precede every nun's name, many nuns adopted their father's name. Sister Miriam Regina, who succeeded Sister Loreto as administrator of St. Vincent, became Sister Helen Marie Smith, adopting her lay name. Sister Mary O'Leary, one of two Sisters of Providence still working at St. Vincent Hospital, adopted her family name. When her mother suggested that she take her father's name, she replied, "I did, mother. I will always be an O'Leary."

While bringing the Church closer to the laity, Vatican II also attempted to bring the laity closer to the Church. "The Church has not been really founded," part of one decree reads, "and is not yet fully alive, nor is it a perfect sign of Christ among men, unless there is a laity worthy of the name working along with the hierarchy."

Many aspects of Catholicism remained unchanged. For example, religious communities such as the Sisters of Providence continued to be subject to the power of their bishop, a decree on missionary work says, but adds ambiguously that the bishop should lead "in such a way that the zeal and spontaneity of those who share in the work may be preserved and fostered."

Perhaps the change that had the greatest impact on St. Vincent Hospital was the decision by Vatican II that nuns could take a more open, proactive role in society. Rather than remain semi-cloistered in a convent at St. Vincent Hospital, they could go out into the world more and perform social work openly, quite literally carrying out the will of St. Vincent, who had said the city streets should serve as cloisters for his Sisters of Charity.

As with any major change, there is an adjustment period. The adjustment period was particularly difficult for the Sisters of Providence and for the people who worked with them. After many years of observing a code of silence, communication did not come easily. The nuns didn't know how to use their new-found freedom and the laity didn't know how to respond to it.

"When we changed, we affected people," according to Sister Adrianella. "We didn't do a good job educating people."

There were fewer sisters to work in the hospitals and more hospital positions to fill, but there were other reasons for bringing laity into management positions. As health care became more sophisticated and more technically challenging, the sisters' brand of hands-on, personalized health care became old fashioned and outdated. Many of the skills handed down by the sisters from one generation to the next became unnecessary. Prepackaged dressings and other ready-to-use medical supplies made the labor less manual and more technical. It was becoming more important to have staff that could use the new equipment; staff that understood the new regulatory environment. Education was becoming increasingly important, and the bedside patient care practiced by the sisters was becoming less important.

An attempt was made to adjust to changing times by better educating nuns placed in supervisory positions, but sometimes nuns left the order once they received special training. While receiving an education, they adjusted to the outside world and found it difficult to readjust to life in a religious community.

Change was inevitable. In the late 1950s, St. Vincent first began hiring lay people for key positions. Lay people took over purchasing and pharmacy work. A personnel office became necessary. Over time, there were lay accountants on staff.

But the mix of laity and religious created new problems. They came from two different worlds, with different rules and different expectations. They didn't understand each other. Like a boy and a girl at their first dance, socialization was slow and awkward. Some of the sisters felt threatened by these outsiders who suddenly had a foothold in the power structure of a hospital the sisters worked so hard to build.

"We all knew we couldn't handle it alone," Sister Adrianella said, "but they didn't know their place there. There was a lot of uneasiness on their part. They didn't know if they had any job security; whether they were just being given a job while a sister trained for it."

There also were financial matters to consider. "The sisters worked for free, and suddenly, they had to pay for help," Sister Adrianella said. "We were afraid to give them a fair price for their work, the amount seemed so big to us, but we learned we couldn't keep good people unless we paid them well."

Further complicating the financial situation, even nuns began to draw a salary in the 1960s. For many years, Catholic hospitals had the benefit of a pool of free labor. But as health insurance became widespread, the hospitals had to pay their nuns, because the hospitals had to show an expense if they wanted to be compensated by the insurance companies. Suddenly, the division between religious life and the laity was not nearly as great as it had been for so many years.

While some of the nuns found it difficult to adjust to their new-found freedom, others adjusted quite naturally. Sister Mary Mercedes, for example, enjoyed talking with the doctors and lay nurses, and kept them informed about what was happening in her order. Because of their ability to talk with the nuns on a more open basis, some of the St. Vincent staff developed close relationships with some of the nuns and have fond memories of them.

Mrs. Darcy, for example, remembers that one time, when she heard the pains of someone in labor, the screams seemed so painful she knelt down and prayed. Sister Mary of Assisi saw her praying. She came to Mrs. Darcy after the baby was born and said, "My dear, you've got to see the baby. Anyone who went through labor like you did should at least see the baby."

Dr. Lambi Adams remembers being comforted by Sister Mary Trinita after one of his grade-school teachers who had become a patient of his died from a rheumatic heart. When she died, Dr. Adams cried, because "she had gone, and I couldn't bring her back. I remember Sister Trinita telling me, 'You are not God.' She made an impression on me. Every time I saw a patient, I asked myself, 'What would Sister Trinita do?'"

Handling these changes might have been easier if the long-established leadership of the hospital hadn't also changed. Bishop Wright was replaced by the Most Rev. Bernard J. Flanagan on September 24, 1959. In 1961, Sister Mary Hildegarde became the local superior, serving until 1967, when she was replaced by Sister Frances Murphy. In 1963, Sister Loreto ended her long reign at St. Vincent. After 26 years, it was time for a change. She was appointed mother general of the order, making way for her assistant of the previous two years, Sister Miriam Regina, to become hospital administrator. At the same time, Sister Agnes Marie left after 14 years as St. Vincent's comptroller to become treasurer general of the Sisters of Providence, and Sister Adrianella became acting comptroller of St. Vincent.

"It's good that I move on," Bishop Wright reportedly confided to a friend after his appointment. "It's time that Worcester had a new face. The people are getting tired of me." While Worcester may not have tired of Bishop Wright, the bishop must have felt that he had accomplished as much as he could in the new diocese and was ready for a new challenge.

The ecclesiastical title of "Bishop" was already familiar to Bishop Flanagan. He served as the first bishop of the Diocese of Norwich, Connecticut, which abuts the Diocese of Worcester, from 1953 until his appointment to Worcester. He also was familiar with his new diocese, having graduated from Holy Cross in 1928. It was only fitting that he should return to Worcester, since some of his Holy Cross teachers influenced his decision to join the priesthood.

Bishop Flanagan grew up in Proctor, Vermont, a town whose population of just 2,500 produced 12 priests, including two bishops. Bishop Flanagan lived on West Street, a street that came to be called "Pope's Row," because most of the town's dozen priests grew up there. His family was deeply religious, and he had an uncle who was a priest, so Bishop Flanagan naturally began thinking about the priesthood at an early age.

After graduating from Holy Cross, he attended the North American College in Rome. He was one of the most promising students at the college and was among the few chosen to write accounts of the class lectures to disseminate to other students. While copying and sharing notes would be disallowed at many schools, it was necessary at the North American College, where the lectures were given in Latin. With students and teachers from all over the world, the language barrier presented many difficulties that could be overcome only by distributing notes explaining the lectures.

His friends recall Bishop Flanagan as a friendly, even-tempered man who enjoyed sports and cigars. In a newspaper interview, the Reverend Cornelius F. Donohue, a friend and classmate of Bishop Flanagan, both at Holy Cross and at North American College, recalled taking many photos of Bishop Flanagan, "and there was only one in which he was not smiling." In that photo, he was smoking a cigar. Later, when a prospective host asked an associate what kind of cigar Bishop Flanagan smoked, he was told, "The answer usually given is, 'Anybody's.' "

Bishop Flanagan was ordained in 1931. In 1940, he was sent to the Catholic University of America and received his doctorate in canon law in 1943. He returned to his home state after graduating from Catholic University to serve as chancellor of the Diocese of Burlington. He served as secretary to two bishops in Burlington before being named bishop of the Norwich diocese.

"He was radically different from Bishop Wright," according to Dr. Kocot. "He did not use the political process. He used the soft-step approach."

Not flamboyant like his predecessor, Bishop Flanagan got things done in his own quiet, unassuming way. Dr. Kocot remembers visiting his father-in-law in the hospital just before he was about to undergo major surgery. His father-in-law had converted to Catholicism, but was never confirmed and wanted to be before his operation.

"He looked at me and said he had promised to be confirmed before he died," Dr. Kocot said. "He remembered that he hadn't fulfilled that promise. I bumped into Bishop Flanagan in the parking lot, and he said he would take care of it. I went to see my father-in-law the next day, and told him what Bishop Flanagan had promised. My father-in-law said, 'He came in last night and confirmed me.'"

Dr. Adams first met Bishop Flanagan early one morning when the bishop was trying to get into the hospital and the door was locked. "I opened the door for him," he said. "I thought he was a priest. He told me he was the bishop. I said, 'You don't look like a bishop to me.' Bishops usually have all of the trappings. He said, 'I'm a poor man's bishop.'"

An athlete and sports enthusiast, Bishop Flanagan developed a reputation for predicting the outcome of sporting events with a good degree of accuracy. A diehard Red Sox fan, he rarely missed a game and was known to break up business meetings to watch or listen to a game.

Suite 558, the Bishop's suite, was no longer used during Bishop Flanagan's service, according to Sister O'Leary. "He was not as involved in the hospital as Bishop Wright. He figured the hospital had people on staff capable of running it."

Still soft-spoken and gentle, Bishop Flanagan recalled that when he came to the Worcester diocese, Bishop Wright already had accomplished the difficult task of establishing the diocese: "I was fortunate to be named to a diocese which, although still young, had been so well organized. It was already on a firm foundation. My only agenda was to use whatever gifts God had given me to build on that foundation."

Likewise, with the hospital still under the supervision of Sister Loreto at the time, he said, "I felt that it was in firm and able hands. The hospital didn't really demand much more than my occasional visit."

In addition to continuing the good work of Bishop Wright, Bishop Flanagan participated in Vatican II. Bishop Flanagan wrote about his experience: "Very few of us, bishops included, realized at the time the Council opened in the Fall of 1962 the significance and future impact of it. I think many of us felt we would be in Rome for only a few weeks in order to give formal approval to decrees already prepared by Council commissions which had been at work for many months.

"But, any such illusions were quickly dispelled. In the very first days following the Council's opening on October 11, 1962, we were made aware that we faced a long, arduous task. The Second Vatican Council was to be no rubber-stamp assembly. It was to continue through four sessions . . . it was to engage in a process of study, discussion, and, often, sharp debate that in the end would result in documents and decisions aimed at renewing virtually every facet of the Church. . . . Future history, I am certain, will record Vatican II as one of the great turning points in the long history of the Church."

Describing Bishop Flanagan's role at Vatican II, Owen Murphy said, "He went to the Vatican Council and saw the old Church turned upside down. He understood it. He was touched by what was going on at the Council. He came back and immediately put everything into practice."

Murphy believes Bishop Flanagan was the ideal successor to Bishop Wright.

"Bishop Wright broke down the walls between the Catholics and the Yankees," according to Murphy. "Bishop Flanagan started to rebuild them in the light of the Vatican Council. The combination of the two bishops was ideal for the diocese."

While the bishop no longer kept a suite at the hospital, the Right Reverend Monsignor Timothy J. O'Connell did, living in Rooms 301 and 303. Although he held the titles of executive secretary and vice officialis to the diocese, Msgr. O'Connell was really the bishop's liaison, his eyes and ears at the hospital. After

Bishop Wright left the Worcester diocese, Msgr. O'Connell played an increasingly important role. He sat on the Executive Committee of the Board of Trustees, and Bishop Flanagan allowed him the flexibility of making day-to-day operating decisions on behalf of the diocese.

"He became very knowledgeable about the inner workings of the hospital," according to Bishop Flanagan. "He was closely connected with many members of the medical staff."

Living at the hospital, Msgr. O'Connell assisted in caring for the sick, but he also was able to watch out for the interests of the diocese. Msgr. O'Connell joined his friend, Bishop Wright, in Worcester in 1950, helping to set up the legal offices of the new diocese. He continued a teaching appointment at Regis College in Weston, and added teaching duties in medical ethics at St. Vincent's School of Nursing from 1950 to 1958. In 1952 he also became a marriage instructor at Anna Maria College after the campus moved from Marlboro to Paxton. In addition, he organized the diocesan marriage tribunal and was its first chief justice.

He was elevated to the rank of domestic prelate by Pope Pius XII in 1952 and was named a permanent member of the Worcester diocesan clergy in 1954. He was appointed officialis of the diocese in 1956.

During the energy crises of the 1970s, Msgr. O'Connell developed a reputation as a crusader for conserving energy. He was so diligent at putting out lights that the guild members complained to the hospital administration, because they were tripping in the dark.

Dr. Jaffee remembers Msgr. O'Connell as "the best-read man I ever met. He was the greatest acquirer of new books I've ever encountered. He read novels, politics, sports stories, biographies, histories. He was very knowledgeable. I loved walking through the hospital talking to him. He was a kind, concerned guy."

Robert C. Maher, a friend of Msgr. O'Connell and a fellow Boston College graduate, said, "He'd read until 2 or 3 a.m. He'd read anything of interest, but especially anything dealing with theology, psychology, psychiatry or politics. He read some pretty deep stuff."

He shared what he read with others, too, regularly mailing newspaper articles to his friends.

"Every day, at least one envelope was in my mail with clippings from newspapers," said Val Mancini. "Anything to do with nursing or health care he'd send me. He never disappointed me."

Given Msgr. O'Connell's reading habits, it's no wonder, perhaps, that he was close to Bishop Wright. He also developed close ties with Sister Miriam Regina, the new administrator of St. Vincent Hospital. But Dr. Mancini may have been the person who was closest to him.

They were already close friends when, one night, when she was working as a shift coordinator, Dr. Mancini heard loud music coming from his suite.

"I walked in and said, 'Monsignor, your stereo's too loud,' " she recalled. "He said, 'Come in and listen with me.' It was an opera, and once he knew I liked it, he started sending me albums. When he became ill, I was devastated. When he died, his lawyer called. He left his stereo and music to me; hundreds of albums. I listen to it and it's sad. I still miss him."

CHAPTER FOURTEEN

A New Administration

"In the acute phase of illness, there is little awareness on the part of the patient even of the existence of the Administrator. At this stage, the doctor is the center of the patient's universe and the nurse is considered an extension of the doctor and the patient's most frequent point of contact. Then the span of attention widens to recognize what is happening in the immediate environment. The food, the housekeeping, the attitude of other hospital personnel, the nursing care and other services are evaluated and classified according to the patient's standards of correctness. It is at this point that there is a realization that somewhere 'management' is responsible for all this." **The Outlook, July 1962**

Sister Regina, born Helen Marie Smith in Pittsfield, Massachusetts, entered the order of the Sisters of Providence in 1936. After graduating from the Boston College School of Nursing, she joined the Sisters of Providence and was appointed as a night nursing supervisor at St. Vincent Hospital. Sister Regina showed a great deal of promise in her position, so Sister Loreto sent her to Xavier College in Cincinnati to earn a master's degree in hospital administration. She completed an administrative residency at St. Elizabeth's Hospital in Dayton, Ohio, before becoming Sister Loreto's assistant in 1962.

Less than two years later, she became the administrator of St. Vincent Hospital. Even if she had time to learn more about managing the hospital, her new post would have been difficult.

She was succeeding a very popular person who was loved by almost everyone, and who had run St. Vincent for a quarter century.

Not only did she have to adjust to a great deal of change within her own order, but she also was stepping in at a time of great change in the field of health care. Where previously the industry was not heavily regulated, during the 1960s, new programs like Medicare and Medicaid were creating tremendous changes in the way hospitals were being run. In the new regulatory environment, Sister Loreto's penchant for making on-the-spot decisions was no longer possible. When the new regulations came in, according to Dr. Howard, "You could no longer just have a person behind a desk saying 'Yes' to everything."

On the whole, she was less accommodating to the medical staff than Sister Loreto. Sister Loreto tended to give the doctors what they wanted, trusting their judgment about what they needed. Sister Regina "had an entirely different attitude toward doctors," according to Dr. William A. Carey, who became a radiologist at St. Vincent in 1964. While Sister Regina was instrumental in supporting many of the same medical programs as the doctors, if she did not agree with the need for a program, she was sometimes confrontational.

Patrick J. Roche, who was appointed as the first lay assistant administrator in 1965 before being named chief operating officer the following year, said Sister Regina gave him a great deal of latitude in his position, but after he disagreed with her on an issue, he fell out of favor with her.

"If she liked you," he said, "she'd trust you 110 percent."

Sister Regina spent more time in the classroom than most of her fellow sisters, but less time in the hospital room. When she was named administrator, she still lacked the practical experience she needed to complement her classroom work, according to Dr. Carey. Sister Loreto had the benefit of being able to grow with the job. When Sister Loreto became superintendent in 1937, hospital administration was still fairly uncomplicated, and she was resourceful enough to adapt to the gradual changes that took place over the 26 years that followed. But Sister Regina began her tenure at a time of revolutionary change in both health-care administration and the Catholic Church. Change was taking place so rapidly, no one could be expected to keep up with it.

At the same time, relationships between the doctors and the Sisters of Providence were being affected by the decrease in the number of nuns on the hospital staff. A few of the nuns, perhaps recognizing how tenuous their hold on the hospital was becoming, tried to exercise their authority, creating rifts with some of the doctors. Where previously relations between doctors and nuns were overwhelmingly positive, some of the doctors began to view the nuns as being out of touch with the rapid changes taking place in health care. Yet it had been the sisters' hospital. They created it and made it succeed, so why, they must have reasoned, should they hand over their authority to the doctors?

The death of Dr. Ware in 1968 made Sister Regina's job even more difficult. In the years to come, a well-established cardiology department became a prerequisite for any hospital that wanted to maintain a reputation as a major hospital. While he lived, Dr. Ware put St. Vincent's Cardiology Department well ahead of practically any other community hospital's cardiology department. But his death left a great void that remained unfilled for many years.

The 1960s was a time of upheaval for the country as a whole. The Vietnam War; the assassinations of John and Robert Kennedy, and Martin Luther King; protest marches and race riots; the first man on the moon. These and other factors created tremendous changes in the American way of life — changes that were sometimes difficult to adjust to and accept.

Few administrators could have made it through the tumultuous sixties unscathed. Still, in her early years as administrator, despite the formidable obstacles she had to overcome, Sister Regina managed to hold things together at St. Vincent, initiating many of the improvements the hospital needed to compete and grow. She worked closely with the guild and supported the hospital gift shop. She oversaw continuing changes and improvements in the hospital's training program, and the restructuring and updating of several departments.

She never achieved Sister Loreto's popularity, but she accomplished much. Bishop Flanagan said, "During Sister Miriam Regina's years, the hospital went through some of its greatest growth."

In 1968, 75 years after the founding of St. Vincent Hospital, Sister Regina oversaw the reorganization of the hospital staff. She was named executive director of St. Vincent Hospital, assuming broader administrative duties than any of her predecessors. By then, she had taken the name Sister Helen Marie Smith. It proved to be a foreshadowing of things to come.

Sister Smith's appointment came at the beginning of a new era in health care. Medical knowledge had evolved to the point where doctors were treating the diseases of the elderly and prolonging life. Medical costs doubled in the 1950s, but third parties were covering an increasing percentage of the costs. These conditions led to a surging demand for medical coverage for the elderly.

Responding to the increasing demand, Congress passed a law in 1960 that extended welfare programs to provide medical insurance for low-income elderly. In 1964, medical insurance for the elderly became the cornerstone of President Johnson's Great Society programs. Congressman Wilbur Mills, the powerful chairman of the House Ways and Means Committee, spearheaded efforts for a Medicare program, tied to Social Security, to provide medical insurance to all elderly for hospital and physician visits. During negotiations in Congress, expanded medical insurance for the poor also was added to the program as Medicaid.

Medicare proved to be a financial boon to the medical industry. As with commercial insurance programs, and Blue Cross and Blue Shield programs, it paid hospitals and doctors on a fee-for-service basis. Hospitals and doctors charged fees based on their costs. The more resources they consumed, the more money they made. In addition, Medicare included provisions allowing hospitals to include accelerated depreciation of their physical assets as part of their costs — a particularly attractive arrangement, especially considering the nonprofit nature of hospitals. Even the earlier Hill-Burton program, which first spurred postwar hospital construction, didn't offer accelerated depreciation as an incentive.

Regulatory checks and balances, such as determination-of-need studies, were still nonexistent, so it was common even for hospitals that were close together to offer overlapping services. The only strategy practiced by many hospitals was to attempt to grow faster than their competitors. While in previous years, massive fund-raising drives and careful planning accompanied hospital expansions, the new arrangements encouraged growth for the sake of growth.

For some time after Sister Smith's appointment, St. Vincent Hospital continued to enjoy the golden period that had begun with the opening of the new hospital. Sparked in part by the new federal legislation, the hospital continued to build new facilities and update existing facilities during the 1960s and early 1970s.

Continuing its history of innovation, St. Vincent became one of the first community hospitals in the country with intensive care beds specially designated for cardiac patients. St. Vincent also became the first hospital in the country to form a joint venture with the ITT-Sheraton Corporation of America, parent company of the Sheraton Hotel chain, to operate an extended care home. The hospital's facilities were enhanced in 1964 with the opening of Saint Luke's Hall and the five-floor east wing, and in 1965 with the opening of the Bishop Wright Pavilion.

St. Luke's, a six-story apartment house for married house officers and their families, was designed to help St. Vincent attract house officers of a higher caliber, since it eased the economic burden for young families, made apartment hunting unnecessary, and kept the young house officers close to both their families and their patients. Before St. Luke's opened, housing of residents and interns was difficult for St. Vincent. For some time, residents literally lived at the hospital. In the 1950s, after the Great Brook Valley housing project was built, Robert Maher, who worked with the St. Vincent Guild and later became president of the St. Vincent Research Foundation, arranged for many of the house officers to live in the project.

St. Luke's solved the hospital's housing problem, providing 31 apartments, each with two bedrooms, a living room, dining room, bathroom and kitchen. As an apartment building specifically for married house staff, St. Luke's was "the first of its kind built in the State of Massachusetts and might be the first in the United States," according to promotional materials prepared by the hospital for the dedication of the building.

St. Luke's reflected changing demographics. Where previously house officers were primarily single men, changing educational requirements resulted in older house officers, who were more frequently married.

"In the past, relatively few medical students were married during medical school or their post-graduate hospital training," according to the hospital materials. "Now, however, hospital training for physicians skilled in modern medicine can extend after a year of internship from a minimum of two up to seven years according to their specialties. This change has resulted in the majority of young doctors being married either during medical school or during their training period in the hospital. The resulting housing and economic problem for house officers is a factor which has an influence on their choice of hospital."

The economic benefit of the apartments was particularly important, since residents at the time earned salaries of just $3,600 to $5,000 a year.

Construction of the east wing was part of a $4 million renovation, which also included construction of the Bishop Wright Pavilion. The five-story addition to the east side of the hospital featured expanded business and administration offices on the first floor, expanded X-ray and heart catheterization facilities and an orthopedic department on the second floor, anesthesiology and a postoperative department on the third floor, an intensive care surgical unit on the fourth floor, and an intensive care medical unit on the fifth floor.

The medical intensive care unit was "fully equipped with an array of exotic equipment to meet virtually any conceivable emergency," according to an article in the *Worcester Telegram*. In addition to two isolation beds enclosed by glass, built-in oxygen and other apparatus for emergency procedures, the unit included the four-bed heart-monitoring section that was spearheaded by Dr. Ware and Dr. Stapleton.

By 1968, coronary artery disease was the leading cause of death in the country, with myocardial infarction, the common heart attack, accounting for more than a half-million deaths. With the opening of the cardiac intensive care unit, St. Vincent's mortality rate for acute myocardial infarction fell to just 15 percent, compared with an average of 20 to 25 percent for hospitals throughout the country.

The heart-monitoring section provided patients with 24-hour monitoring, an innovation at the time. By the time the heart-monitoring section opened, researchers had discovered the importance of providing constant attention and care to the patient during the first three to five days after a heart attack. During that time, a heart-attack victim's heart may stop beating or start beating so rapidly it pumps almost no blood. Unless the problem is detected and treated within about four minutes, the patient dies. The heart-monitoring section was designed to prevent such deaths. The American Medical Association estimated at the time that heart-monitoring sections, if developed at hospitals throughout the country, could prevent 35,000 deaths each year.

"To provide this second-by-second observation essential to the recovery process," the *Worcester Telegram* reported, "the St. Vincent unit has a combination heart monitor and pacemaker a little larger than an old-fashioned table-model radio mounted over each of four beds. Running from it are several small wires, topped by electrodes which will be placed on a patient's chest and, in some cases, also around his arms and legs to sense the little pulses of electricity that the heart produces as it beats.

"The monitor in the apparatus will show, by blips on a TV-like screen, whether the heart is beating as normally as can be expected. The pacemaker portion will stand in reserve, ready to take over and 'pace' the heart through small electrical shocks if monitoring shows that the patient's heart is not pacing itself properly."

In addition, monitors were set up in a central nurses' station. Alarms on the monitors alerted the nurses if a patient's condition worsened. A defibrillator was on hand in the unit at all times to shock a heart into producing regular rhythm patterns, and a portable, battery-operated pacemaker was available for use if a patient had to be moved out of the intensive-care unit.

The heart-monitoring section was designed not only to save lives, but to help the hospital operate more efficiently. Before the monitoring section was set up, a nurse had to stay with a single patient watching a bedside monitor.

The Bishop Wright Pavilion, an even larger project, opened the following year. While the influential bishop was gone, the memory of his Worcester years was commemorated in a three-story, white-brick addition built to expand the psychiatric unit, maternity ward and surgical patient care services. The new, 90,000-square-foot wing added nearly 150 beds to the hospital, including 52 for short-term psychiatric care, 45 for maternity use and 52 for surgical nursing, bringing the total number of beds in the main hospital building over 600.

Appropriately, the maternity ward was located in the Bishop Wright Pavilion. When he first came to Worcester, Bishop Wright lived in the old maternity ward. He also had a special fondness for children. In the new maternity ward, as in the old one, fathers were given their own room to await the birth of their children. With maternity services moving from Providence House, the old "1898" hospital, St. Vincent was finally ready to operate completely with 20th-century facilities.

After the psychiatric unit moved into the Bishop Wright Pavilion, St. Vincent established an innovative 36-bed self-care unit on the sixth floor, where the psychiatric unit was located. The self-care unit, a precursor to today's subacute care units, was designed for patients who were well enough to get along with minimal medical attention. Patients in the unit made their own breakfasts, took lunch and dinner at the hospital cafeteria, and reported to the nursing station at an appointed time for their medication. In doing so, patients had an opportunity to reduce their hospital costs by $6 to $8 a day. The idea of the unit was not only to reduce expenses, but to give patients an opportunity to recover in a home-like setting. The rooms in the unit were furnished more comfortably than other rooms at the hospital.

"There is nothing more traumatic for a person who isn't seriously ill than the constant sight of serious illness around him," Sister Mary Ann, director of nursing services, said when the unit opened.

In 1968, a $500,000 addition to the St. Vincent School of Nursing was dedicated. The 12,000-square-foot addition jutted out toward Spurr Street like the leg of an "L." The addition was designed with a large open area that could be used for recreation, or as an auditorium large enough to accommodate the entire student body. It also could be partitioned into three classrooms. The addition included a kitchen for nutrition classes, and science laboratory and office space.

The following year, the Anderson Building was constructed on Winthrop Street as a data processing center for the newly computerized hospital. Appropriately, the $200,000 computer building and residence hall was named for Sister Agnes Marie Anderson, the first chief accountant and later the controller of St. Vincent Hospital. In those days, computers were still enormous and required a large amount of space — enough space to warrant a separate building. The Anderson Building included 5,000 square feet of ground-floor space for the computer and living quarters for 24 unmarried residents and interns on the second floor.

Initially used for payroll, billing, census reports and accounts receivable, by 1973, the hospital's IBM 360 Model 40 computer was also tracking patient information. The November 1973 issue of *The Outlook,* a hospital publication, comments: "The ability of the new patient information system to retrieve information boggles the mind. Let us suppose that Mrs. K has just arrived at the admitting desk. The admitting clerk needs only Mrs. K's full name. By keying up one of over 75 different forms available on the tube, the clerk 'asks' the computer if Mrs. K has been a patient in the past five years. The computer scans over 135,000 patient records going back for 5 years. In about 3 seconds, the answer is typed out on the screen. . . . Whole words and sentences appear almost instantaneously. 'Yes,' says the computer, 'Mrs. K was a patient in June of 1968 when she entered through the Emergency Room.' The computer goes on to give the patient's full name, address, age, telephone number, next of kin, and all other pertinent material on Mrs. K."

The hospital spent two years planning the computer system and about 10,500 man-hours programming it. Twenty terminals linked to the computer were set up in admitting, preadmitting, outpatient admitting, the emergency room, the business office, medical records, radiology, the pharmacy, chemistry, hematology, housekeeping, dietary offices and data processing.

By 1974, house officers were using a program set up in the emergency room to improve their medical knowledge. In addition to providing general information about 19 different medical subjects, the program provided the computer operator with a limited amount of information about an imaginary patient and asked the operator to diagnose the case and treat the patient. If the operator chose incorrectly, the computer told the operator why he was wrong and what would have happened in a real-life emergency.

With the additions St. Vincent made in the 1960s, it became the second largest private hospital in New England, second only to Massachusetts General Hospital in Boston.

When Sister Smith was a student at Xavier University, she became a friend of James Martin, director of the graduate program in hospital administration. Martin later left his post and became director of ITT-Sheraton's new program for establishing "convatels," which combined the features of convalescent centers and hotels.

In the late 1960s, hotel chain executives were looking for new business opportunities, and thought they saw a link between their services and the personal medical care provided by hospitals and continuing care facilities. As Philip L. Lowe, then president of the Sheraton chain, saw it, hotels and hospitals were both in the "people" business. "We both treat, house and feed people," he said at a luncheon in Worcester, "only hospitals do it in periods of adversity. These centers are a natural extension of the hotel business."

The Holiday Inn chain began operating its Medicenter at Boston University Hospital in 1968, and soon after, ITT-Sheraton began construction of a stand-alone, for-profit convatel in Burlington, Vermont.

Even then, the idea of a nursing home had a negative connotation. The nursing home was, as one administrator said, a "place where people went in and didn't come out." Rather than providing medical care for elderly, chronic patients, the convatel was designed to provide what is today called subacute care — care for adult patients well enough to leave the hospital, but not yet well enough to return home. Richard Boonisar, who was chairman of ITT-Sheraton, described the convatel as "sort of a half-way house," providing an intermediate stop between the hospital and the patient's home.

In addition to providing medical care more appropriately suited to recovering patients, the convatel was designed to lower the costs of health care, because less equipment and fewer people were required for each patient. These expected efficiencies were supposed to produce a profit for ITT-Sheraton. James F. Coggins, director of finance for St. Vincent Hospital, predicted in 1969, when plans were first announced, that rooms at the convatel would cost about half as much as rooms in the hospital. Semi-private hospital rooms cost $44 a day at the time.

Recognizing that by linking a convatel directly with a hospital, the convatel could benefit from a steady flow of patients,

Martin contacted his friend, Sister Smith. Sister Smith must have seen the convatel as a perfect solution to her own problem. Providence House was too old and outdated to function much longer as a home for the chronically ill. Having already moved the maternity ward into the Bishop Wright Pavilion, the convatel gave her an opportunity to replace her chronic care facility with a potentially more financially rewarding convalescent care facility. Under the agreement with ITT-Sheraton, the land for the convatel was leased from the hospital. The hospital's medical staff treated the patients.

The St. Vincent board accepted the concept, Msgr. O'Connell was appointed to head a building committee and plans advanced for a $2 million, 152-bed facility with 84 rooms. The five-story Sheraton Continuing Care Center was built on hospital land on Providence Street and was connected by a tunnel to the Bishop Wright Pavilion so that patients could conveniently be transported from the hospital. It was one of the first convatels in the country, and the first to be physically connected to a hospital.

Despite the underground link and an architectural design complementing the hospital, the convatel had a deliberately noninstitutional look inside. It featured wall-to-wall carpeting, soft lights and reproductions of art works "from Wyeth to Warhol." A dining area was included on each floor, and a recreational director developed crafts and games. With its physical therapy, speech therapy and occupational therapy programs, the center quickly developed a reputation for providing a high quality of care.

It didn't take long for ITT-Sheraton to recognize that the concept of a convatel was flawed. While linking the facility to a hospital provided a steady flow of patients, it did not provide the projected flow of income. Most of the patients were insured under the new federal Medicare program, and Medicare, which was generous for reimbursing hospital services but not nursing home services, did not provide a large-enough reimbursement for ITT-Sheraton to recover its costs, let alone make a profit. The hotel chain also discovered quickly that there were differences between operating a hotel and operating a health-care facility. While ITT-Sheraton managers were accustomed to generous compensation, the revenues generated by the convatel were insufficient to pay such high salaries. ITT-Sheraton also found that operating the convatel required more staffing than expected.

"The convatel was a tremendous vision that ITT-Sheraton had," according to Thomas J. Cullinane, who now serves as vice president, extended care at St. Vincent. "At the time, the cost reimbursement system was set up so there was no incentive to move people out of the hospital early. With today's DRG system, it would have been the most successful model around."

During its first three years operating the Worcester and Burlington convatels, ITT-Sheraton lost $2.5 million. In 1974, just a few years after predicting that convatels would be established across the United States, Sheraton announced that it was abandoning the business.

By 1972, less than two years after opening the Sheraton Continuing Care Center, ITT-Sheraton put the convatel up for sale. It took three years to sell it. In 1975, the People's Church Nursing Home, Inc., which operated a 160-bed nursing home next to City Hospital and an 80-bed home at 25 Oriol Drive, purchased the convatel and renamed it Providence House, the same name used earlier for St. Vincent's chronic care home. People's Church Nursing Home was operated by the Greendale People's Church, a nondenominational church.

As St. Vincent Hospital grew, so did the war raging in Vietnam. As U.S. involvement increased, so did the involvement of those on staff at St. Vincent. The shortage of priests serving in Vietnam was particularly severe, and Dr. Jaffee played an unintended role in addressing that problem.

Like many of St. Vincent's doctors, Dr. Jaffee participated in the U.S. Army Reserves and spent many of his weekends in training. Many of his fellow reservists expressed an interest in having a priest on hand to say Mass for them. Although he is Jewish, being on the staff of St. Vincent, he knew he could find a priest to say Mass for them.

"I said, 'I'll get you a priest,' " he recalled. "I went to Father Dan, a St. Vincent priest, who was also a priest for the Worcester police and fire departments, and asked him to say a Mass one Sunday a month. He said, 'Fine.' A month later, he got a letter from Cardinal Spellman in New York, saying, 'In this era, when some priests are burning draft cards, you enlist in the military. You deserve more. I've activated you as a chaplain and you'll receive your orders for Vietnam within a week.'

"I hadn't heard from him in some time, and the next thing I know, I get a postcard from him in Alaska. He was involved in an earthquake. He sent me a postcard and asked me, 'Did you do that, too? Signed, Father Dan.' "

Vietnam was half a world away and did not have a direct impact on the operation of St. Vincent Hospital. The hospital continued to evolve, and changes were made to reflect the profession's growing emphasis on education. One of the improvements made during Sister Smith's tenure was the creation of the position of full-time medical director. The medical director was to have a broad range of duties, and was responsible for the quality of patient care, medical education and research.

In seeking a suitable candidate, Dr. Jeghers was contacted for his advice. Dr. Jeghers, who had a special fondness for St. Vincent Hospital, since he helped the hospital establish its medical training program, recommended a suitable candidate — himself.

Students for Life

**"The next best thing to knowing something is
knowing where to find it."**
Samuel Johnson

*O*ne day Dr. Jeghers asked if he could have dinner at the
home of one of the doctors on his staff at Georgetown. The doctor, of course, was happy to have his chief joining him for dinner. He didn't even mind when Dr. Jeghers requested that they
stop by his house first.

After arriving at the Jeghers home, Dr. Jeghers gave his visitor several medical journals to read and told him he would soon
be ready to leave. The visitor sat down and waited, and a few
minutes later he heard a lawn mower outside. He looked out the
window and saw Dr. Jeghers mowing his lawn.

Ten minutes later, Dr. Jeghers shut off the lawn mower and
they went off to dinner. Explaining himself to his befuddled
guest, Dr. Jeghers said, "My lawn is so big, mowing it is a terrible job. That's why I do one seventh every day."

It was then that the doctor noticed the varying height of Dr.
Jeghers' lawn.

Dr. Jeghers had a method for just about everything he did.
Knowing the Dr. Jeghers method for lawn mowing lends cre-
dence to Dr. Jeghers' explanation for why he accepted the medical director's position at St. Vincent. In accepting, Dr. Jeghers
gave up a plum appointment most doctors would envy. As chair-

man of the Department of Medicine at the New Jersey College of Medicine, he had a prestigious and powerful academic position that seemed ideally suited for a man as interested in medical education as Dr. Jeghers.

So why did he give it up? Having just changed its name from the Seton Hall College of Medicine, there is some conjecture that the school was going through internal changes that may not have benefited Dr. Jeghers. Perhaps Dr. Jeghers was merely taking his lifelong interest in community teaching hospitals — and especially in St. Vincent — to its logical next step.

Or perhaps, as Dr. Jeghers explained to Dr. Blute, "My philosophy is to do all I can in a place for 10 years and then leave," the thought being that after a decade, it would become difficult to initiate fresh ideas and it would be time to move on. True to form, he stayed a decade each at Boston City Hospital, Georgetown and Seton Hall, and spent 11 years at St. Vincent before moving on to become a professor at the Northeastern Ohio Universities College of Medicine in 1977.

There is, however, another plausible explanation for his departure from the New Jersey School of Medicine. The school may have run out of room for Dr. Jeghers' medical index.

Dr. Jeghers accepted his position at St. Vincent under the condition that he could bring along his files. When he told the hospital board he needed space for his files, the board told him that, of course, he would be given space. What the board failed to realize is that Dr. Jeghers' medical index consisted of 36 file cabinets filled with medical articles. Dr. Jeghers' files "took up half of the basement of the hospital," according to Dr. Massarelli.

Dr. Jeghers began saving medical articles in the late 1920s, when he was a student at Case Western Reserve University College of Medicine.

"I was interested in teaching by Socratic methods," he told a reporter for the *American College Physicians Observer* in 1985. "And I found that I could educate myself by reading journals. . . . I had a little money from working on the ambulance squad my senior year, so I began to buy journals."

Initially, he stored his journals in a trunk. After moving to Boston for his internship at Boston City Hospital in 1932, he began to cut up the articles, staple them together, send for reprints and file everything according to a system he established. He also began spending time in the medical library at Boston City Hospital, reading through journals to which he did not subscribe. Photocopiers did not exist then, so Dr. Jeghers jotted down notes, references and bibliographies.

In 1939, Dr. Jeghers and other doctors at Boston City Hospital studied the relationship between skin pigmentation and internal polyps. Their work resulted in the article, "Generalized intestinal polyposis and melanin spots of the oral mucosa, lips and digits." Their work described the condition in which patients with pigmented spots developed intestinal polyps, which came to be known as Peutz-Jeghers syndrome. Dr. Jeghers' article was so thorough and so well researched, Dr. William J. Pomidor used it as the basis for an article on how to prepare manuscripts for medical journals.

With the help of his wife, a graduate nurse at the hospital, Dr. Jeghers filled eight complete file cabinets with his medical articles by the time he moved on to Georgetown in 1946. While at Georgetown, he refined his index. He began to review the quality of the articles, making certain those not up to his standards never made it into the index. He also began to cross-reference information in a card file, so that medical students and doctors researching a subject could find information buried in a related article.

His single-minded devotion to his medical index and to medicine in general was such that he talked about little else. While at Georgetown, he confided to Dr. Stapleton that he was disappointed with the college cafeteria, because during lunch the other doctors preferred to talk about golf instead of medicine.

Dr. Jeghers' files were so extensive, Georgetown hired a librarian and secretaries to maintain the index, and favored medical students — Dr. Stapleton among them — were assigned as "reading residents" to read and assess potential index articles. Dr. Jeghers began to require interns to research their patients' ailments in his index and to present the appropriate information during rounds the following morning. By the time he moved on to Seton Hall, he had filled 22 file cabinets.

Dr. Jeghers wrote, "A major attraction for me going to Seton Hall was the opportunity to integrate more effectively the use of the medical library into the curriculum structure," since Seton Hall was a new school with no medical library. During Dr. Jeghers' tenure, many of the students were inspired to start personal medical libraries. Dr. Jeghers brought pliers with him when he lectured students on how to prepare a medical index, so he could teach them the proper way to remove staples from the medical journals.

While at St. Vincent, Dr. Jeghers perfected his medical index. The Jeghers Medical Index System, as it came to be called, by then contained articles from more than 200 English-language journals that met Dr. Jeghers' quality requirements. The articles were filed in 15,000 folders, arranged and referenced in a manner to promote self-education by both doctors and students.

"These folders are classified by an open and evolving vocabulary of key words suggested by clinical 'patterns' in the literature," according to an article cowritten by Robert Cheshier, director of the Cleveland Health Sciences Laboratory at Dr. Jeghers' alma mater, Case Western Reserve University. "By thinking in these patterns, physicians learn to use problem solving strategies characteristic of an expert clinician."

The article points out that the busy physician does not have time to read every article written on a subject, and notes, "the amount of information in each folder is manageable and thus represents a consensus of the significant and classic literature on any subject published during the past 50 years."

Reflecting on a visit with a small group of people from Ohio who came to Worcester to see how the system works, Cheshier told a reporter, "The system was absolutely mind-boggling. . . . It looked to all of us like this guy was the most obsessive-compulsive individual we'd ever met. He had all these damn articles and he tore up journals and he put them in cabinets all according to some system he developed."

"In other words," the reporter concluded, "he was awed."

The shelves in Dr. Jeghers' home library were empty. His journals were broken down and added to the index, which was made readily available to the St. Vincent staff.

"If you needed literature on any subject," according to Dr. Blute, "you'd go to Dr. Jeghers. He'd give you every article ever written all the way back to the '20s."

One time, for example, an attorney came to see Dr. Blute about a worker's compensation case. An exploding light bulb had perforated a worker's eye, and the physician prescribed Diamox® to relieve pressure. The worker developed kidney stones, and the attorney wanted to show a link between the use of Diamox® and the kidney stones. Dr. Blute asked Dr. Jeghers for the background information, and early the next morning he found a two-inch stack of articles on his desk. The mere sight of the volume of information on Diamox® was enough for the injured worker to win his case.

As extensive as his files were, Dr. Jeghers seemed to be intent on reading and learning everything that went into them.

"He read every book in the library from AAA to ZZZ," according to Dr. Carroll. "He had a photographic memory. He could give you the 60 causes of coughing up blood without looking them up."

One time, on a trip to Boston with another physician, he stopped by his home and left the doctor waiting in the car. After a time, the doctor went in the house and found Dr. Jeghers so absorbed in his reading, he had forgotten about the trip to Boston.

Dr. Jeghers' lifelong devotion to his medical index was in line with his philosophy that every doctor must be "a student for life." During and after World War II, medical research expanded rapidly, resulting in greater growth in medical knowledge than had ever before been seen.

From World War II to the 1960s, when Dr. Jeghers was formulating his ideas for community teaching hospitals, medical knowledge was growing by an average of 9 percent a year.

"As a consequence," he wrote in the *New England Journal of Medicine,* "what was learned during the formal period of basic training steadily becomes less useful and must continually be replenished. Even more troublesome is the need to replace old knowledge, an educational process more difficult for the practicing physician than for students and house officers."

The students and house officers have the advantage of being presented the latest medical knowledge when it is fresh and new, while the older practicing physician has to discard his old ideas while at the same time absorbing new knowledge. Yet unless the practicing physician keeps up with new information, over the period of a decade, his students will enter practice knowing more than he does, according to Dr. Jeghers. That's why, in Dr. Jeghers' mind, even the most experienced doctor on a hospital's medical staff is still a student.

"The span over which graduate and postgraduate education is needed is tenfold longer than the undergraduate period of four years," he wrote in the *Journal of the American Medical Association.* "The great need is to make the postgraduate education period a lifelong process and equal in quality with the present high standards of undergraduate education."

Dr. Jeghers recognized that physicians at community hospitals, in particular, were in need of educational opportunities. After World War II, funding from government agencies, foundations and private sources helped to bring the large university-affiliated and medical-school-affiliated hospitals up to new levels of sophistication. They succeeded not only in absorbing new medical knowledge, but in creating it.

The community hospital, meanwhile, "places a higher priority on the application of newer knowledge to improved patient care rather than creation of new knowledge," Dr. Jeghers wrote in 1974 in St. Vincent's *Outlook.* "New knowledge only accrues to improvement in medical care through the medium of medical education."

Essentially, to keep up with changes in medical practice and to keep their hospitals competitive, Dr. Jeghers believed, all doctors had to become lifelong students.

Some people didn't quite know what to make of Dr. Jeghers. He was a creative thinker and he drove a Porsche, but he was anything but flamboyant. One physician remembers him falling asleep in mid-conversation during a dinner with the medical staff.

"He could give a lecture and not realize that everyone had already gone," according to Dr. Levinson.

At six-foot-three, he was so big, he earned the nickname "moose." Yet he was so shy around women that, while eating breakfast at Dr. Stapleton's house one morning, instead of asking Mrs. Stapleton for bread, he asked Dr. Stapleton, "Does she have any bread?" Another time, while at a medical conference, he called Dr. Harvey's hotel room and Mrs. Harvey answered the telephone. Dr. Harvey was taking a shower, so Mrs. Harvey asked if she could help him.

"No," Dr. Jeghers said, "it's something I have to discuss with him."

When they met later that evening, Dr. Harvey asked Dr. Jeghers what he wanted to discuss that was so important. Dr. Jeghers asked him for his telephone number.

Dr. Jeghers is credited with regenerating the medical program at Georgetown University, and with helping to make the medical education program at St. Vincent a model program for community hospitals throughout the country. In the 1965–1966 academic year, St. Vincent received 20 applications from potential interns and appointed six. In 1973–1974, St. Vincent received 73 applications and appointed 13 interns. The following year, St. Vincent received more than 100 applications.

Dr. Jeghers also helped attract key doctors to the St. Vincent staff. When he came to St. Vincent, the shine on the new hospital had dulled somewhat. Certain departments needed to be updated. He saw what had to be done, and began making broad changes, beginning with the internal medicine and radiology departments, the areas of the hospital he knew best. According to Dr. Levinson, Dr. Jeghers understood that he could attract top-quality doctors to St. Vincent only if he provided the right environment. That meant giving them not only the opportunity to care for their patients, but also the proper equipment to create a sense of "academic excitement."

Dr. Jeghers succeeded in attracting a great number of top-quality doctors to St. Vincent, including Dr. Levinson; Dr. Earle B. Weiss, who wrote a leading book on asthma; Dr. Snyder; Dr. Jiri Palek, associate director of hematology; Dr. Burton D. Rose, a nephrologist, or kidney doctor, whose textbooks are known throughout the world; Dr. Murray L. Janower, chief of radiology; Dr. Gilbert H. Friedell; and many others.

But his attempt to revamp the existing equipment and to hire top-quality specialists ran counter to the natural frugality of the nuns and of Msgr. O'Connell. The Sisters of Providence had made the hospital successful by saving money whenever possible, and they saw no need to change direction.

Still, Dr. Jeghers had enough authority to maintain a degree of flexibility. To recruit doctors, he invited them to come to the hospital as consultants, then he offered them positions. While opinions differ over how much authority Dr. Jeghers had in setting contracts for individual doctors, some believe he was responsible for setting contract terms that varied widely. For some, it created animosity and resentment. Dealing with the internal political situations that arose was not Dr. Jeghers' strong suit.

While he was generally well liked and recognized for his dedication and his honesty, he was also considered to be, one doctor said not unkindly, "a blundering apostle." Although people skills were not Dr. Jeghers' strong point, Patrick Roche said Dr. Jeghers was "a man of great vision. He's one of the men I would hold in the greatest respect. He was always five to 10 years ahead of everybody else in their thinking."

Dr. Jeghers was already 73 when he left St. Vincent in 1978 to accept his position at Northeastern Ohio Universities. Determined to find a permanent home for his medical index, he worked with Northeastern Ohio Universities, St. Elizabeth Hospital in Youngstown and the Cleveland Health Sciences Library to move the index to permanent quarters at St. Elizabeth. By then, the Jeghers Medical Index System consisted of 99 full file cabinets. Medical students at St. Elizabeth's continued to use and add to the index, maintaining an ever-growing memorial with more than a million articles.

St. Vincent's reputation as one of the country's leading community teaching hospitals was enhanced even further with the opening of the Philip and Mary Rose Diagnostic and Research Wing. Construction began in 1970 and the wing was opened and dedicated in 1972.

The link between the Roses, a prominent Jewish family, and New England's largest Catholic hospital was made indirectly through their son-in-law, Haskell R. Gordon. Gordon's son, Gary, enrolled in a summer internship program at the St. Vincent Research Foundation and found the experience of studying under Dr. Lee to be inspiring and rewarding. So much so that he introduced his father to Dr. Lee.

"Ever since Gary introduced me to you a few weeks ago, I have been stimulated with the idea that your research foundation needs lots more help," Gordon wrote in a letter to Dr. Lee in September 1967. "I have been struck with the basic concept that your research team is developing on a broad base to help many people overcome their medical problems in the not too distant future. Nobody is much more aware than I am that basic and applied research can be quite humbling and costly before useful results come about."

He enclosed a check for $100, and asked Dr. Lee to have the foundation contact him each year, because "hopefully I can add larger sums in the future." He proved to be true to his word. Gordon started the Rebecca and Samuel Gordon Memorial Fund with a $500 donation in 1968. He continued his involvement with the foundation, and, equally important, convinced other family members to contribute.

The $6.2-million Rose Wing benefited from many fund-raising efforts, including a concert by Arthur Fiedler and the Boston Pops that was sponsored by the Guild of Our Lady of Providence. But the project's success was ensured with the help of a $250,000 contribution made in memory of Philip and Mary Rose by their children, Mr. and Mrs. Ralph Rose, Mr. and Mrs. Sidney Rose and Mr. and Mrs. Haskell R. Gordon. In addition, $4.8 million of the project was financed by floating a tax-free bond through 25 financial institutions in the Worcester County area.

Philip Rose was a 16-year-old immigrant when he started a contracting business that resulted in the establishment of the Standard Paint Store in 1924 and eventually the Fair Discount Department Stores in 1954. The Fair developed into a chain of stores throughout Central Massachusetts.

The Rose children's memorial to their parents proved to be a tribute that benefited the entire community. The 83,000-square-foot addition included space for 200 professional and technical specialists. The five-story reinforced concrete structure is attached to the west end of the main hospital by a three-story connector. The wing was designed with 80 percent of its space to be used for diagnostic work and 20 percent for research.

Speaking at a dedication ceremony for the new wing, Bishop Flanagan said, "May I pledge for us all a new dedication to our common goal . . . the finest health care for all, plus a continuing enthusiasm and imaginative broadening of our medical and scientific horizons through research."

The Rose Wing brought St. Vincent's diagnostic equipment together in one area for more efficient operation. The new wing included laboratories for gastroenterology, nuclear medicine, electroencephalography, biochemistry, hematology and coagulation, pulmonary physiology and pathology. Among the advanced diagnostic equipment in the laboratory was a sequential modular analyzer, which could analyze a dozen chemical tests simultaneously and provide a computer printout, and an atomic absorption flame photometer, which provided rapid analysis of blood gases. A tumor registry, an early computerized medical data base, was located in the Rose Wing to tabulate information about the care of cancer patients.

"As predicted last year," Dr. Jeghers wrote in 1974, "this Diagnostic and Research unit has had a remarkable effect on uplifting the quality of clinical diagnostic services available to the medical staff in management of their patients, improving our teaching potential, and stimulating our full-time staff members to look for creative clinical research opportunities when encountering puzzling consultative problems. The presence of this unit in a community hospital has had a profound and favorable impression on every physician who has visited The St. Vincent Hospital. It has likewise enormously enhanced our ability to recruit house officers, who see in it, the diagnostic sophistication they are familiar with in a university hospital but feared would not be present in a community hospital."

With sophisticated facilities and professional staff that were much more advanced than most expected at a community hospital, St. Vincent succeeded in building on its reputation, attracting new staff and new grants.

In 1971, the year the country proclaimed "War on Cancer," the National Cancer Institute established cancer projects at some of the country's leading medical facilities. St. Vincent Hospital became one of three research centers in the country to serve as headquarters for a major cancer research project. St. Vincent Hospital was chosen as headquarters for the National Bladder Cancer Project. At the same time, the M. D. Anderson Hospital and Tumor Center in Houston, Texas, was chosen to coordinate colon-rectal cancer research and the Roswell Park Memorial Institute of Buffalo, New York, was chosen to study prostate cancer. A fourth project, for the study of breast cancer, was coordinated directly by the cancer institute.

As the project director for the bladder cancer project, Dr. Gilbert H. Friedell, the chief of pathology at St. Vincent who later replaced Dr. Jeghers as medical director, was responsible for managing research and disbursing $2 million a year in grants to other research centers. Project directors approved grants in six areas, including epidemiology, prevention, detection, diagnosis, prognosis, treatment, and establishment and study of animal models. For its part, St. Vincent received a three-year project grant of $450,000.

In addition to heading up the bladder cancer project, St. Vincent received a grant from the institute to research breast cancer.

Until the construction of the Rose Wing, St. Vincent Hospital's cancer research laboratories were located in the old Providence House, which was forced to close its program to provide care for the elderly and chronically ill in 1969, because it failed to meet the modern standards set by the state's Joint Commission on Hospital Accreditation. The building was adapted for use as a laboratory, but the Rose Wing was more conducive to fruitful research, and the cancer laboratory moved right in.

Finally abandoned, Providence House was deemed to have outlived its usefulness. Having served St. Vincent Hospital for three quarters of a century, the building was demolished in 1973. The only piece of equipment left after the demolition was the bell, which was moved to its new home on top of St. Vincent Hospital. Before the move, it was inscribed as follows: "Over the years the bell has tolled the angelus at 6 a.m., noon and 6 p.m., its sweet, pure notes ringing across the hill and over the valley. To patients, to nurses, and to those working and living in the homes that climb the hill, the St. Vincent Hospital bell has been a friendly companion."

By the early 1970s, despite its new research facilities, equipment and full-time staff, certain departments still were in serious need of updating. Dr. Jeghers started with the radiology department, one of the departments he knew best. He hired Dr. Janower to run the department and in 1974, he oversaw a major revamping, including the purchase of $2 million worth of equipment and an increase in the staff of radiologists from two to seven.

The new radiology department was part of a two-floor, $4 million addition that also featured a new emergency room. Called "radical and unusual" by Charles A. Bianchi, administrative and technical assistant to Dr. Janower, the new radiology department was based on a European design. The department space was square with two parallel "H" shapes forming corridors that pass through it and divide the department into quadrants. A different function was assigned to each quadrant — general radiography, emergency procedures, fluoroscopy and special procedures, such as diagnosis using catheters. The purpose of the design was to increase the efficiency of the department and to provide patients with as much privacy as possible. Film-developing chemicals were supplied to 14 processors from central tanks.

The radiology department included a new mammography section featuring an $18,000 "soft" X-ray machine for detecting breast cancer. A soft X-ray penetrates breast tissue, but, unlike a traditional X-ray machine, does not penetrate bone tissue. A new viewing room also was included, where physicians could view up to 80 X-rays at a time on eight different viewing units. In contrast, the old viewing room allowed radiologists to look at only four X-rays at a time. A special room also was built for taking X-rays of children. The children's room featured a plastic holding device for babies and a giraffe that children sat on so they would stay still during X-rays.

As part of the project, a four-million-watt linear accelerator was installed underground in a former storage area behind the Bishop Wright Pavilion. The first linear accelerator in Central Massachusetts, the machine was designed to provide radiation treatment for cancer patients. A niche was blasted into the rock ledge of a wall to provide a natural protective barrier, saving the cost of shielding the equipment.

Much like today's laser surgery equipment, the linear accelerator could aim a beam at a tumor with a great deal of accuracy and deliver quick bursts of energy to minimize damage to healthy tissue surrounding the cancerous tumor. The accelerator, which was much more accurate than competing cobalt equipment of the day, was operated by remote control. The operator of the accelerator stayed behind a thick concrete wall and observed the patient through a series of television cameras, communicating instructions by microphone.

With its new facilities in place, St. Vincent quickly became a leader both in radiology and radiation therapy, which was organized as a separate department chaired by Dr. Sidney P. Kadish. Under Dr. Janower's leadership, the Radiology Department was the first in Central Massachusetts to provide lung scans, the first to use ultrasound for pregnancy, and one of the first in the state to use mammography. The department was the first outside Boston to use CAT scans, and the first in the area to use CAT scans for the whole body.

At the same time the Radiology Department was upgraded, the emergency care area also was upgraded. Upgrades included a new enclosed and heated three-bay ambulance dock, new entrances for walk-in emergency room patients and a new registration desk. Dr. Howard S. Schwartz, director of emergency medical services at the time, explained that the renovated emergency medical services area would provide quicker treatment to critically ill patients, because the ambulance dock led directly into the cardiac and trauma resuscitation area.

Some last-minute changes were made in the plans for the emergency services to keep them from overlapping with services provided by the new University of Massachusetts Medical Center.

"In 1970, when we first planned this, we had no knowledge the medical school planned to have an emergency department," David Hannah, assistant director for laboratories, told a reporter for the *Worcester Telegram.*

✤ ✤ ✤

While the upgrades were bringing St. Vincent Hospital back into the vanguard of health care, they also were costing money. As the costs of the new equipment became evident, Dr. Levinson said, "The administration seemed to lose its nerve. They decided there were things that we shouldn't try to be."

When an RFP circulated for a trauma center, St. Vincent's administration had to be prodded by the attending staff to submit a proposal. The hospital also lost time in reactivating its cardiac surgery program, because the administration refused an invitation from the chief of surgery at UMass to join the university in a combined program.

"For a while, because we lacked a cardiac surgery program," Dr. Levinson said, "we couldn't even do a coronary angioplasty — one of the most important advances in interventional cardiology — even though Dr. Richard Myler, our former cath lab director, was one of the pioneers of coronary angioplasty."

As these examples show, according to Dr. Levinson, St. Vincent lost its momentum after Dr. Jeghers left, and "the administration decided it didn't want to try to be first."

Difficult Times

"Medicine, like many other American institutions, suffered a stunning loss of confidence in the 1970s. . . . The economic and moral problems of medicine displaced scientific progress at the center of public attention. Enormous increases in cost seemed ever more certain; corresponding improvements in health ever more doubtful." Paul S. Starr in
The Social Transformation of American Medicine

The post-World War II era was an exciting time for the health care industry. Encouraged by the limitless possibilities of medical treatment that were just beginning to be unveiled, the country was willing to pay more and more for health care. Nationally, medical expenditures increased from $12.7 billion in 1950 to $71.6 billion in 1970. Health-care costs as a percentage of gross national product increased from 4.5 percent to 7.3 percent over the same period.

The cost of medical progress was relatively low in the 1940s. Inflated in part by the building excesses of Hill-Burton, health-care costs doubled in the 1950s. In the 1960s, the focus for advancing health care shifted to new equipment. Machines such as isotope scanners and linear accelerators may have helped to advance medical treatment, but they cost much more than a dose of penicillin.

Other factors also were driving up the cost of health care. Doctors were paid on a fee-for-service basis. Treatment in a hospital was especially lucrative, so there was a financial incentive for doctors to hospitalize their patients. With private insurance and federal programs paying most of the country's medical bills, prices were allowed to rise considerably before the cost of health care became a public issue. But by the end of the decade, the vast spending programs that were spurred by government funding had escalated out of control.

By 1970, the American public was in no mood to accept further price increases. With the country continuing to fight a costly war in Vietnam, inflation was running high. President Richard M. Nixon's solution was to institute price controls. But hospitals do not operate in a static environment. The price controls applied to hospital services, but not to hospital suppliers. By September 1973, when the president's economic stabilization program finally allowed St. Vincent to increase its room rate by $7 a day, the hospital already had been forced to absorb a 50 percent increase for the year in the cost of bed linen, a 25 percent increase in the price of fuel and a 12 percent increase in the price of food.

The unprecedented regulatory burdens placed on hospitals in the early 1970s aggravated the hospital industry's financial difficulties. For the first time, society began to view medical care as a basic right. Extending the already costly Medicare and Medicaid programs, Congress passed a series of new laws that imposed restrictions, added to paperwork and made it difficult for hospitals to operate profitably.

St. Vincent Hospital, like every other hospital in the country, was forced to absorb new costs, but at the same time could not charge more for its services. St. Vincent was faced with absorbing the cost of its recent expansion projects in addition to its rising payroll costs. Where previously the hospital relied on virtually free labor from the Sisters of Providence, by the 1970s the number of nuns serving the hospital had dwindled dramatically. At the same time that the hospital was forced to add lay staff to keep up with the growing complexities of running a hospital, the cost of hiring new staff was increasing.

St. Vincent also faced more competitive pressures than most community hospitals. In 1893, when St. Vincent Hospital was built, Worcester had just one hospital bed for every 700 people. By 1970, Worcester was being served by 1,800 hospital beds — about one bed for every 100 people — and the area's seventh hospital, the University of Massachusetts Medical Center, was preparing to open.

While price controls and increasing regulation were having a profound impact on the hospital industry across the country, a very personal, very private decision by Sister Smith had an even deeper impact on St. Vincent Hospital. Sister Smith's decision was meant to affect her own life, but it affected an entire institution, forever changing the history of St. Vincent Hospital. It was a decision that sparked the beginning of a new era, creating a change that everyone knew must someday come, but which was never openly discussed or considered.

In April 1973, Sister Helen Marie Smith became Helen Marie Smith. Miss Helen Marie Smith. After 36 years with the Sisters of Providence, she decided to leave the order.

Mary Darcy, her personal secretary and the hospital's director of public relations, drove her to the Mother House in Holyoke on the day she left the order. "I told her I didn't want to go in," Mrs. Darcy said. "I waited in the car." Sister Smith walked in, left behind her crucifix and the ring she wore on her right hand to symbolize her "marriage" to Christ and emerged as Helen Marie Smith.

"She seemed to have a mixed feeling about it," Mrs. Darcy said. "I think she hoped she was doing the right thing. I'm not sure she was all that convinced." Afterward, they went to see Miss Smith's sister in nearby Springfield, and during the drive there was no discussion of the decision. "She was very quiet," Mrs. Darcy said. "It was a closed book."

"Why she left the order was a personal and private decision that she never discussed," according to Dr. Kocot. "All she ever said was that she could be more effective as a lay person."

Roche conjectured, "It may be that she was trying to prove something to herself. She was very visceral. A lot of gut instincts steered her."

She may have concluded that independence from the order would give her more control over her job as hospital administrator. Because her position made it difficult for her to participate fully in the activities of the order, she may have felt that she no longer belonged with the Sisters of Providence. Or she simply may have found it impossible to separate her daytime hospital position from her nighttime responsibilities in the convent.

"She'd come in during the day and be the boss," Dr. Howard said. "Then she'd go under the tunnel and wash dishes. She'd have to answer to a Mother Superior."

Miss Smith's decision had a stunning impact on the hospital. While many nuns were beginning to leave their religious orders, the idea of a hospital administrator leaving the order was so unexpected, no one was prepared for it.

Roche, who was then associate director, took over for several months while the Board of Trustees decided what to do next.

For many, the board's decision was as shocking as Miss Smith's. The board voted to reappoint her, though her title changed from administrator to executive director. Regardless of her title, it was still her job to run the hospital, and she was the first lay person to be given that responsibility.

"Historically, she was the first lay person to be a CEO," Dr. Kocot said. "It caused quite a furor. It was inferred that there would always be a Sister of Providence at the helm."

"It was a very difficult decision for our board," Bishop Flanagan said. "In the end, we made a very sensitive, and what proved to be a very successful, decision to retain her as administrator."

Some believe the support of Bishop Flanagan and Msgr. O'Connell was a key factor in her reappointment. Others say she was simply the most qualified candidate for the position, and that there were no other sisters in the order qualified to replace her. The board undoubtedly believed it was merely hastening the unavoidable. A lay administrator would run the hospital eventually, so why not reappoint the one person with the necessary experience?

If Miss Smith had thought out the reaction to her decision to leave the order, she may have continued her life as a nun. The Sisters of Providence were upset to have control of the hospital they worked so hard to build taken out of their hands. But, as Bishop Flanagan maintains, the change was inevitable.

"It was the beginning of a kind of natural separation," according to Bishop Flanagan, "because so few from the community continued to work in the hospital. I'm not sure most of them were pleased to see the leadership of the hospital no longer in the person of a member of the community, but you can still have a Catholic hospital if good lay people are running it. That does not have to change as long as the goals and the philosophy are the same. There are committed Catholic lay people who can carry out the Catholic philosophy and its goals."

Even though she was no longer a nun, Miss Smith was still a committed Catholic, who continued to manage St. Vincent Hospital in a manner worthy of the hospital's namesake, according to Bishop Flanagan.

The months after she left the order were difficult for Miss Smith.

"I didn't see her all summer after she left the convent," Dr. Blute said. "We had a meeting and all the chiefs were there and Helen came in. There was a silence. She sat down before the meeting, and I said to her, 'Helen, how was your summer?' She said, 'It's like that old story about when they asked Mrs. Lincoln how the play was.'"

The decision to reappoint her drove a wedge between the hospital and the Sisters of Providence. As rational as the decision to reappoint her may have been, the sisters could not abide the reappointment of a person who had rejected the order. The reinstatement of Helen Marie Smith "was a turning point in our relationship with St. Vincent," according to Sister Adrianella. "She was very efficient, very capable, but her relationships with the Community (the order) were very awkward."

Roche noticed a difference between Helen Marie Smith and Sister Helen Marie Smith. Without the protection of the order behind her, she seemed more guarded, less secure. More than ever, she isolated herself from anyone or anything she viewed as a potential threat to herself or to St. Vincent Hospital.

She remained a very religious person, according to Margaret L. McKenna, vice president, human resources, but she changed her lifestyle dramatically. She bought a house on Cape Cod and commuted to work every day in her new Mercedes. "She liked nice things," Mrs. McKenna said, "and she seemed to be compensating for her years as a nun."

"Talk quieted down after she returned," Mrs. Darcy said. "Things were back to the way they had been." But Sister Miriam Regina remained a part of Helen Marie Smith for many years afterward. Mrs. Darcy recalls her saying on occasion, "I'm not sure I ever should have left."

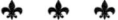

The management role of the Board of Trustees at St. Vincent always has been atypical, perhaps even unique. The board always has balanced the interests of the nuns, the bishop, the community and the medical staff.

Where other Catholic hospitals typically are owned and operated either by an order of nuns or by a diocese, St. Vincent's control, and even its ownership, has been loosely defined. The balance on the board also has been subject to change, but history has shown that the diverse groups have worked amazingly well together to create a hybrid that is both a Catholic hospital and a community hospital.

For more than 75 years, the Board of Trustees of St. Vincent Hospital was made up primarily of clergy, doctors and nuns. There were often businessmen on the board, but they tended to be people like George Crompton and Stephen Salisbury III, who were expected to help raise funds for new projects, not to manage the hospital. In the 1950s, Bishop Wright was clearly a dominating force. In the 1960s, the makeup of the board gradually changed. By the 1970s, the board was more business-like, and its decisions clearly reflected the business perspective of the board members.

The decision to reappoint Miss Smith, for example, seems to have been based on sound business judgment. She had experience managing the hospital, and she had kept St. Vincent on firm financial footing despite the difficult environment of the early 1970s. But earlier boards most likely would have weighed other factors into their decision, including the impact that the decision would have on relationships with the Sisters of Providence.

In 1973, Bishop Flanagan was still president of the board and the Sisters of Providence were still represented on the board by their superior general, Sister Mary Caritas, and by Sister Smith until she left the order. Cardinal Wright, the former bishop of Worcester, was still an honorary board member. Msgr. O'Connell, the Rev. Msgr. John F. Gannon, pastor of St. John's Church in Clinton, and Msgr. Francis J. Manning, pastor of St. George's Church in Worcester, also served on the board, but other board members were businessmen. They included William J. Cadigan of Shrewsbury, president of the Massachusetts Electric Company; Edward B. Coghlin, Sr., president of Coghlin's, Inc.; John J. Curran, president of Bay State Savings Bank; Michael J. DiPierro, owner of Amoco Chemicals Corp.; William L. Fox, president of the Worcester Bus Company; Jeremiah F. Gallo, owner of Gallo Motor Sales and chairman of the Worcester Housing Authority; Richard J. Harris of Shrewsbury, treasurer of the Coca-Cola Bottling Co. plant there; Francis S. Harvey, president and treasurer of Harvey & Tracy & Associates, Inc.; Louis C. Iandoli, president and director of Iandoli's Supermarkets, Inc.; James B. Kenary, Jr., secretary and treasurer of Kinsley & Adams; Leo W. Malboeuf, president of Harr Motor Company; James J. Marshall, Jr., president and treasurer of the Daniel J. Marshall Insurance Agency; Cosmo E. Mingolla, president of Baver & Mingolla Industries; and Robert

C. Reidy, a partner in the real estate firm of Maurice F. Reidy & Co.

On June 14, 1973, while the hospital was without a permanent administrator, the board's Executive Committee made another business decision. It voted to close St. Vincent's maternity ward. Actually, it turned out that the committee as a whole had discussed the idea in January and had decided to close the ward, though no formal vote was taken at the time. The committee vote was 7-2, and Msgr. O'Connell was the most vocal defender of the decision. Bishop Flanagan and Harvey voted to oppose the closing.

Financially, it was unavoidable that St. Vincent Hospital cut back or consolidate some services. It was clear that for Worcester's hospitals to remain on firm financial footing, they needed to reduce the overlap in their services.

St. Vincent's Executive Committee reacted with a decision that was outwardly logical. In voting to close the maternity ward, the committee was following a decision that already had been made by most other hospitals in Central Massachusetts. Since the mid-'60s, eight other hospitals in Central Massachusetts already had closed their maternity wards. Even with fewer maternity wards in the area, St. Vincent was picking up little new business. Most of Worcester's babies were being born at Hahnemann Hospital and Memorial Hospital. St. Vincent's child births dropped from 1,500 in 1968 to fewer than 850 in 1972. At the time, state guidelines recommended that hospitals with fewer than 1,500 births close their maternity wards. Because St. Vincent delivered fewer than 1,500 babies a year, the hospital was in danger of losing third-party payment accreditation from Blue Cross and Blue Shield, and Medicaid. In addition, the hospital was running the maternity ward at a deficit of more than $100,000 a year.

At the same time, St. Vincent's pediatric services were thriving. St. Vincent officials figured they could give up maternity services to Memorial, if Memorial gave up pediatric services to St. Vincent. Owen Murphy, who covered the issue closely as editor of *The Catholic Free Press,* said St. Vincent may have wanted to use the maternity ward space for a critical care unit.

When Roche announced publicly that the maternity ward would close as soon as all expectant mothers in the program gave birth, he said the decision was necessary, "because of low occupancy, certificate-of-need legislation, governmental regulations and pressures being brought to bear on all health facilities for efficient and economical operation in the delivery of health care."

The decision may have been financially logical, but it was not well received by the doctors, the Catholic leaders or the Sisters of Providence. Just months after the U.S. Supreme Court ruled in the famous *Roe* v. *Wade* decision that women had a right to abortion, the Board of Trustees had closed the one maternity ward in the city that symbolized the Catholic view opposing abortion. As the area's only Catholic hospital, St. Vincent did not provide abortion or contraceptive counseling to women.

While Blue Cross and Blue Shield of Massachusetts hailed the decision to close the ward, the hospital's doctors, who were predominately Catholic, did not. Dr. Kocot and Dr. Paul H. Martin, an internist at St. Vincent Hospital, discussed the Executive Committee's decision to close the maternity ward and decided to do something about it. They initiated a petition among the St. Vincent doctors and collected $400 to take out a full-page ad in the *Worcester Telegram*. The ad, which was signed by a majority of the medical staff, read: "We the doctors of St. Vincent Hospital, do hereby proudly join the Sisters of Providence in protesting the decision of the Executive Committee of the Board of Trustees to discontinue maternity services. As a matter of public record, in April 1972, a motion was passed by the Staff Physicians of St. Vincent Hospital encouraging the promotion and continuation of maternity services at St. Vincent Hospital. In May 1973, a similar motion was again passed (unanimously) by the Executive Committee of the Medical Staff of St. Vincent Hospital."

The doctors prepared the petition, Dr. Kocot said at the time, because "this is not just the concern of obstetricians. This is a problem which concerns all doctors and, indeed, all citizens of Worcester. The decision to close the maternity section is very frightening to those of us who feel that certain principles cannot be equated in terms of dollars and cents."

The doctors also convinced the nurses to run a full-page ad, and they met discretely with clergy and others who opposed the closing to develop a strategy for overturning the Executive Committee's decision.

After hearing of the decision to close the ward, Cardinal Wright, who was still an honorary trustee, asked that his name be removed from the board membership, that his name be dropped from the Bishop Wright Pavilion and that the statue of St. Vincent be removed from the hospital.

Members of the Guild of Our Lady of Providence also spoke out against the closing. Among the past guild presidents interviewed by *The Catholic Free Press,* Mrs. John B. Butts said, "A Catholic hospital should have a maternity unit to take care of women who would like to have their babies in Catholic surroundings. I think the people responsible for the decision didn't think far enough ahead. If a woman is having a baby in a hospital and is impressed with the care, she will keep going back for other things."

Directors of the Diocesan Council, the service agency for parish councils in each of the 131 parishes and three missions in the diocese at the time, sent a telegram to the Executive Committee saying, "Pro-Life proponents need St. Vincent's maternity ward. Please reconsider your decision." In addition, Attorney Francis P. O'Connor, a Worcester attorney and St. Vincent incorporator, raised legal questions about whether the 12-member Executive Committee had the authority to act for the full 24-member Board of Trustees.

At a follow-up meeting with the Executive Committee, Msgr. O'Connell defended the committee's position and said that, because of the hospital's financial situation, any services that did not contribute more income than they cost should be eliminated. "Then you've just eliminated the chapel," Dr. Kocot responded. "And the (City of Worcester's) Police Department and the Fire Department."

The outpouring of opposition was so great that less than two months after the Executive Committee voted to support the closing, the entire committee reconsidered and decided to keep the ward open. On July 30, 1973, the board voted unanimously to keep the service open. The reason for the change in the vote, according to Bishop Flanagan, was "the strong support expressed by the staff, the public and the diocese." After the vote was taken, he said, "I breathed a sigh of relief."

Dr. Mancini, who was a nurse in the maternity ward at the time, said that before the decision to close the ward was rescinded, "it was like the grieving process" was taking place in the ward. When Dr. Philippe W. Ouellette, chief of obstetrics and gynecology, informed his staff that the ward was going to remain open, "we all jumped up and down we were so happy. We were re-energized. The threat of the closing made it so real to us, we did some grassroots recruiting, and if we heard about anyone who was pregnant, we tried to get them to use the maternity ward."

The maternity staff hung a sign in the nursery after the incident was over that read: "Welcome all you lucky babies with a new lease on life. A big thanks to all responsible for helping us stay open."

Responding to the decision to rescind the vote, Miss Smith said it was up to the medical staff to determine the future success of the maternity ward. Miss Smith said the decision was made to close the ward, because, with an occupancy rate of just 36 percent in 1972, "there was no demonstration that we were meeting a community, or a Catholic, need."

"We are counting on the good will of those who expressed their opposition to our decision to close the unit," Miss Smith said. "I am very happy with the decision to maintain the maternity section here. We always had one and we do want it."

If St. Vincent had gone through with the maternity ward closing and instead concentrated on pediatric care, "it would have been a financial nightmare," according to Dr. Kocot. Soon after the decision was made to keep the maternity ward open, pediatrics began to evolve into more of an outpatient specialty. By 1981, St. Vincent eliminated 18 of its 68 pediatric beds, because they were no longer needed.

Meanwhile, business in the maternity ward picked up, in part, perhaps, because the widespread publicity over the closing drew so much attention to the hospital's maternity ward. In 1974, St. Vincent worked with Memorial Hospital to create a joint neonatal unit at Memorial for high-risk newborns. Soon after, St. Vincent formed an agreement with City Hospital to provide maternity services to patients referred by City Hospital.

In addition, St. Vincent began to offer more innovative maternity services. In 1975, the hospital added birthing rooms and Lamaze classes to train new parents about natural child birth. The same year, St. Vincent became the first hospital in Central Massachusetts to introduce the Leboyer method, an alternative delivery method more commonly known as "birth without violence." The delivery method, which seeks to replicate the uterine environment for the newborn, calls for lights to be dimmed immediately after the birth of the baby. The baby remains in a nesting position on the mother's stomach for several minutes before the umbilical cord is cut, then the baby is bathed in warm water for several minutes to restore the floating sensation of the womb.

One of the reasons for the fall-off in births was the shortage of obstetrical staff at St. Vincent. During the early 1970s, only a dozen physicians had obstetrical privileges. After deciding to keep the ward open, St. Vincent worked at building up its obstetrical/gynecological and family practice staffs, recruiting some of its physicians by the late 1970s from the University of Massachusetts Medical Center. By 1980, the St. Vincent maternity ward had 26 doctors with obstetrical privileges and was busier than ever, with a record 152 babies delivered in the month of May alone — an average of five babies a day.

✤ ✤ ✤

The 100th anniversary of the opening of the Holyoke mission by the Sisters of Providence was proving to be the order's most difficult year. The sisters survived their first harsh winter at the Bartlett farmhouse and had, during the 80 years since then, built St. Vincent into the second largest private hospital in New England. They survived epidemics of malaria, typhoid fever, influenza and polio. They survived natural disasters, two World Wars and the Great Depression.

But suddenly, a few simple business decisions, made over the course of just a few months, threatened their existence at St. Vincent. In December 1972, the hospital adopted new bylaws that dropped Sister Caritas, major superior of the Sisters of Providence, from the Executive Committee. In April, Miss Smith left the order. In June, the Executive Committee voted to close the maternity ward. By then, only 36 of the 1,800 staff positions at St. Vincent — just 2 percent of the total — were filled by Sisters of Providence. After the closing of the maternity ward, Sister Caritas said the order was considering ending its affiliation with St. Vincent Hospital.

So it was under difficult conditions at best that the sisters were commemorating their 100th anniversary. During an anniversary Mass in September 1973, Bishop Flanagan addressed the sisters' problems and concerns without specifically naming them: "We are aware of the painful experience which our sisters, along with almost every other religious community, have undergone in these past few years. Their ranks are thinner, new aspirants to take the place of the aging are greatly reduced in number. . . . This is not the first time in history when the Sisters of Providence have faced trials and crises.

"It is reassuring to note, as they confront the particular problems of this moment, they do not give way to pessimism or discouragement. Rather, they come forward with this beautiful dissertation on the signs of hope, seeing in the trials of the moment a time of testing and asserting a determination to press forward, doing the work of the hour, spurred by a living faith and fired by a hope that is aware of the vast promises of God to those who are faithful in his service."

The Sisters of Providence did press forward, however cautiously, and the order continued its affiliation with St. Vincent Hospital. But the sisters' days of running the hospital had ended. Their numbers continued to decrease and by 1979, fewer than a dozen sisters occupied the convent. On November 3, 1979, the Sisters of Providence announced that they were moving out. After living on the grounds of St. Vincent Hospital for 86 years, the sisters closed the convent and the 11 sisters remaining at the hospital left.

The convent was converted for use by St. Vincent's anesthesiology program, the alcoholism clinic and the bladder cancer research program.

Without the sisters, who had run the hospital so frugally, it was that much more difficult to run the hospital. And with financial conditions as tight as they were, St. Vincent had to take a much more business-like approach to its operation.

"The days of philanthropy are essentially gone," Jim Coggins, who was then the assistant hospital director in charge of fiscal affairs, said at the hospital's 1974 annual meeting. "Now all hospitals have to charge patients to remain in the black."

St. Vincent Hospital finished the 1972–1973 fiscal year with a loss of $250,000. Because of tight budgeting and a small rate increase, St. Vincent finished the following year with a surplus of $82,925, a tiny, barely perceptible profit, considering the hospital's $28 million annual budget.

To operate more efficiently, St. Vincent sought approval to consolidate its surgical and medical intensive care services, but the state refused to allow the consolidation. As cost controls became necessary, the length of hospital stays began to shorten considerably, not just at St. Vincent, but at hospitals throughout the country.

One response to keep St. Vincent profitable was to increase outpatient services. In the 1973–1974 fiscal year, the hospital saw 19,000 patients, an increase of more than 6 percent from the previous year, and 8,000 of the patients used the hospital's services on an outpatient basis. By 1975, St. Vincent had 22 different outpatient clinics.

St. Vincent also announced the addition of its first satellite office in 1974 in South Grafton, which was perceived as being an underserved market. The Grafton Family Health Care Center used the additional services of residents and nurse practitioners to examine patients on an outpatient basis. Members of St. Vincent's medical staff would supervise the program and be available to provide inpatient care when needed.

Two New Entities

"Worcester rejoiced. Educators, civic leaders, medical professionals and Worcester area residents proudly accepted the congratulations that poured in from all over the state."

1982 Annual Report, UMass Medical Center, recalling the state legislature's decision to locate the medical school in Worcester

That the University of Massachusetts Medical Center opened at all is testament to the tenacity of its supporters. That it opened in Worcester is remarkable.

Talk of a new state-supported medical school began in 1948 when J. John Fox, chief executive secretary to Massachusetts Governor Paul Dever, put forth the idea. Little happened, though, until 1961, when the state legislature responded to a nationwide shortage of doctors by creating a commission to study the feasibility of a new medical school. The commission recommended the creation of a four-year medical school as part of the University of Massachusetts, and suggested that the school's trustees appoint a dean and select a site for the school. The legislature approved the commission's recommendations in 1962.

Dr. Lamar Soutter, a chest surgeon at Massachusetts General Hospital, was appointed dean by the trustees. Dr. Soutter, who had sailed to the North Pole, organized one of the country's first blood banks and flown into the Battle of the Bulge on a glider, was about to face one of his greatest challenges — approval of a site for the new medical school. Only two of the 22 UMass

trustees were from Worcester, and the city was seen as an under-
dog in the competition. Boston politicians and doctors lobbied
for a site in Boston or the Boston suburbs. Others supported a
site in Amherst on the existing UMass campus. A committee of
65 community leaders, including Dr. Richmond and Bishop
Flanagan, was assembled by Worcester's Chamber of
Commerce to lobby for a Worcester site. The Worcester area
also was well represented in the legislature at the time by powerful political figures who played a major role in the building of
the medical school. But the person who probably played the
greatest role in influencing the selection process was Major
General John McGuinness, one of the two UMass trustees from
Worcester.

Although Worcester's overabundance of hospital beds was
never a central topic of debate, initially there was some opposition to the Medical Center by the Worcester District Medical
Society, which argued that the need for another medical school
in the state had not been demonstrated. Some local doctors saw
the medical school as unwelcome competition. Others supported
it, believing it would increase the quality of both house officers
and doctors practicing in the Worcester area, and provide new
opportunities for existing doctors.

Dr. Soutter met with medical groups throughout Worcester
and placated their fears about UMass, telling them that UMass
would offer only noncompeting specialized medical services.
According to Dr. Kocot, "Dr. Soutter did not present the hospital
as it was already on the blueprints. Suspicions were heightened
when the hospital was built, because it already had all of these
competing entities in place. You can't fault the university for
what it did. If it hadn't been presented that way, it probably
never would have been built."

A consultant hired to review sites across the state issued a
report ranking Worcester fourth out of five sites. But Maj. Gen.
McGuinness and other supporters were undaunted. In 1965,
when the trustees finally voted on the site, no clear winner
emerged on the first ballot. Amherst received nine votes to
Worcester's seven. After four ballots, Amherst and Worcester

were deadlocked at 11–11. Between votes, Maj. Gen. McGuinness approached a trustee he did not know and struck up a conversation. Maj. Gen. McGuinness learned that the trustee was supporting the Amherst site, but the trustee confided that he held a grudge against someone in Amherst.

"Now's your chance to get even," Maj. Gen. McGuinness told him. The Worcester site was selected on the next ballot by a vote of 12 to 10.

It was still many years before the Medical Center was built, because funds had to be appropriated to build the school. By the end of 1968, with the help of state and federal funding, $70 million was available to finance the project. But, during the years since planning began, cost estimates increased to $124 million. In 1969, Gov. Francis W. Sargent, who opposed the Worcester site, expressed concern about the escalating cost and promised to take a close look at the project. Gov. Sargent ordered project studies first from a consultant at the Massachusetts Institute of Technology and then from a group of out-of-state doctors. At the time, he said the purpose of the studies was to determine the best approach for the school. But with a record budget to balance, and a purported interest in killing the project so that state aid could instead be funneled to medical schools at Tufts University and Boston University, Gov. Sargent was accused of attempting to stall or sabotage construction of the medical school and hospital. However, before the year ended, Gov. Sargent approved plans for the new school in Worcester.

In 1970, the new University of Massachusetts Medical School opened in temporary quarters in a converted tobacco warehouse. Groundbreaking for the first building at the UMass campus at 55 Lake Avenue North also took place in 1970. At the time, the school had 16 students and 23 employees. In 1971, the school became affiliated with St. Vincent Hospital and used St. Vincent's existing training facilities. With a local medical school as a training partner, St. Vincent dropped its affiliation with Georgetown University.

Gov. Sargent finally approved construction of the new hospital portion of the Medical Center in Worcester in 1972. At the same time, he approved three other hospital projects that had been delayed, including a $1.75 million expansion of the radiology department at St. Vincent. Other projects at Memorial Hospital in Worcester and Burbank Hospital in Fitchburg were approved, but scaled back.

In 1973, the school moved into the newly completed basic and clinical sciences building at the Lake Avenue site. Construction of the accompanying Medical Center hospital was completed and the hospital saw its first patient in 1976. The $130-million University of Massachusetts Medical Center gradually built up to its 400-student, 400-bed capacity.

Writing about the health-care industry in the Worcester area in 1975, *Worcester Telegram* reporter Jon Towne concluded that having seven hospitals serve the area was like having seven restaurants on the same street. To survive, he wrote, the hospitals "not only have to get along with their employees and patients, they have to get along with other hospitals. And hope that they all don't sell Chinese food."

Expressing frustration with what she saw as the public's failure to understand that running a hospital was indeed a business, Miss Smith spoke with Towne about the public perception of the health-care industry, concluding, "I think everybody keeps singling us out, and I don't know why we are different. We are trying to pay competitive salaries and provide work. But our product is different. It is human life."

At a time when the public was becoming angry about rising hospital rates, she said that without rate increases, the hospital would go bankrupt, adding, "I'd hate to think what people would say if I walked out front and put up a sign that said, 'Closed.' "

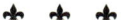

The health-care industry is unlike any other. As Miss Smith said, its product is human life. It is also the only industry where the most important employees are allowed to work for competing companies. Doctors usually are not hospital employees, so to speak. Although some practice full-time at a single hospital, many become affiliated with two or more hospitals at the same time. The Fallon Clinic doctors, for example, were affiliated with St. Vincent Hospital, but many also taught or practiced at the UMass Medical Center.

Not only was it not unusual for some of St. Vincent's best doctors also to be on the UMass staff, but the opportunity to affiliate with the new medical school was one of the attractions of St. Vincent to many physicians.

The medical staff at St. Vincent Hospital was ambivalent about the creation of the University of Massachusetts Medical Center, according to Dr. Massarelli. While they were concerned about having yet another hospital to compete with St. Vincent, many of the St. Vincent doctors also recognized that it would provide new opportunities for both teaching and learning. And there was a feeling among many that when a successful medical school is located nearby, it increases the quality of medical care at other hospitals in the area.

Soon after the medical school opened, St. Vincent and other Worcester-area hospitals lost some of their most prominent staff to the new school. Dr. H. Brownell Wheeler, for example, left his position as chief of surgery at St. Vincent to become chief of staff of the new medical school, while Dr. Barry Hanshaw became chief of pediatrics, leaving a similar position at St. Vincent.

Others held positions at St. Vincent, but taught at UMass. Dr. Stephen M. Ayres, for example, joined St. Vincent as chief of medicine in 1974 and also served as a professor at UMass. A nationally known heart and lung specialist, Dr. Ayres was national chairman of the American Lung Association's Anti-Smoking Committee and was a member of the U.S. Surgeon General's subcommittee on the cardiovascular effects of smoking. He left St. Vincent in 1975, less than two years after coming to Worcester, to accept a post as chairman of the department of internal medicine at the St. Louis University School of Medicine. Before leaving, Dr. Ayres spoke out against what he saw as an overlap between services planned at UMass and those already provided by St. Vincent and other area hospitals.

"We need the medical school and a lot of us would not be here without it," he said. "But we have to be able to work with it and cannot let one institution dominate others."

He questioned the need for emergency care services at UMass and concluded that the 400 beds at the new hospital would siphon patients from other Worcester hospitals. He also recommended a change in the salary structure for doctors teaching at UMass and practicing at other hospitals. At the time, the salaries for teachers at UMass were paid completely by the hospitals where the doctors were affiliated. Dr. Ayres urged that UMass not duplicate existing services at St. Vincent, adding that in some cases St. Vincent's services already were highly sophisticated.

"We are a tertiary hospital with tremendous care capability and a large group of division chiefs who are extremely well trained," he said. "They are leaders in their specialties, write articles and regularly speak around the world. When a person walks in the door, we can take care of anything that is wrong with them, except cardiac surgery."

A week earlier, Miss Smith had been the first official of any local hospital to voice her concerns about UMass.

"I get the feeling," she said, "that the teaching hospital is becoming more interested in primary care and is duplicating the efforts of community hospitals. This is one way it will be in direct competition with community physicians and hospitals."

Also citing the Medical Center's planned emergency room service, Miss Smith said there appeared to have been a "change in philosophy" by the hospital administration, and that, rather than relying on referrals from St. Vincent and other area hospitals for its patients, the hospital was gearing up to be a competitor.

The concerns of Miss Smith and of other Worcester hospital administrators were addressed by the creation of the Affiliated Hospital Consortium, which included representatives from the five hospitals that had affiliated with UMass — St. Vincent, Memorial, City, Hahnemann and Springfield's Wesson Memorial Hospital. The consortium was developed to work with UMass to ensure that the new hospital would not threaten the already precarious health-care environment in Worcester. Miss Smith said she did not expect the consortium to solve every problem, but "we will never get anywhere if we feel threatened all the time."

Dr. Wheeler said at the time that the creation of the consortium "has not solved the problem, but it has relieved the tension."

UMass followed Dr. Ayres' advice to branch into areas that were not already being offered. That year, UMass began offering coronary artery bypass operations.

By the mid-1970s, it was a given that the best hospitals had fully developed cardiac surgery programs, and UMass wanted cardiac surgery to be its flagship operation. Dr. Ware had given St. Vincent a head start over other community hospitals, but his death in 1968 brought the program to a sudden halt. Despite efforts to revive the program, it was too costly to carry out, particularly in the frugal health-care environment of the early 1970s.

Miss Smith "was convinced we could start our own," Dr. Blute said, "but it wasn't to be."

In 1972, St. Vincent became one of the few hospitals in the country to own a special heart pump designed to sustain life in a heart attack victim while waiting for surgery. The pump encased the patient's legs in a water-filled jacket and, by compressing the legs, pushed blood back into the heart, easing its work load. In 1974, St. Vincent received a more advanced balloon pump that was inserted directly into the heart by a catheter. By inflating and deflating in synch with the patient's heartbeat, the pump increased the efficiency of the patient's circulatory system. The $15,000 machine was donated by Francis A. and Jacquelyn H. Harrington.

As advanced as the new heart-pumping equipment may have been, it was useful only for preparing patients and keeping them alive until they were transported to another hospital.

UMass, on the other hand, benefited from the expertise of a team of experienced surgeons from Massachusetts General Hospital led by Dr. Mortimer J. Buckley, Jr., a Worcester native and renowned surgeon, and Dr. Gerald Austen.

St. Vincent did not succeed in restarting its own cardiac program until 1985.

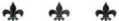

UMass Medical Center was not the only successful new health-care entity to start up in Worcester during the 1970s. The other new major force, the Fallon Community Health Plan, later played an even greater role in the future of St. Vincent Hospital.

Fallon Community Health Plan, one of the country's first health maintenance organizations (HMOs), was a surprisingly successful outgrowth of Fallon Clinic. The clinic itself had achieved substantial growth by following Dr. Meyers' strategy of providing comprehensive medical services through a single group practice.

In 1966, the clinic moved from Institute Road to 630 Plantation Street, an office still widely used by the clinic. The two-story building more than tripled the floor space the clinic had at 10 Institute Road. By then, Fallon Clinic had about 40 employees, but its real era of growth was just beginning. By the early 1970s, Fallon Clinic was the second largest group practice in the state, smaller than only the Lahey Clinic in Burlington. Even the new Plantation Street site was soon filled to capacity, and, in recognition of Dr. Meyers' contributions to the success of the clinic, the Meyers Wing was opened at the site in 1973.

Even with Dr. Meyers' proven success at predicting the future of health care, his fellow doctors at Fallon Clinic thought he was fantasizing when he predicted that prepaid group health plans, what we now call HMOs, were the wave of the future. His ideas were not without foundation. Henry J. Kaiser's Kaiser Permanente, established in 1942, had caught on in California, proving that prepaid plans limiting enrollees to designated group practices could work effectively.

In 1971, President Nixon proved Dr. Meyers right. With an election on the horizon and continuing financial upheaval in the health-care industry, President Nixon sat down with his top advisors to plan a national health-care strategy. And the centerpiece of their plan was the HMO.

In the Nixon Administration's terms, an HMO was either a prepaid insurance plan offered by a group practice, or prepaid coverage offered through a group of independent doctors. HMOs were expected to help control health-care costs because, by paying doctors straight salaries rather than on a fee-for-service basis, doctors would no longer have an incentive for performing unnecessary procedures. In addition, because patients would pay only a small charge for every doctor's visit, they would be more likely to take preventive measures and see their doctors before developing serious health complications requiring hospitalization. President Nixon's plan was to offer grants and loans as incentives for HMO start-ups. When President Nixon announced his plan, there were only 30 HMOs operating throughout the United States.

While Dr. Meyers formulated his ideas about HMOs in the 1960s, Fallon Clinic's first step toward forming an HMO came in 1970, when Fallon Clinic, St. Vincent Hospital and Massachusetts Blue Cross and Blue Shield studied the idea of "contract medicine," as it was then called. The idea of the plan, according to a Blue Cross newsletter, was "to coordinate the activities of the physicians, the hospital, and the health insurance operation. The plan will provide routine preventive medicine to a large segment of the people in the Worcester area, with an emphasis on ambulatory care. It is aimed at reducing the incidence of hospitalization. In addition, a sort of medical 'troubleshooter' has been named to help coordinate the service of the three agencies, thus providing a more efficient use of the combined facilities."

Fallon Clinic's new coordinator, or "troubleshooter," for the program, Alan M. Stoll, was given the responsibility of matching patients with the services and facilities best equipped to meet their needs.

"Through the Community Health Plan," Dr. Meyers is quoted as saying, "it is safe to predict that the physician will be able to spend more of his time in treating the health problems of the patient, because many essential but nonmedical responsibilities will be taken off his shoulders by the coordinator."

In 1973, the U.S. Congress passed the HMO Act. The new law required employers with more than 25 employees to offer their employees a choice between traditional health insurance and an HMO, if there were an HMO close enough to the workplace certified by the federal government. While the new law created a ready market for start-up HMOs that achieved certification, it also imposed restrictions on the HMOs. They could not, for example, impose preexisting conditions or restrictions that prevented anyone from joining the plan. They had to offer an open enrollment for at least one month a year, and charge the same "community" rates to all subscribers, instead of basing rates on a group's or individual's medical experience.

Despite the formation of the Fallon Community Health Plan, the Nixon Administration's 1971 commitment to HMOs and the 1973 HMO Act, little happened for several years. The initial project Stoll was hired for lasted about six months, after which he was hired as administrator of Fallon Clinic. In 1972, Fallon was one of six clinics to receive funding from the American Association of Medical Clinics to study the idea of establishing an HMO for its group practice. The idea of HMOs was still so unpopular, Stoll said, "they had a tough time coming up with six that wanted to participate."

While St. Vincent and Blue Cross continued to discuss the idea of an HMO with Fallon, their interest was minimal. Given that an HMO reduced hospital use, its goals were at odds with St. Vincent's, according to Stoll, so it made sense for St. Vincent to remain relatively uninvolved with the Fallon plan.

Like many others at the time, Miss Smith opposed the idea of an HMO. "It was a new idea and she didn't feel comfortable with it," Roche said. "She decided she wanted nothing to do with it. Accepting it could have created some difficulty. The predominant mode of physician practice was still private practice; group practice was still alien then."

In 1975, the Fallon Community Health Plan's efforts resulted in a federal grant of $49,585 to study whether an HMO should be formed in Central Massachusetts. By then, the Fallon Clinic had grown to include 26 physicians, all affiliated with St. Vincent Hospital, and 90 employees. Once Fallon had a grant in hand and the potential for additional federal funds, Blue Cross again showed interest in working with Fallon. In December 1976, Fallon Clinic received another grant, for $690,000, to purchase equipment and hire administrative personnel needed for the new HMO. The Fallon Community Health Plan finally began operation in 1977 in cooperation with Blue Cross. Under the terms of the plan, subscribers received coverage at a cost of $36 a month for individuals and $97.50 a month for families. An additional $2 was charged for each visit.

The Fallon plan grew rapidly, from 300 subscribers during February 1977, its first month, to 2,500 subscribers after six months, 600 more than expected. By April 1978, the plan had 4,000 subscribers and more than 80 Worcester-area employers offered it to their employees. But it was still a long way from the 18,000 subscribers it was projected were needed for the plan to break even.

In November 1978, a competing HMO to Fallon was formed. Central Massachusetts Health Care, which was started by a group of local physicians, received state approval to operate. Unlike Fallon, CMHC was not attached to a group practice. Subscribers chose a family physician from among the doctors in the plan, but the plan doctors did not operate in a central location.

The same month, the Fallon plan received an important boost. By becoming certified by the federal government, Fallon ensured that employers with 25 or more employees had to offer

Fallon enrollment as a health-care option. Between 1977 and 1979, membership tripled and the number of participating employers increased to more than 360.

In 1980, the Fallon Community Health Plan became the first HMO to receive a special contract for Medicare recipients through the U.S. Health Care Financing Administration. For $22.50 a quarter, elderly subscribers supplemented their Medicare coverage with Fallon coverage that included charges of $1 per prescription. Fallon's "Senior Plan" served as a national model for other health-care programs for the elderly. The Senior Plan exceeded even Fallon's expectations and, as the population has continued to age, it has accounted for an increasing portion of its market.

Spurred by the success of its new health plan, Fallon Clinic also continued its rapid growth.

After being approached by Westboro officials, who wanted to establish health-care services for their growing town, Fallon's first satellite office opened at 95 East Main Street in Westboro in 1977. The 6,800-square-foot building included examination rooms for two full-time internists, a pediatrician and an obstetrician-gynecologist. The clinic also included a medical laboratory, an X-ray suite, an electrocardiography unit and conference rooms. The office expanded in 1981, 1984 and 1988.

A second satellite office was opened in 1980, when Fallon Clinic purchased the bankrupt Auburn Medical Center at 35 Millbury Street. The renovated building was opened in November and offered complete ambulatory care, primary care, pediatrics, internal medicine, urgent care and specialty services, including orthopedics, obstetrics and ophthalmology.

The clinic's expansion continued unabated through the 1980s. While St. Vincent struggled with limited success to continue its growth and to adapt to the changing health-care environment, Fallon Clinic thrived, boosted by the success of the Fallon Community Health Plan. It was in the right place at the right time.

The Era of Limits

"This is no time for nostalgia."
Helen Marie Smith, in the
1980 St. Vincent Hospital Annual Report

$\mathcal{I}$n a world without government regulation, the management style of the Sisters of Providence could make St. Vincent Hospital the most financially successful hospital in practically any market. Every nun, and every nurse trained by the nuns, learned to use hospital resources as efficiently as possible.

But the regulatory environment of the 1970s and 1980s turned the benefits of economic efficiency upside down. State and federal regulations created an environment where hospitals were rewarded for practicing a philosophy of "the more you spend, the more you make." In this environment, a hospital that recycled sheets into bandages, put virtually all of its surplus funds into building maintenance, and paid cash for capital improvements was at a distinct disadvantage.

Beginning in 1975, the Massachusetts legislature approved a series of cost-containment regulations and for the first time set the amount of revenues a hospital collected from patient care. St. Vincent adjusted to the restraints of the new regulations, but St. Vincent's regulatory problems escalated in 1981, when the state decided to use hospital costs for that year as a base for future spending, according to William W. George, vice president, finance.

"Using 1981 as a base year, St. Vincent's efficiencies became detrimental," George said. "St. Vincent participated in a voluntary wage freeze. In the early 1970s, St. Vincent sold off its trust funds to pay for the new radiology and ambulatory care units. The Sisters of Providence paid cash so they would not have to pass the interest expense on to the community."

John L. Nespoli, who is now St. Vincent's chief operating officer, called the decision to pay cash for the $20 million in capital improvements "one very, very critical mistake" that later threatened the survival of the hospital. With wages frozen and almost no debt in 1981 as a result of its past frugality, St. Vincent was locked into its 1981 spending habits. Spending in years to come had to be based on St. Vincent's 1981 expenditures. In addition, St. Vincent had to factor in productivity improvements each year. As a result, St. Vincent's competitors, which had been less frugal, could spend more money and still meet the productivity targets with little effort. St. Vincent, meanwhile, had to be more frugal than ever to meet state-mandated targets.

Essentially, St. Vincent was being punished by the state for practicing the type of frugal fiscal behavior the state wanted other hospitals to practice.

Legislative cost-containment efforts culminated in 1983 in a federal law that altered the Medicare reimbursement system. Under the diagnosis-related group (DRG) system created by the federal law, hospitals are reimbursed based on the diagnosis of each patient. The DRG system was designed to provide incentives opposite to those inherent in the traditional fee-for-service system. When hospitals and physicians are reimbursed based on the services they perform, there is an incentive for them to provide as many services as possible. The DRG system, by setting reimbursement based on the diagnosis of the patient, provides an incentive for doctors to minimize medical procedures.

Because St. Vincent was locked into very low spending limits, the hospital spent very little on capital improvements. As a result, when Nespoli came to St. Vincent from the UMass Medical Center as vice president of planning in 1987, "It looked as though the hospital had neglected itself. It had stopped capitalizing itself." While the hospital still had much to offer, according to Nespoli, it was in great need of an update.

✤ ✤ ✤

Physicians who practiced in the glory days of medicine could be excused for being nostalgic during the fiscal crises of the 1980s. They had experienced the boon of penicillin and other breakthroughs. They had seen their profession revered as something special, elite, even sacred. They had chosen as a profession the healing of people and the saving of lives, and expected the status that came with the responsibility. People put their lives in the hands of their doctors, called upon them to make split-second decisions, to act with a superhuman clarity of mind and to cut with machine-like precision. They were expected to work long hours without making mistakes; human error could cost a life. Yet, increasingly, their authority was being questioned.

Dr. Robert D. Ouellette, president of the medical staff, wrote in St. Vincent's 1980 annual report, "Medicine, one of the most glamorous professions, has lost some of its sparkle." He goes on to explain not only why the role of the doctor changed, but how the health-care industry, and St. Vincent, were addressing their changing environment:

"Physicians in early times were revered to the point of holiness; they could do no wrong. Their judgments were non-negotiable and who would have thought of suing them? Doctors brought patients to the Hospital and their diagnosis, length of stay or medical records were never questioned. How that has changed! Hospital Administrators at one time would never question a physician. Then we witnessed a sudden turn-about where disagreement was seen. Decisions were made with little input from the Medical Staff; criticisms were offered by both Administration and the Medical Staff. However, that soon gave way to a mutual effort, more united than ever, in the face of the common external forces pressuring from all sides.

"The Trustee of a generation ago and today's Board Member differs markedly. The role has shifted from one type of status-seeking token position to that of an individual who is knowledgeable, politically astute, appreciative, supportive of the institutional goals, health care needs of the community and perceptive of the need for quality control.

"This metamorphosis has been achieved against the onslaught of mighty forces — the heat and pressure of consumerism, the financial interest of third-party payers, revised interpretation of accountability, liability, the demands of new technology, the changing reimbursement system and, last but not least, competition by other institutions, both old and new. All this means we must work together more so than ever before. It has never been more important than now that Administration, Trustees and the Medical Staff work together as a cohesive unit."

Perhaps this introspective longing for earlier days provided a necessary catharsis, but, as Miss Smith concluded in the same report, it was "no time for nostalgia." The issues of the day had to be dealt with, including government regulation, cost containment, malpractice suits and technological changes that were taking the doctor further away from the patient. These issues had become part of every hospital's existence. Reminiscing did not solve the problems of the day.

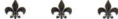

The massive hospital expansion that began after World War II with the Hill-Burton program and continued through the 1960s with Medicare came to a screeching halt during the 1970s. The bills for years of rapid growth were coming due. The costs of maintaining the huge monuments to health care that were built in the previous decades were draining hospital budgets. While earlier legislation encouraged expansion for the sake of expansion, new regulations made it mandatory for hospitals to justify any new building projects. If the need for a new project existed, the hospital would have to go through a long and tedious process to prove it.

That was fine with St. Vincent Hospital. With the additions of the Bishop Wright Pavilion and the Rose Wing, and the construction of St. Luke's Hall, Providence House and the Anderson building, St. Vincent's Board of Trustees saw no need for any new building projects. The board was looking to minimize capital expenditures and was determined that if money was going to be spent on the hospital's physical plant, it should be used to maintain the current hospital, which was beginning to show its age.

But Dr. Kocot had other ideas. St. Vincent Hospital had made medical education a major priority during the 1950s and 1960s, but it was clear to Dr. Kocot during the decade that followed that two things were lacking. First, the hospital needed an amphitheater for lectures, conferences and orientation meetings for students, house officers and the medical staff. Second, it needed a more modern, more extensive medical library. He saw the abandoned convent, which was adjacent to the hospital and connected by an underground tunnel, as the ideal location for the project.

While the necessity of the proposed upgrades was clear to Dr. Kocot, it was not clear to the hospital's Board of Trustees. When Dr. Kocot first approached the board, he was quickly turned down. The hospital had just spent a half-million dollars on new windows, and the trustees didn't think they could afford another large expenditure. Dr. Kocot argued, to no avail, that, without the proper educational facilities, the hospital was "a Cadillac with a flat tire."

Most people would have stopped there, but Dr. Kocot's "Polish obstinacy" kept him going. Figuring that the trustees would take him seriously if he backed up his ideas with money for the project, he began raising funds by soliciting contributions from the St. Vincent staff. Having served at St. Vincent beginning as an intern in 1957 and then as a cardiologist beginning in 1960, Dr. Kocot was well known and well liked, and he had a proven ability to get things done. Even though his practice would not have been affected by the closing of the maternity ward, he was a leader among the members of the medical staff who helped convince the Executive Committee to keep the ward open. Devoted to both his religion and his medical practice, Dr. Kocot had a long and loyal career at St. Vincent, serving as president of the medical staff in 1978 and 1979. If anyone could see the amphitheater project through to completion, it was Dr. Kocot.

The board found out just how serious Dr. Kocot was about the project when he showed up at a board meeting with $400,000 already pledged. Stunned that he was able to raise such a large sum of money, the board gave its approval for him to proceed.

Dr. Kocot calls his fund-raising project "one of the most satisfying things I've ever done. The entire hospital family became involved. It was a group effort. I was very, very proud of the support they had given us."

Pledges came from throughout the hospital. From part-time cafeteria workers on up, practically everyone contributed. The Guild of Our Lady of Providence, the Fallon Clinic, the University of Massachusetts Medical Center and the St. Vincent medical staff each made substantial contributions.

"The Guild was monumental in its response," Dr. Kocot said. "Betty Iandoli was president when I approached her. Before I knew it, they had pledged $100,000 (and eventually pledged a total of $167,000). That energized me for a long period. Then Dr. Meyers helped with Fallon Clinic. They gave $100,000."

To obtain a Determination of Need certificate, Dr. Kocot also had to convince the Central Massachusetts Health Systems Agency and the state Public Health Council that the project was worthwhile and necessary. Before receiving approval for a three-story addition to the former convent, hospital management had to show that the amphitheater and library could not be built within the main hospital building. The project was approved, but only under the condition that all funds be raised from private donations, and that the project be scaled back from a projected cost of $1.5 million to $1.2 million.

From in-house fund raising alone, Dr. Kocot eventually raised $642,000. Over several years, the entire sum eventually was raised through various foundations, canvassing of former patients and other efforts. A three-story addition to the former convent and the addition of the 256-seat amphitheater began in 1983, and the project was completed and dedicated in 1984. A satellite was installed in 1991 that gives the amphitheater the ability to pick up more than 150 channels, providing the ability for St. Vincent to participate in major medical conferences throughout the world. Video equipment is also hooked into the hospital, so medical students can observe medical procedures up close, from the surgeon's point of view.

The amphitheater project was an exception, though. Speaking at the 1982 annual meeting, Miss Smith made it clear that the efforts of St. Vincent Hospital would focus on financial restraint, not further building. She concluded that "instead of managing the growth of our institution, we must now manage for financial stability and sometimes for survival itself." This change in focus was common to hospitals throughout the country. While federal and state legislation sparked a period of tremendous expansion that lasted from the end of World War II through the 1960s, the 1970s began a period of cost containment and even more government regulation. Cost containment became an even greater issue in the 1980s. "The national mood has changed now from the 'health care is a right' of the 1970s," she said, "to the 'era of limits' of the 1980s."

Her concerns were shared by others. Dr. Friedell, medical director at the time, concluded, "It has become increasingly apparent that the state and federal governments are more interested in the cost than in the quality of care provided." Dr. Edward Mason, who became president of the medical staff in 1982, wrote in the annual report for the year that the physician's "therapeutic enthusiasm" was being constrained by the government and the third-party payor, and that "budgetary requirements compel hospital administrators to negotiate a veritable governmental obstacle course in an effort to provide its physicians with the newest and best equipment."

Bishop Flanagan added that St. Vincent "has a real and demonstrable human element not visible to those who attempt to put a dollar sign on our product, which is the life of the patient."

As a first step toward adjusting to the "era of limits," St. Vincent instituted a Quality Assessment Program in 1980. Its purpose, according to the bylaws of the Quality Assessment Committee, was "to develop an ongoing program of objective analysis of important aspects of patient care" and to discover "recognized deficiencies." The committee's leaders would then bring the deficiencies to the attention of the unit directors "for appropriate correction."

The next step was alluded to at the 1982 annual meeting when Raymond Cisneros, a health-care planner in the Boston office of Touche Ross & Co., addressed the need for increasing sources of hospital revenues. To respond to decreasing philanthropic donations and to cost-containment efforts, he recommended that the single corporation that ran St. Vincent Hospital be split into multiple corporations as a way to avoid some government regulation. St. Vincent Hospital followed his advice.

In 1983, St. Vincent Hospital became St. Vincent Healthcare System, Inc., a corporate parent for St. Vincent Hospital, Inc., St. Vincent Management Corp. and SVH Services, Inc. St. Vincent Management was established to provide management services under contract to St. Vincent, with the idea that it eventually would branch out to other health-care groups. SVH Services was established to provide a variety of services, such as data processing and laundry, both to hospitals and to other types of businesses. Unlike the nonprofit hospital and St. Vincent Management, SVH Services was established as a for-profit subsidiary.

The reason for the changes, according to Kevin J. Carroll, legal counsel for the hospital, was "to gain flexibility, maximize opportunities and realize cost savings, and regain some of the self-determination the hospital once had." In other words, because the management and services companies were split from the hospital, they did not have the same regulatory constraints as the hospital. The restructuring also provided important tax advantages.

In 1984, the first year after its massive reorganization, St. Vincent Healthcare System showed signs of recovering, netting a \$3.5 million profit, up from \$1.9 million in 1983. The hospital seemed to have adjusted to cost-containment formulas, and actually held its billing \$2 million below what the formula allowed the hospital to charge.

Under the reorganization, Miss Smith was named chief executive officer of St. Vincent Healthcare System, Inc. and president of St. Vincent Hospital, Inc., and Coggins was named executive director of the hospital.

Coggins' role steadily increased in importance at the hospital as increasing regulation focused attention on financial issues. A native of Rochester, New York, who earned his degree in business administration from Boston College, Coggins was an auditor for Blue Cross and Blue Shield of Massachusetts in 1966 when he wrote to Sister Agnes Marie and asked her if there was room for him on the staff of St. Vincent. A devout Catholic, he was attracted by the idea of working for a Catholic community hospital.

Familiar with the quality of his work, and seeing the value his experience could bring to the hospital, Sister Agnes Marie saw to it that he was hired as the assistant controller. Soon after, he was promoted to controller, and then to director of finance. In 1977, he was appointed associate director, a position second only to executive director. In 1981, Coggins was named chief operating officer, taking over responsibility for the day-to-day control of the hospital. While Coggins' open personality contrasted with that of Miss Smith, for the most part, they worked well together.

"He was scrupulously honest," according to Dr. Kocot. "He attended Mass daily. He was an individual who could be approached by anyone, and they would receive the truth." Roche added that, because of his government experience, Coggins "knew how to work the Medicare formulas."

He also was very decisive, according to Tom Cullinane, who worked for Coggins at the time. He describes Coggins as "a very black-and-white guy. There were no grays with him. You always knew where you stood with him." Cullinane also remembers Coggins for the pride he took in his athletic abilities. Using a St. Vincent softball game to play a trick on Coggins, "the guys in data processing painted a grapefruit to look like a softball. He creamed it and soaked himself."

Mrs. McKenna remembers Coggins most for his dedication to his family, recalling, "He didn't talk about sports. He talked about his kids." When Coggins' oldest son, Jimmy, died of a heart attack, "he was devastated," according to Mrs. McKenna. He died just a few months later, in October 1985, at the age of 58. Coggins served as executive director for just two years.

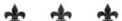

Another change at the time was the appointment of Bishop Timothy J. Harrington to replace Bishop Flanagan, who retired effective March 31, 1983. Bishop Harrington, who had served as the diocese's first auxiliary bishop for 15 years, already had been an active participant in efforts to keep St. Vincent's maternity ward open, and he was involved with St. Vincent's clinics for low-income people when he worked for the new Worcester bureau of Catholic Charities in the 1960s.

A graduate of Holy Cross College, Bishop Harrington was ordained in Springfield, Massachusetts, in 1946 and assigned as an assistant at St. Bernard's Church in Worcester. After the new Diocese of Worcester was formed in 1950, he assisted in establishing Catholic Charities in the new diocese. He obtained his master's degree in social work from Boston College in 1952, and the same year was named chaplain of the Nazareth Home for Boys in Leicester. By 1957, he became director of the House of Our Lady of the Way, a shelter for homeless men, and in 1960 he has named to head Catholic Charities.

Bishop Harrington always saw himself as a social worker. In fact, he earned the title "Bishop of the Bowery" in the days when he had to take off his clothes and shake out the cockroaches after visiting Worcester's poor. Given his background, his first contact with St. Vincent Hospital was surprising, at least to him. During the 1950s, he was called on by Bishop Wright to teach social psychology to St. Vincent's nursing students. He did not relish the idea of teaching, nor did he feel qualified to teach social psychology, given, as he said, that, "I never even heard the term before I was asked to teach it."

But the letter he received from Bishop Wright, which he can still recite precisely, was quite compelling. It said:

Dear Father Harrington:

Enclosed is a letter from Sister Mary Loreto, administrator of St. Vincent Hospital, and she asks you to take on the duty of teaching social psychology to pre-clinical students.

I hereby give you permission to take on this extra assignment.

I think you can and hope you will.

Bishop Harrington could have read just the last two words — "you will" — and known what the letter meant. He took the assignment.

When he was named auxiliary bishop in 1968, he was so surprised, he thought the letter announcing his appointment was sent to the wrong person. Since being named bishop, his role, like that of Bishop Flanagan, has been primarily to represent the interests of the diocese on the Board of Trustees.

From the building of the new St. Vincent Hospital in 1954 to the 1970s, few would dispute that St. Vincent Hospital was the leading health-care institution in Central Massachusetts, and was, in fact, one of the most progressive community hospitals in the country.

But the changing health-care environment in the 1970s and 1980s, particularly in Massachusetts, favored the growth of two other Worcester institutions — the University of Massachusetts Medical Center and the Fallon Clinic.

Miss Smith increasingly was concerned about the rapid growth of UMass and Fallon. Her response was to "build a moat around the hospital," according to one manager. Actions taken by UMass only added to her feelings. Some believe that in its early years, UMass failed to live up to its promises to St. Vincent and to the hospital consortium.

With its major teaching affiliation with UMass, St. Vincent saw a significant percentage of UMass students, but some hospital officials thought the affiliation should have been stronger. By the 1979–1980 academic year, about half of the 100 fourth-year medical students at UMass had one or more electives at St. Vincent and a third of the third-year students served month-long clerkships at St. Vincent. In addition, a third of the UMass pediatric residents and a fourth of the surgical and orthopedic residents were based at St. Vincent. But there was still a feeling that UMass was not sending as many interns as it might have to St. Vincent's. UMass by then was affiliated with Memorial Hospital, City Hospital and many other institutions throughout Massachusetts. St. Vincent was the city's largest hospital, but it wasn't being given any special treatment.

Even more important, the problem of overlapping services worsened. In 1982, St. Vincent announced plans to expand its radiation therapy program by purchasing a 12-million electron volt linear accelerator at a cost of $1.6 million. At nearly the same time, UMass publicly announced the $1.4 million radiation therapy program it had long been planning.

The biggest disagreement between the two hospitals, though, was over St. Vincent's plans to reestablish its open-heart surgery program. By 1979, St. Vincent was the first hospital in Central Massachusetts to offer angioplasty, a procedure to improve circulation in arteries narrowed by cholesterol deposits, through its cardiac catheterization laboratory. But St. Vincent's cardiac patient care was glaringly incomplete as long as the hospital lacked the ability to offer open-heart surgery.

Both UMass and St. Vincent wanted cardiac surgery to be the flagship of their respective institutions. Having a cardiac surgery program in-house enhanced a hospital's reputation. It was necessary for any hospital that wanted to be thought of as a major hospital. Cardiac surgery also served to draw business for other heart-related services. Patients would likely go to the same hospital for angioplasty, CAT scans and other services that they went to for open-heart surgery. In addition, cardiac surgery gave hospitals a reason to have the best and the latest equipment and laboratories. And after all, on top of all of these other reasons, it was St. Vincent, not UMass, that started the region's first cardiac surgery program. Some believed that Dr. Ware's groundbreaking work entitled St. Vincent to take the lead in cardiac surgery.

Without its own cardiac surgery program, St. Vincent had to refer patients to other hospitals, losing revenue at a time when the hospital was barely operating in the black. In 1978, St. Vincent referred 150 open-heart surgery cases to other hospitals. By 1981, the figure rose to 230. In the meantime, the UMass cardiac program had become enormously successful. UMass introduced its program in 1976, and by the early 1980s UMass was performing 700 procedures a year.

St. Vincent first began planning to reestablish its open-heart surgery program in 1978, but held off because of a "gentlemen's agreement" with UMass, according to Dr. Alan C. Brewster, St. Vincent's new medical director at the time. At a determination-of-need hearing before the state Public Health Council in 1982, Dr. Brewster charged that UMass had reneged on the agreement. Dr. Brewster said an agreement was reached when UMass first opened, stipulating that St. Vincent would wait to reestablish its program until the new Medical Center's cardiac surgery program was firmly established. In return, after a few years, UMass would share the market with St. Vincent. The agreement unraveled in 1982, when UMass officials stipulated that all cardiac surgery at St. Vincent be performed by UMass surgeons.

Miss Smith maintained that St. Vincent was willing to cooperate with UMass, but that, "after a while, you don't hold hands when you're boxing, and that seems to be the point we're at." She said that surgeons at Massachusetts General Hospital had agreed to assist St. Vincent in reestablishing its open-heart surgery program, just as they had assisted UMass, but that UMass pressured them to not become affiliated with St. Vincent.

Dr. Robert E. Tranquada, chancellor and dean of the UMass Medical Center at the time, responded that UMass faculty had told the Massachusetts General surgeons that it was "not consistent" for St. Vincent to seek assistance from them "to do something in Worcester that we have indicated our faculty is interested in doing, particularly when St. Vincent is a fully affiliated hospital of UMass. This can in no way be construed as blocking St. Vincent from having its own cardiac surgery program."

There were other factors behind the disagreement. Miss Smith charged that UMass did not want St. Vincent to start its own program because St. Vincent's cardiac surgeons would be better compensated than its own surgeons. Even though St. Vincent planned to charge a maximum of $11,800 for each operation, she argued at the time that the St. Vincent surgeons would be better compensated than the UMass surgeons, because, instead of being paid on a fee-for-service basis, the UMass surgeons were part of a faculty group practice and were paid a negotiated salary.

Another issue was the unwillingness of St. Vincent doctors to refer their open-heart surgery patients to UMass. Some doctors were afraid that if they referred patients to UMass for open-heart surgery, their patients would go to UMass for all of their medical needs.

With the UMass program expanding to capacity, directors of the Central Massachusetts Health Systems Agency agreed in November 1982 to allow St. Vincent to reopen its open-heart surgery program, despite a recommendation by the agency's staff that approval be denied. Approval was granted under the condition that St. Vincent perform no more than 260 operations during its first year and that the cost per operation not exceed $11,800 for each patient, barring complications. A determination-of-need certificate was granted by the state Public Health Council in 1984, and St. Vincent's open-heart surgery program was reestablished in 1986.

In November 1985, just after Miss Smith's retirement, Dr. Kocot announced St. Vincent's affiliation with the

Massachusetts General cardiology department. Under the agreement, Massachusetts General surgeons practiced at St. Vincent and offered educational conferences, grand rounds and opportunities for St. Vincent staff to observe at the Boston hospital.

Under the leadership of Massachusetts General's Dr. Willard M. Daggett, the program grew, and in April 1986, Dr. Jeremy N. Ruskin of Massachusetts General was appointed director of the new clinical cardiac arrhythmia and electrophysiology service at St. Vincent. Dr. Ruskin was a pioneer in electrophysiology and the use of implantable cardioverter defibrillators to treat irregular heartbeats. A defibrillator stimulates the heart with electricity through electrode catheters placed in the heart. A cardioverter defibrillator is implanted under the patient's skin and delivers a shock to normalize the heartbeat when it senses an abnormality.

Even before the St. Vincent program began, Dr. Daggett had built a strong relationship with St. Vincent and its cardiology staff. Many of the referrals from St. Vincent went to Dr. Daggett, so "it was a natural for him, by virtue of this long-standing association, to help the St. Vincent program to succeed," according to Dr. Kocot.

While the reintroduction of the cardiac surgery program would help expand its patient base, St. Vincent's continuing financial health was more highly dependent on the number of its referring physicians. St. Vincent's response to the increasingly competitive health-care environment was to appeal to the area's independent primary care physicians.

The Grafton Family Health Care Center became the home base for Primary Care Physicians, P.C. with Dr. William T. O'Connor as president. Soon, other offices opened in Holden, Sturbridge and downtown Worcester. While Primary Care Physicians remained tiny compared with Fallon Clinic, it was able to grow throughout the 1980s and to have 23 physicians at 14 locations throughout Worcester County.

At the same time, St. Vincent continued to build relations with other independent physicians by allowing the establishment and then the expansion of the Vernon Medical Center at 10 Winthrop Street. The center was built on two-and-a-half acres of land adjacent to what had been Providence House. The land was sold by St. Vincent Hospital to Medical Associates, a group of doctors who often referred patients to St. Vincent Hospital. The $1.5 million professional building, which included offices for 30 doctors, opened in 1975 and later expanded.

St. Vincent continued to appeal to the area's independent physicians by forming the St. Vincent Physician Alliance in 1988. The alliance banded the various physicians affiliated with St. Vincent into an independent practice association that could contract as a unit with new health plans entering the market. The alliance, which quickly contracted with the Tufts Associated Health Plan, was established to bring a wider choice of health care plans to the area while providing a unified health-care system.

While St. Vincent Hospital was experiencing an "era of limits," no such limits were placed on the growth of Fallon Clinic. In the early 1970s, Fallon Clinic was merely a successful group practice. Its nearly two dozen doctors were important to St. Vincent Hospital, but still accounted for a fairly small part of the hospital's business. But by the mid-1980s, its subsidiary, Fallon Community Health Plan, was one of the most successful HMOs in the country. It had become, according to Dr. Kocot, "the driving force behind St. Vincent's census. Every time Fallon added a doctor, it became more powerful."

The relationship between St. Vincent and Fallon historically was symbiotic, though for most of its history, St. Vincent was the more powerful of the two entities. Fallon was dominated by Catholic doctors, and, through much of its history, the doctors would have found it difficult to practice in non-Catholic hospitals, which sometimes still harbored prejudices against Catholic doctors. St. Vincent brought Fallon an accessible hospital and, through its teaching program, a steady flow of new doctors, while Fallon brought St. Vincent a significant percentage of its business.

Fallon's tremendous growth caught the St. Vincent administration by surprise and upset the balance between Fallon Clinic and the hospital. As Fallon grew, it was seen as a threat by some. Many of the area's independent doctors who were affiliated with St. Vincent were afraid of being overpowered by Fallon.

As the Fallon plan grew, Miss Smith felt threatened not only because the increasing size of the Fallon plan made St. Vincent Hospital ever more dependent on Fallon, but because the concept of managed care as practiced by Fallon created disincentives for hospitalizing patients at a time when St. Vincent needed more patients. Fallon also had developed its own diagnostic facilities, cutting into an important source of revenues for the hospital.

By 1985, Fallon Community Health Plan had 60,000 members. Its membership was growing faster than Fallon could handle at its current sites. In 1984, Fallon added a site in Paxton, and in 1986, two additional sites opened in Worcester and one opened in Leominster. The Worcester and Leominster sites were renovated at a cost of about $1.5 million each. The Leominster site was located at the former Branch Motor Express trucking terminal on Mill Street. Worcester sites included a converted Big D grocery store at 95 Lincoln Street and a two-story Medical Center at Fairlawn Hospital.

As Worcester's smallest hospital, 94-bed Fairlawn Hospital was able to adapt to the changing health-care environment of the early 1980s by developing a niche as a same-day surgery center. Fairlawn Hospital created a strong relationship with Fallon with construction of the two-story Medical Center called Fallon Medical Center West. Robert S. Schedin, president of Fairlawn, called it "a new step in our continuing collaboration with Fallon," and said it would lead to "a more important integration of Fairlawn Hospital into their HMO."

That integration came in 1986, when Fairlawn rejected overtures from Memorial, and instead chose to convert to an acute, inpatient rehabilitation hospital affiliated with Northeast Medical Alliance, which was itself an affiliation formed between UMass and Fallon. In 1988 and 1989, Fallon continued its consistent growth, expanding its branches in Auburn, Leominster and Westboro, constructing a new Medical Center in Milford and opening a newly renovated $3 million specialty care center on Gold Star Boulevard in Worcester. By the end of 1988, Fallon had 140 physicians at seven clinics throughout the county and 94,000 subscribers in its HMO.

Squeezed between the growth of Fallon and UMass, Miss Smith's isolationist strategy proved to be her undoing. Recognizing, at last, that even St. Vincent could not survive a battle with Worcester's two fastest growing health-care institutions, she retired in November 1985, just a month after Coggins' death. After Coggins' death, Miss Smith knew it was time to leave, according to Mrs. McKenna. "She came in and cleared out her office, and said, 'Everyone's time comes.' "

Msgr. Edmond T. Tinsley, who ran the local Catholic Charities office, was appointed to replace Miss Smith temporarily as chief executive officer of St. Vincent Healthcare System and president of St. Vincent, while Dr. Kocot was named to serve as temporary executive director of the hospital.

Fixing Things

"It's fair to say that over the past 20 to 25 years, hospitals have traditionally offered services based upon what the hospital wanted to offer. Today we're seeing hospitals paying more attention than ever before to what consumers expect as far as programs, services and up-to-date facilities."
                                        Richard A. Pozniak,
                                    Director of Public Relations
                                Massachusetts Hospital Association

$\mathcal{D}$r. Kocot describes his tenure running St. Vincent Hospital with Msgr. Tinsley as "short in terms of time, but long in terms of what had to be done."

With Coggins' death, Miss Smith's resignation and the financial pressures that had faced the hospital during the preceding years, "the institution was in emotional chaos," according to Dr. Kocot. "Many people were terror stricken, because they thought we might clean house. We decided there and then that our biggest challenge was to regain the emotional peace."

Dr. Kocot and Msgr. Tinsley agreed to make no major changes. Even Miss Smith's closest associates kept their positions. Dr. Kocot met with St. Vincent staff and reinstituted Mother Loreto's open-door policy.

A search committee was established almost immediately and in January 1986 chose William D. Harkins, president of St. Mary's Medical Center in Evansville, Indiana, to take over as chief executive officer of St. Vincent Healthcare System and president of St. Vincent Hospital, beginning his new job in

March of that year. Harkins had been the first lay administrator of St. Mary's, which is operated by the Daughters of Charity. His experience in helping a hospital make the transition from operation by a religious community to operation by a lay staff, while maintaining a Catholic philosophy of medical practice, was seen as a beneficial experience to bring to St. Vincent.

Bringing in an outsider who was not part of the politically tumultuous decade that preceded his appointment also proved helpful. According to Dr. Kocot, "Bill Harkins could see things objectively."

Harkins' experience overseeing a $38.7 million expansion of St. Mary's also was important. St. Vincent was built in the 1950s based on architectural plans prepared before World War II, and hospital trustees recognized that St. Vincent required a significant upgrading in the not-too-distant future.

Harkins had other hospital management experience, too. Serving in the U.S. Army, he managed hospitals in Vietnam and in Fort Riley, Kansas. He served as the assistant administrator of Manchester Memorial Hospital in Manchester, Connecticut; as administrator at Connecticut Family Health Care Center in Bridgeport, Connecticut; and as associate administrator at St. Mary's Hospital in Waterbury, Connecticut.

Harkins described his management philosophy by stressing that "good leadership is a reflection of participation by all key elements of an organization," and he sought participation from his board, doctors and administrators. Harkins was fond of saying, "I hire people who like to fix things." True to form, he brought in a whole team of turnaround specialists to help bring St. Vincent back to its formerly exemplary financial condition.

Harkins acted quickly, updating many of the hospital's services and making St. Vincent Hospital a more visible part of the community. Discussing the low profile the hospital took in the community in the years preceding his appointment, Harkins said, "I intend to change that in rapid fashion. I expect . . . that key management personnel will assume a more active role in the community."

For Harkins, increased visibility meant not only a greater involvement in the affairs of the City of Worcester, but greater visibility within the health-care community. One of Harkins' first steps was to patch up relationships with UMass and Fallon Clinic.

In January 1987, Harkins reviewed the progress being made at St. Vincent Hospital in *The Evening Gazette* and discussed the hospital's improved relationship with UMass, writing, "Rather than directly competing with the University of Massachusetts, we perceive the medical school as a partner for positive change and development in health care for Central Massachusetts. As a major teaching affiliate of the university, we have benefited by the influx of medical students, residents and physicians. The university has benefited in turn, from the expertise of our staff in the area of clinical medicine, and the large patient base."

The partnership Harkins discussed manifested itself in 1988 when St. Vincent and UMass announced the affiliation of their cardiac surgery program. Dr. Thomas Vander Salm, chairman of cardiothoracic surgery at UMass, was named to direct cardiothoracic surgery at St. Vincent and Dr. Thomas Pezzella, associate director of the program at St. Vincent, assumed administrative, clinical and teaching responsibilities for the program.

The cardiac surgery affiliation was one of many joint business relationships St. Vincent formed at the time.

Affiliations between various hospitals for specialized services, such as cardiac surgery, have been common since before St. Vincent Hospital existed. The affiliations between hospitals, and the tendency for doctors to affiliate with more than one hospital, weakens the boundaries between competing hospitals.

Working together, sometimes competing hospitals can both benefit. During medical emergencies, such as the polio epidemic and the aftermath of the tornado that struck Worcester during the 1950s, Worcester's hospitals have put aside their competitiveness when necessary. As the 1980s approached, hospitals increasingly realized the need to cooperate for mutual economic benefit. Despite Miss Smith's fear of being overpowered by UMass and Fallon, St. Vincent management recognized the benefit of cooperating with other health-care institutions on many fronts.

In 1979, St. Vincent formed an association with the much smaller Fairlawn Hospital to share medical and administrative services, and equipment. The alliance was formed with the idea of a possible future merger. In the years that followed, the two hospitals shared computer and laundry services, biomedical engineering services and joint medical staff privileges.

The merger was never realized and Fairlawn converted to a rehabilitation hospital. However, Fairlawn continued its same-day surgery program as a source of cash flow, leasing it to St. Vincent Hospital beginning in 1987. In 1988, St. Vincent formed a new Division of General Ambulatory Medicine and integrated same-day surgery into the ambulatory care program. Same-day surgery was moved from Fairlawn to a newly renovated wing of St. Vincent. By 1989, it was the largest same-day surgery service in Central Massachusetts, serving 5,000 patients a year with five operating rooms, a preoperating section, adult and pediatric recovery suites, and a modern nursing station.

In another joint agreement, St. Vincent, City and Memorial joined with 23 medical clinics in 1985 to form the Elder Health Consortium, which was designed to bring health-care services to housing projects for the elderly.

The same year, the state approved a nonprofit consortium between St. Vincent, UMass, Memorial and Hahnemann for the construction and operation of a $3 million magnetic resonance imaging (MRI) center. When it opened in 1987, the Central Massachusetts Magnetic Imaging Center (CMMIC) received national media attention, including a *CBS Evening News* feature by Dan Rather, for the diagnosis of a blood clot in the brain of its first patient — a bald eagle. Since then, CMMIC has treated thousands of patients, including many professional athletes and a second bald eagle. Initially, the center had the ability to visualize a patient's soft-tissue areas, such as the central nervous system, by placing the patient in a magnetic field and bouncing radio signals off of him. More recently, the center has developed the ability to image blood vessels and can provide a noninvasive angiograph.

In 1986, St. Vincent Hospital joined the Health Front Alliance, a regional organization that is part of Voluntary Hospitals of America. The hospitals in HFA can take advantage of national programs for capital formation, joint purchasing, health insurance and other programs that provided economies of scale.

Unique among Worcester's hospitals, St. Vincent also developed ownership and affiliation agreements with a network of home-health-care agencies — Certified Nursing Services, District Nursing of Millbury and Pernet Family Health — to provide on-site coordination of continuing care of patients at home. St. Vincent also developed an agreement with the city's Commission on Elder Affairs to manage 15 outreach clinics throughout the city to provide nursing care, nutrition counseling, and other medical and social services to people who are elderly or disabled.

In 1988, through a joint venture with Burbank Hospital in Fitchburg, St. Vincent converted its clinical laboratory into an independent commercial laboratory called CliniTech Services, Inc. and moved it off site to a highly automated facility at 100 Barber Avenue in Worcester. The consolidated laboratory markets its services to hospitals, physicians, insurance companies and other health-care organizations.

These various relationships established by St. Vincent were a sign of the times. Because regulatory pressures had created financial difficulties for the hospital industry, hospitals increasingly were looking for new sources of income and opportunities that would help them operate more efficiently. Joint agreements, such as those that St. Vincent participated in, often helped.

✤ ✤ ✤

Increasing the various business agreements between St. Vincent and other health-care institutions was just one step taken by Harkins to transform St. Vincent Hospital. Soon after his appointment, Harkins and his board developed a strategic plan and instituted surveys not only of patients, but of the community, to determine the public perception of St. Vincent Hospital.

"Bill wanted to be a change agent," according to Nespoli. "He quickly organized the first strategic planning process the hospital had for many years. He developed about 20 planning teams to assess the strengths and weaknesses of the hospital. What came out of the process were several areas of emphasis. One area was vertical integration — providing health care at all levels. Another conclusion was that managed care would be the future of health care. We also concluded that we needed to create a partnership between St. Vincent, the Fallon medical staff and the non-Fallon medical staff."

The strategic plan also pinpointed medical areas for St. Vincent to concentrate on, based on its expertise and on market needs. St. Vincent announced plans in 1987 to expand seven designated "centers of excellence," concentrating resources on programs for treatment of cancer, treatment of the elderly, psychiatry, maternal and child care, orthopedics, neuroscience and cardiovascular care.

Another conclusion of the strategic plan was to recognize the upgrading of St. Vincent's physical plant as a high priority. While the hospital had been updated with various additions in the 1960s and 1970s, its core was still a building that was designed nearly 50 years earlier. Bishop Harrington commissioned a strategic planning committee chaired by his close friend Richard Flynn, a retired executive of Norton Company, a Fortune 500 abrasives company based in Worcester. After 18 months of work, the committee filed a Determination of Need application for the hospital with the Central Massachusetts Health Systems Agency in September 1987.

The project, which had a projected cost of $35 million, would not add to the hospital's 578 beds. In fact, the renovation was designed to take 140 beds out of St. Vincent Hospital. Nearly half of the money was earmarked for a triangular extension that was designed to jut out between the hospital's two wings. The extension was to feature a new admitting area on the ground floor, eight new operating rooms on the second floor, and 16 critical-care beds on the top floor. The proposal also included funds to modernize the intensive care unit, the emergency room, the cancer center, rehabilitation therapy, and surgical and critical-care support areas.

With the completion of the strategic plan and the filing of the Determination of Need application, Nespoli said, "We finally had a direction; a sense of where we wanted to go."

While St. Vincent's management had a "direction," the direction changed pretty quickly. Through its strategic planning process, and through discussions with Fallon Clinic about a potential joint venture, St. Vincent management began to explore the possibility of an integrated medical campus.

Nespoli wanted to find out what kinds of health-care facilities were being developed in other parts of the country, so he contacted Dr. Ken Quickel, president of the Joslin Clinic and a former executive vice president of the Geisinger Health Care Center, a practice inspired by the Mayo Clinic. Nespoli began his career at Geisinger after graduating from the University of Michigan in 1976. Dr. Quickel referred him to a small developer in Dallas called Medical City.

A group of St. Vincent managers met with Bob Wright, a principal of Medical City, who explained the concept behind Medical City. Nespoli liked what he saw. The Dallas Medical City was designed with an atrium at the center of the campus. The atrium was the center of activity, and the building was designed to be colorful and welcoming, unlike the traditional hospital. Nespoli was struck by the efficiency of the building, which was designed so that all services were easily accessible.

He also recognized that it would be difficult to pursue the Medical City concept in St. Vincent's existing facility.

While pushing the Medical City concept forward, St. Vincent Hospital's management recognized that building a new facility would require a great deal of financial support from the community.

As a community hospital, St. Vincent had always depended on the financial support of the community to survive and to grow. From the first fund raiser by the Washington Social Club to the modern-day efforts by the Guild of Our Lady of Providence, St. Vincent Hospital flourished because of organized efforts to raise funds. In 1986, St. Vincent professionalized its fund-raising efforts, establishing its Careholder Program, a special club that recognizes its members for their regular philanthropic contributions. St. Vincent also consolidated its fund-raising efforts by creating the Saint Vincent Development Foundation, which evolved from the St. Vincent Research Foundation, to address long-term needs for community support.

At the same time, the Guild of Our Lady of Providence continued to play an important fund-raising role at the hospital. In recent years, it has provided funding for major upgrading of maternity care, cancer treatment and critical care. The guild's financial support made it possible to open two new rooms for LDRP maternity care, providing labor, delivery, recovery and post-partum care all in one room. In 1988, guild funding made it possible for St. Vincent to modernize its inpatient cancer unit. The following year, the guild's contribution paid for several noninvasive, peripheral monitors in the Critical Care Department. The monitors, which measure heart rates, blood pressure, and oxygen and carbon dioxide levels in the blood, have improved patient comfort and safety while allowing the nursing staff to work more efficiently.

✤ ✤ ✤

Another change that came early during Harkins' administration was the closing of St. Vincent's School of Nursing in 1987.

As nursing has become more sophisticated, hospital-based nursing programs have generally been abandoned. Today's nursing students spend an increasing amount of time in the classroom and less time at the patient's bedside. Where in earlier days, the St. Vincent nursing student began her first day on the job working with patients, by the 1980s, the typical nursing student completed an academic education before regularly spending time treating patients. In the early 1980s, hospital-based nursing schools were closing with great frequency. Memorial's program, for example, closed in 1980.

St. Vincent Hospital reacted in two ways. First, the hospital changed the focus of its nursing program, adopting a primary nursing philosophy in 1986. Primary nursing focuses on patients instead of tasks, with the goal of making nursing care more personal. Nurses began following a case-management approach, spending their time on bedside care, discharge planning and patient education, instead of on housekeeping duties. A new program called "guest services" was added in 1989 to provide an opportunity for routine personal-care services to be performed by non-nursing staff, freeing up nurses for more specialized medical care duties.

Second, St. Vincent announced plans to discontinue its nursing school because of falling enrollment. Leominster Hospital closed its nursing school the same year, leaving City Hospital and Hahnemann as the only remaining Worcester hospitals with undergraduate nursing schools. Soon after, the City Hospital and Hahnemann programs closed as well.

"People thought I wouldn't support the closing, because I was a graduate of the school," Dr. Mancini said. "Philosophically, I couldn't support keeping the school open. It was inadequate. It was wrong, even if it was ours."

While today's nurse needs to spend much more time in the classroom, Dr. Mancini said a clinical component is still necessary. She is an advocate of internships for nursing students. A nine-month program has been developed for operating room nurses, and a similar program is expected to be developed for critical-care nurses.

Ironically, the nursing school closings came at a time when there was a severe shortage of nurses. From the early days of medical care, nursing was one of the few careers open to women, but, during the 1970s and 1980s, other career options became available and fewer women chose to become nurses.

At the time, St. Vincent Executive Vice President John F. Tighe, a nurse himself, said about 10 percent of openings for nurses were going unfilled. He attributed the shortage to the poor image many people had of nursing, the limited opportunities for professional and financial growth, and the lack of professional autonomy for nurses.

"True professional autonomy means that nurses must have decision making authority at all levels of administration," he wrote in *Hospital News*. "We must restructure the nursing practice system away from staffing 'floors' to staffing 'patients,' a theory we call 'case management.' This allows us to more appropriately use staff for patient care rather than the household duties of managing a unit."

He argued that nurses must have a greater say in the overall management of the patient, as well as budgeting, and control of expenses.

UMass reacted to the nursing shortage in another way. To attract and retain a quality nursing staff, UMass increased the level of pay for its nurses, which, according to Bill George, "created a bidding war for the high-end positions."

St. Vincent also re-entered the nursing home business when, in 1990, it became the owner of three nursing homes. During the 1970s and 1980s, nursing homes were affected by regulatory changes at least as much as the hospitals were, and attempting to comply with the ever-changing regulations drove some nursing home managers out of the business.

"Other than the nuclear power industry, long-term care is the most regulated industry in the country," according to Tom Cullinane, vice president, extended care, who adds that regulation grew because of the prevalence of fraud in the industry.

"For nursing homes, the regulatory environment changes with the wind," according to George. "You can't plan what you're going to get paid. Medicaid has a budget crisis, and they change the reimbursement regulations retrospectively."

The volatility of the industry made it difficult for the Greendale People's Church to continue operating Providence House. In the early 1980s, the Diocese of Worcester took over operation of Providence House, which is now known as Providence Extended Care, and expanded its operation with the purchase of the Smith Nursing Home in Millbury and Liberty House in Southbridge, renaming the two homes Providence House of Millbury and Providence House of Southbridge.

In 1989, the diocese turned over control of the nursing homes, which have a total of 528 beds, to St. Vincent Hospital. The transfer made St. Vincent Hospital the largest operator of nursing homes in Central Massachusetts. St. Vincent has since begun to refocus the operation of the nursing homes to reflect the regulatory environment of the 1990s, George said. Providence Extended Care, for example, has been the first nursing care center in the area to emphasize Level 1 nursing care, also known as subacute care. Level 1 care provides interim treatment for patients who are well enough to leave the hospital, but who are not yet well enough to go home. Level 1 care was developed to lower health-care costs while providing the appropriate level of care, since nursing home care costs less than hospital care. According to Cullinane, Level 1 care resembles the type of care ITT-Sheraton had in mind when it opened its convatel next to St. Vincent.

By operating its own system of nursing homes, St. Vincent Hospital has an opportunity to provide care to its elderly patients on an ongoing basis.

Despite the numerous internal and external changes affecting St. Vincent, the hospital generated a surplus every year during the 1980s except 1985, when the cost of re-establishing the open-heart surgery program left the hospital with a small loss.

The financial state of the health-care industry at the end of the 1980s is summarized in the St. Vincent annual report for 1990: "Imagine a business in which three out of four stores are losing money. Each customer has different needs and is charged a different price. One out of ten customers is broke, but demands full service. Your largest payor tells you how much money you can earn, but someone else orders the supplies. He also tells you what services you must provide, but won't pay for many of them, and then may dispute a bill he paid five years ago. Other businesses blame you for charging too much and being inefficient. Such a business does exist. It's called health care."

From a Hospital to a City

"We have changed our environment more quickly than we know how to change ourselves."
Walter Lippmann

$\mathscr{T}$he affiliations, joint ventures and strategic alliances so common in the early 1980s evolved by the end of the decade to the logical next stage. Hospitals throughout the Commonwealth began to merge. Worcester Hahnemann Hospital, Worcester Memorial Hospital and Holden District Hospital merged to become the Medical Center of Central Massachusetts. The University of Massachusetts Medical Center acquired the financially ailing City Hospital. Fairlawn Hospital was purchased by a consortium that includes UMass, Fallon Clinic and the New England Rehabilitation Hospital of Woburn, now called Advantage Care.

The financial pressures applied by new regulations continued unabated in the late 1980s, especially in Massachusetts, where regulations left the health-care industry so battle scarred, the state became widely known as "the Beirut of medicine." With Medicare payments being squeezed because of the federal budget deficit, insurance companies keeping tight control over reimbursements, and the costs of technology and salaries sending many budgets out of control, many of the area hospitals that served small communities were no longer able to overcome the financial obstacles of running a hospital alone and were looking to become acquired by larger, more stable hospitals.

With regulations favoring hospitals that were controlling costs, St. Vincent and Fallon began to explore the idea of establishing a regional health-care center. In April 1989, St. Vincent announced plans to discuss an affiliation with the 164-bed Marlboro Hospital. Under the agreement, Marlboro was to continue as a locally managed institution offering a full range of acute-care services, but was to refer patients to St. Vincent if they could not be cared for at Marlboro Hospital. Meanwhile, St. Vincent was to help fill the shortage of physicians at Marlboro Hospital. The two hospitals also talked about reopening Marlboro's maternity ward, which had been closed since 1976.

By June, St. Vincent was discussing a similar affiliation with Mary Lane Hospital in Ware. Soon after, financially troubled Clinton Hospital was added to the discussions. In each case, discussions broke off because of differences in strategic objectives. Increasingly, St. Vincent was being drawn in a different direction.

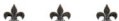

In the meantime, St. Vincent began to rethink its plans for updating its aging facility on Vernon Hill. Although St. Vincent already had received a Determination-of-Need certificate allowing the hospital to spend up to $33.3 million for renovations, through its collaborative planning with Fallon, St. Vincent determined that more ambitious plans were in order.

In August 1989, St. Vincent Healthcare System proposed a $100 million "medical mall" that was supposed to be jointly developed with Fallon at Routes 290 and 140 in Shrewsbury near the Boylston town line. The site was chosen after reviewing 30 different potential locations. The medical mall was to be built, Alan Stoll said at the time, "in cooperation" with Fallon Clinic, though Fallon's role remained ambiguous. The plan called for construction of a 266-bed hospital, a medical office building for Fallon doctors, an office building for non-Fallon doctors, and an atrium for centralized access to services such as admitting, billing and a pharmacy.

Plans called for the new hospital to be used primarily for surgery, with an emphasis on cardiac services, but it also was intended to serve as a stand-alone, full-service primary care facility, offering obstetrics, pediatrics and critical-care services. Under the plan, the Vernon Hill campus was to be extensively remodeled as a separate full-service hospital with 281 beds and special services for cancer treatment, orthopedics, neuroscience, psychiatry and elder care. The new site was planned to be modeled after the Medical City Dallas complex, Harkins announced, and the hospital's previously announced renovation plans were to be shelved.

Calling the plans for construction in Shrewsbury central to St. Vincent's vision for the future, Harkins said in 1989, "This facility will embody the hospital's philosophy of pluralistic medicine, regional networking, cooperation with the Fallon Clinic, and convenience to the physician and patient. By structurally integrating physician offices, the Fallon Clinic and outpatient services, Saint Vincent will create a synergistic entity that will attract new physicians and patients to its health-care system . . . Saint Vincent's vision is ambitious. It is also necessary. It is a logical and realistic response to the community's complex, rapidly changing health-care needs."

At the same time St. Vincent and Fallon announced plans for the medical mall, The Medical Center of Central Massachusetts announced a $125 million expansion project and UMass announced a $179 million expansion project, which later was scaled back to a $123 million project.

The same year the medical mall was announced, Fallon Clinic announced a merger with Primary Care Physicians (PCP).

As Fallon grew, referrals by its physicians accounted for an ever-increasing percentage of St. Vincent's business. Initially, PCP was expected to balance St. Vincent's relationship with Fallon by providing another source of referrals.

PCP also was growing, though not as quickly as Fallon. By 1989, PCP had 23 doctors in 14 locations. In comparison, Fallon had 140 doctors in seven locations and 94,000 subscribers throughout Central Massachusetts. As it grew, PCP, which was becoming an increasingly important source of business to St. Vincent, required more capital to function in the new managed care, competitive environment.

PCP first approached St. Vincent as a potential funding source but the hospital rejected the idea. According to Dr. O'Connor, "PCP needed to achieve a critical size to become large enough to negotiate with new managed care products. When it became obvious that the hospital would not be able to financially support our growth, we turned to Fallon with whom we had already established a good relationship as a non-Fallon Clinic provider to its health plan."

PCP's size made it attractive to Fallon, which needed a new source of primary care physicians to continue to fuel its growth. PCP was especially attractive, because it had located in many of the small towns where Fallon had not yet established a presence.

"It was an opportunity for Fallon Clinic to gain 20 to 24 primary care physicians and solidify its strategic position in the smaller sites, like Sterling, Spencer, Leicester and Whitinsville," according to Dr. FitzGerald, who was a member of Fallon's PCP Negotiation Committee, as well as serving as vice president of hospital affairs.

After the purchase, Dr. Podbielski, president of Fallon Clinic, said, "Primary Care Physicians will enable us to deliver care more conveniently at more locations. It's convenient to the subscribers."

But the purchase also made Fallon the source of a majority of St. Vincent's patients. After the purchase, 55 to 60 percent of St. Vincent's patients were being directed to St. Vincent by Fallon doctors.

After Fallon merged with PCP, St. Vincent Hospital and Fallon depended on each other more than ever. If Fallon's ever-growing base of doctors sent patients elsewhere, it would be a great loss for St. Vincent. Likewise, St. Vincent provided an important base for Fallon's doctors.

Individually, the two institutions were leaders in the health-care industry. But, as their relationship progressed, management of both institutions recognized that St. Vincent Hospital and Fallon could do even more together than they could apart. Because they could provide all aspects of health care, from pre-natal care to elder care, from the routine patient check-up to open-heart surgery, from nursing home care to sports medicine, they reasoned that they could provide better, more efficient patient care by working together. Together, they realized, the two organizations could provide a complete, integrated, seam-less health-care delivery system.

They were finally brought together during the planning of their integrated medical campus in Shrewsbury. The boards of Fallon and St. Vincent disagreed over how much control each party would have over the project. Fallon insisted on 51 percent control of the project, according to Nespoli.

"As the pressure escalated, St. Vincent's board said, 'If you want that kind of input, it is appropriate that you have the responsibility for running the hospital,' " Dr. FitzGerald said.

In February 1990, the two nonprofits, St. Vincent Health-care System and Fallon Community Health Plan, announced plans to merge. The Fallon Foundation, Inc., a charitable trust, was then reorganized as the parent company with Dr. Podbielski, president of Fallon Clinic, becoming president of the foundation.

"By merging, we now have all of the components of a health delivery system under one umbrella," George said. "We have the area's largest group practice, a hospital and an insurance plan. It puts us in a position of controlling our business thoroughly. It's true managed care."

The merger also signaled a trend toward a more doctor-oriented approach to the management of the hospital, with the idea that by better responding to doctors, who are closer to the patients and understand their needs better than administrators, St. Vincent can improve the quality of health care.

"Saint Vincent believes that increased cooperation between the hospital and physicians is critical to its abilities to function effectively," according to the 1989 St. Vincent annual report, which discusses the merger. "Toward this end, physicians share in the governance and administration of the hospital, helping to define its direction and manage its scarce resources. The merger incorporates an inclusive, rather than exclusive, arrangement with an open medical staff comprised of Fallon physicians, and physicians in other groups and solo practice.

"To ensure that this integrative task is accomplished, the hospital will continue to work with solo practitioners, Fallon clinicians, and full-time faculty, our affiliated hospitals and their respective staffs."

According to Dr. FitzGerald, the merger was in the best interest of both St. Vincent and Fallon. "The interests of The Fallon became totally aligned with the interests of the hospital," he said. "We became like two people on the same side of the table. With that stability St. Vincent and Fallon could look forward to the future together with even greater confidence and assurance."

During the same month that Fallon and St. Vincent merged, Mary Lane Hospital merged with Bay State Health Systems of Springfield. Leominster Hospital and Burbank Hospital in Fitchburg also announced a merger. Clinton Hospital's financial condition continued to worsen, and eventually the hospital filed for Chapter 11 bankruptcy protection.

During merger negotiations, St. Vincent and Fallon recognized the importance of continuing St. Vincent Hospital's century-old tradition of operating as a Catholic institution. A covenant was signed as part of the merger to ensure that the hospital will continue to follow the ethical direction of the Catholic Church. The Bishop, his designee, and the president of the Sisters of Providence of Holyoke or her designee continue to sit on the board. A chapel continues to offer services, and a pastoral care department counsels and consoles patients and their families.

The Diocese of Worcester sought the services of a Catholic canon lawyer and Catholic moral theologian during negotiations to ensure that St. Vincent Hospital continued to meet the requirements of Catholicity after the merger. The hospital continues to be guided by *Ethical and Religious Directives For Catholic Health Facilities,* published by the National Conference of Catholic Bishops.

Former Bishop Flanagan sees the hospital succeeding in continuing its Catholic mission.

"Many people in the community were concerned about whether the hospital would continue to be committed to the same goals and ideals as it had been under its former constitution," Bishop Flanagan said. "From my perspective, it seems to be unchanged. As long as the people in charge are committed to the principles and goals of a Catholic hospital, the future is in good hands.

"A Catholic hospital is one that's committed to the teachings of the Catholic Church with respect to the dignity and sacredness of life," he said, "and that mission can be carried out not just by a religious staff, but by a lay staff."

Addressing the issue in *The Catholic Free Press,* Bishop Harrington wrote, "The creative affiliation which has been crafted to bring about this new era for St. Vincent Healthcare System will preserve the Catholicity of St. Vincent Hospital. That is a necessity for me, for the members of the Board of Trustees of St. Vincent Healthcare System, and for the Board of Directors of the Fallon Community Health Plan. All are single-minded in that goal."

Harkins was an early supporter of the merger between Fallon and St. Vincent Hospital. With no endowment and the need for a substantial updating of its physical plant, he recognized that regulatory forces and cost-containment measures would weaken the hospital unless it joined forces with Fallon.

But the merger with Fallon also probably hastened his departure. After the merger, he stayed on as president and chief executive officer of St. Vincent Healthcare System for several months, and Dr. FitzGerald was named chairman. In November 1990, he announced that he had accepted a position as executive vice president of Ancilla Systems, a multihospital corporation based in Chicago. He was named president the following year. After Harkins' departure, Dr. FitzGerald was named St. Vincent's president and chief executive officer.

Dr. FitzGerald was the logical choice for the position. The son of Dr. Arthur FitzGerald, former president of the St. Vincent medical staff, Dr. FitzGerald grew up in a Catholic family and spent much of his childhood in the corridors of St. Vincent Hospital. He was immersed in his father's medical practice from the day he was born.

"For a long time, my dad ran his office without a secretary," he said. "Mom answered 40 to 50 telephone calls a day, and dad would make 20 to 30 house calls in a 24-hour period. He was a guy you couldn't see doing anything else, his life was so tied up in his profession and his family. It was a part of him, and his patients were like an extended family."

Growing up with his father as a role model, Dr. FitzGerald was inspired to follow his father into medical practice. Dr. FitzGerald became an apprentice researcher under Dr. Oscar Feinsilver and Dr. Morse before pursuing an internship at St. Vincent in 1967, when his father was president of the medical staff. After serving in the Navy, he worked as an ophthalmologist in a solo practice before joining the Fallon Clinic staff in 1977.

At Fallon, he was given administrative responsibilities, first as chief of the Department of Visual Services. As Fallon grew, so did his administrative responsibilities. He added the title of administrative director of the Obstetrics and Gynecology Department in 1982 and chief of the Surgical Division in 1983. He became administrative director of the Orthopedic Department in 1985 and joined Fallon's Medical Advisory Board in 1986.

Explaining his decision to join the administration, he said, "You can try to help people one-on-one, or you can try to influence a lot of people, making it easier for them to be helped. I do miss the personal one-on-one care, but, on balance, I can have more of an impact on more people."

In 1987, Dr. FitzGerald pursued his master's degree in health administration at the University of Colorado and in 1989, he became Fallon's vice president for hospital affairs. He also served on various Fallon negotiating committees, helping to manage the conversion of Fairlawn Hospital, the merger with Primary Care Physicians and the final merger agreement between St. Vincent Healthcare System and Fallon Community Health Plan.

Dr. FitzGerald's appointment as CEO was equally beneficial to both Fallon and St. Vincent. The Fallon and St. Vincent boards needed someone with a link to and an understanding of both institutions to step into the delicate role as head of the hospital. Dr. FitzGerald brought to the position an understanding of not only the Fallon doctors but also St. Vincent's non-Fallon doctors, many of whom felt threatened by the merger. As a Catholic, he was sensitive to the Catholic tradition of the hospital and felt comfortable carrying that tradition forward. Because of his experience, he combined administrative, financial and managerial abilities, and understood St. Vincent's tradition of placing the patient first.

Dr. FitzGerald saw St. Vincent as an equal partner in the merger. Because of his lifelong link to the hospital, he had the ability to keep St. Vincent culturally intact. In addition, many on the medical staff liked having a CEO who was not a career administrator. As a former ophthalmologist, he understood the physician's perspective and endorsed the physician's strengthened role in determining patient needs.

"We're very, very fortunate to have Dr. FitzGerald as a CEO," said Dr. Howard, president of the medical staff. "My mission is satisfying the needs of the medical staff, and our missions are right on direct course with each other. The level of communication is up front and out front."

One of the first steps taken after the appointment of Dr. FitzGerald was an upgrading of St. Vincent's residency program. Dr. Levinson, who headed the residency program until 1985, was reappointed.

Just as the appointment of Dr. FitzGerald sent a clear signal that Fallon was interested in maintaining a strong role for St. Vincent Hospital, the reappointment of Dr. Levinson in 1991 to head St. Vincent's residency program sent a clear signal that Fallon was interested in recreating a leading residency program. Dr. Levinson, a strong advocate of primary care practice, had many of Fallon's and St. Vincent's present doctors as his former students.

Dr. Levinson said on his return, "I have a great deal of emotional investment in St. Vincent. I had been here nine years. I found that roughly 50 doctors here practicing internal medicine were trained by me. That's very seductive to a teacher to work with those you trained."

With the merger completed, Fallon/St. Vincent Healthcare System could turn its attention back to the planned Medical City in Shrewsbury and Boylston.

After reviewing the site closely, though, Fallon/St. Vincent decided that the site presented too many problems. Costs for the planned construction began to soar and a separate development project, a corporate center in Boylston proposed by Digital Equipment Corporation, encountered a great deal of local opposition. Fallon/St. Vincent officials decided instead to concentrate their efforts on updating the Vernon Hill campus.

"After the merger, we looked at what we could do, and we came to the conclusion that the Shrewsbury–Boylston location was not viable," Dr. FitzGerald said, "and that we should consider building on the hill."

Preliminary plans were drawn up for renovations to the Vernon Hill campus, and Fallon/St. Vincent officials met with city officials in April 1991 to present them.

With Central Massachusetts in the midst of a recession, Fallon/St. Vincent officials expected the development plans for Medical City to be embraced enthusiastically by city officials. But Mayor Jordan Levy saw a development of the scale of Medical City as not fitting well with Vernon Hill's residential setting. He said it would create traffic problems. He also saw an opportunity for using Medical City as a catalyst for development in downtown Worcester. At the time Medical City was proposed, downtown Worcester was languishing. Building projects ranging from a new hotel to the conversion of the city's Union Station into a convention center had been proposed then abandoned. Plans were being formulated to renovate a downtown shopping mall, but the mall was having difficulty attracting tenants. Downtown Worcester was at a low point and badly needed an economic boost. Coincidentally, one of the few downtown projects to be carried out was the opening of a new office for the Fallon Clinic at 100 Central Street.

Although Fallon/St. Vincent officials initially were skeptical about the city's ability to find a suitable site, they agreed to consider a downtown location — if the city could find one. Michael S. Latka, the city's assistant city manager for development, contacted them with a site a couple of weeks after the meeting, but the 17-acre site was deemed to be insufficient. He returned soon after with a 21-acre site bordered by Worcester Center Boulevard.

The city agreed to assemble the parcel of land, taking 25 parcels by eminent domain. City officials said they would obtain environmental clearance, demolish the buildings on the site and complete other site preparation work. They pledged to do work with a total estimated cost of $42 million, but at a cost of just $5 million to Fallon/St. Vincent. The city and state agreed to float a bond to make up the $37 million difference. Suddenly, Fallon/

St. Vincent officials were no longer skeptical about the downtown location.

St. Vincent officials also recognized that the downtown site offered advantages to both the hospital and the city. It would be more accessible and more visible than the Vernon Hill site, while at the same time providing an economic boost to downtown Worcester by bringing, potentially, one-and-a-half-million people a year downtown.

In April 1991, the downtown plan was presented to the medical staff, Nespoli said, "and the medical staff said, 'Go for it.' They are incredibly committed to the city of Worcester."

Fallon/St. Vincent modified and refiled its Determination-of-Need application for the project in July 1992 and later that month the City Council voted to borrow $40 million for site preparation costs. City projections showed that the project will be virtually revenue neutral for the city; that additional taxes generated by the development and state funding will pay off the bond.

Msgr. Griffin, Sister Ursula and Mother Mary of Providence could scarcely have imagined a century ago that their work, and the work of thousands of others, would culminate in the St. Vincent Hospital of today.

St. Vincent Hospital continues to enjoy its reputation as one of the most advanced hospitals in Massachusetts, a state known around the world for its advanced health-care facilities. With planning for Medical City moving forward, the St. Vincent Hospital of tomorrow promises to be even better.

In spite of the ambitious scope of its future plans, St. Vincent Hospital is not standing still, waiting for the future to happen. The hospital is continuing to grow at its present quarters. St. Vincent's Emergency Department is one of only two designated trauma centers in Central Massachusetts and serves more than 40,000 patients a year.

Complete cardiology services are available at St. Vincent. Each year about 400 patients undergo open-heart surgery at the hospital, and about the same number undergo angioplasty. Cardiac services include an extensive noninvasive cardiac laboratory, a comprehensive cardiac rehabilitation program, a cardiac catheterization laboratory and an electrophysiology laboratory for studying arrhythmia and implanting pacemakers.

In November 1992, reflecting the success of St. Vincent's revived open-heart surgery program, the hospital opened two new cardiac surgery suites with a combined cost of $1.5 million. The new suites include specially designed air conditioning that allows them to be cooled down below 60° F. within a few minutes for optimal surgical conditions. The project was partially funded by the St. Vincent Development Foundation and the Guild of Our Lady of Providence. The suites were dedicated in memory of Dr. Ware.

Nearly 3,000 babies are delivered each year at St. Vincent Hospital, four times the number that were delivered two decades ago, when the hospital considered closing its maternity ward. With the decision in 1990 of Lincoln OB/GYN Associates, Inc. to shift deliveries by its physicians to St. Vincent, the hospital's maternity services have expanded to accommodate an additional 800 new births a year. The closing of Hahnemann Hospital's maternity ward after Hahnemann's merger into The Medical Center of Central Massachusetts also resulted in an increase in business for the bustling St. Vincent maternity ward.

In 1992, St. Vincent admitted 21,702 patients for a total of 122,698 patient days. St. Vincent surgeons performed 12,599 procedures. There were 40,499 emergency room visits and 21,638 outpatient visits. A total of 122,358 X-rays were taken. The hospital finished the year with $131,591,674 in operating revenues and a surplus of more than $3.5 million. St. Vincent has a 600-member medical staff and a 75-person full-time house staff. The hospital employs more than 2,000 people.

St. Vincent also has taken control of its costs to a greater extent than its local competitors, and is now the low-cost provider in the Worcester market, according to Nespoli.

New technological breakthroughs continue to yield new surgical techniques, and St. Vincent continues to be a leader in adopting new, improved surgical procedures. Laparoscopic cholecystecomy, for example, is revolutionizing gall bladder operations at St. Vincent, and laparoscopic techniques are being extended to a wide range of surgical procedures. What would Msgr. Griffin and Mother Mary of Providence think about the fiber-optic and laser technologies being used today at St. Vincent — technologies that have taken a great deal of the stress and some of the cost out of many operations?

100 Years Later

"Dr. Ware came to see me and asked if I'd be his emissary. He asked me to deliver a sizable gift to a person who was going to lose his house. I said, 'This place is hard to find,' so he took me and showed me where it was. During the trip, he was telling me how he was going to Mass. General to operate on dogs one or two days a week. I thought to myself, 'This guy's a dreamer.' But then I thought, 'What's wrong with being a dreamer? This nation is built on dreams.'"

Bishop Timothy J. Harrington

St. Vincent Hospital is built on dreams. Dreams that, in many cases, have been realized. The Sisters of Providence were certainly dreamers, thinking they could build a modern hospital when all they had was a drafty farmhouse and a dozen blankets. Dr. Michael Fallon practiced sewing cloth with his eyes closed and dreamed of stitching wounds and saving lives. Dr. Ware operated on dogs but dreamed of curing defective human hearts. When Dr. Meyers talked about prepaid managed care health plans, everyone thought he was a dreamer — until the Fallon Community Health Plan succeeded.

Today St. Vincent's dream is to be an integral part of a new kind of health-care system which provides the highest quality and most affordable care to the patients and the community it serves.

Dr. FitzGerald believes that "to succeed in the 21st century, health-care institutions will have to break down the barriers and align the interests of physicians, hospitals and insurers — the three corners of what we call The Golden Triangle. Once The Golden Triangle is brought together, the patient will benefit from a higher quality of health care provided in a financially efficient manner. That is what we expect to accomplish with a horizontally and vertically integrated health-care delivery system."

The Fallon/St. Vincent vision is to provide a continuum of care for patients from birth to death. The Fallon/St. Vincent system foresees a system that provides each patient with "the most appropriate level of care in the most clinically effective setting using the most cost-efficient methods available," according to Dr. FitzGerald.

In an age when technological, regulatory and organizational change has made health care increasingly impersonal, the Fallon/St. Vincent system will give each patient's personal physician the responsibility to determine the most appropriate care for the patient. Plans for the new Fallon/St. Vincent system also call for "patient empowerment," placing the patient at the level of being not just a customer, but a fellow health-care provider.

"In the old days, the doctor didn't have many of the medical tools we have today," Dr. FitzGerald said. "What he really had was a caring attitude, sympathy and guidance. Technology moved health care from the home, now it seems to be moving back. In the future, care is going to be high tech *and* high touch. It's going to be delivered in the home almost at the same level that it is being delivered in the hospital today."

With the passing of a century, it is not surprising that the St. Vincent Hospital of today bears little resemblance to the St. Vincent Hospital of 100 years ago. But there has been one constant element in the 100-year history of St. Vincent Hospital —

the Catholic philosophy, a philosophy that holds a reverence for life and, therefore, a reverence for the patient.

Reflecting on St. Vincent's ties with the Catholic church, Bishop Harrington said, "One thing the Church stands for is the Christian conviction of the dignity of a human person. The human is made in the image and likeness of God. That is why life is sacred. Whether you're well endowed or poorly endowed; whether you're weak or strong, firm or fragile, it's sacred.

"St. Vincent was founded on that philosophy and tries to teach it without imposing the theology of Catholic Christianity upon those who use its services. One hundred years later, we look back and have change and more change, and the only thing that hasn't changed is God and the love of God, expressed in human hearts and human hands."

Bibliography

Almagno, R. Stephen, O.F.M. *Cardinal John Joseph Wright: The Bibliophile.* The Pittsburgh Bibliophiles, 1980.

Ashley, John. *Can Spring Be Far Behind?* New York: Vantage Press, Inc., 1973.

Behrman, S.N. *The Worcester Account.* New York: Random House, 1946.

Bergin, Dr. Paul F. "History of a Hospital: St. Vincent Hospital, 1894–1967." Brochure, St. Vincent Hospital, 1967.

Bergin, Dr. Paul F. "History of the Worcester District Hospitals and Allied Medical Societies." Manuscript, Worcester District Medical Society, 1953.

Bhawan, Jag, et al. "Lobomycosis: An Electronmicroscopic, Histochemical and Immunologic Study." *Journal of Cutaneous Pathology,* 1976.

"Bishop Officiates At Funeral of Mother Mary of Providence." *Holyoke Transcript,* January 29, 1943.

Caccamo, Dr. Leonard P., et al. "The Jeghers Medical Index Comes To Ohio." Manuscript.

The Catholic Free Press, various issues.

The Catholic Mirror, March 1943.

The Catholic Observer, Centennial issue, 1970.

Coile, Russell C. *The New Hospital: Future Strategies For a Changing Industry.* Rockville, Md.: Aspen Publishers, Inc., 1986.

Erskine, Margaret A. *Heart of the Commonwealth: Worcester.* Woodland Hills, Calif.: Windsor Publications, Inc., 1960.

The Evening Gazette, various issues.

"Fallon Clinic Gets Clearance, Locates Here." *Auburn News,* November 18, 1980.

"Fallon Clinic Opens." *The Westborough News,* July 27, 1977.

Fallon, Dr. John M. "Essays on Occupations: Surgery." *The Tomahawk,* College of the Holy Cross, October 23–30, 1946.

Fallon, Dr. Michael F. "An Anatomical and Surgical Study of Pericecal Membranes." *Medical Communications of the Massachusetts Medical Society,* Vol. 24, June 10, 1913.

Fallon, Dr. Michael F. "The Heritage and Reckoning of the Surgeon." *The Boston Medical and Surgical Journal,* September 14, 1922.

Fallon, Dr. Michael F. "Instruction For House Officers." Fallon Clinic.

Fallon, Dr. Michael F. "A New Era in Medicine." Undated manuscript.

Fallon, Dr. Michael F. "Resume of a Three Months Surgical Service." Address presented to the Worcester District Medical Society, December 14, 1905.

Fallon, Dr. Michael F. "Sepsis." Address presented at St. Vincent Hospital, April 13, 1916.

Fallon, Dr. Michael F. "Some Present Day Problems in Surgery." *The Boston Medical and Surgical Journal,* March 23, 1916.

Fallon, Dr. Michael F. "Symposium on the Mayo Clinic." Address presented to the Worcester District Medical Society, January 10, 1912.

Farnsworth, Albert, Ph.D., and O'Flynn, George B. *The Story of Worcester, Mass.* Worcester, Mass.: Davis Press, Inc., 1934.

Fiftieth Anniversary of St. John's Parish. Worcester, Mass.: Harrigan & Kay Printers, 1896.

FitzGerald, Dr. Denis J. "The Fallon Story." Report presented to American College of Physician Executives, National Conference on Medical Management, Toronto, Canada, May 21, 1991.

"Fortieth Anniversary: Guild of Our Lady of Providence." St. Vincent Hospital, June 1990.

"Golden Jubilee, 1900–1950." Booklet, The St. Vincent Hospital School of Nursing, June 10, 1950.

Grinney, Ellen Heath. *The Hospital.* Chelsea House Publishers, 1991.

Dr. Harold J. Jeghers Symposium, tape, June 18, 1993.

Harper, Wyatt E. *History of Holyoke.* City of Holyoke Centennial Committee, 1973.

"Historically . . . ." Brochure, St. Vincent Hospital.

Impulse, various issues, St. Vincent Hospital.

"In Four Short Years . . . A Progress Report." Brochure, Saint Vincent Hospital Research Foundation, 1966.

"John Fallon, M.D.: Surgeon, Bibliophile and Poet." *New England Journal of Medicine,* Vol. 271, #24, December 10, 1964.

Law, Sylvia A., et al. *Blue Cross: What Went Wrong.* New Haven, Conn.: Yale University Press, 1976.

Loreto, Sister Mary. "There Were Only Minor Flaws in St. Vincent's Disaster Plan." *Modern Hospital,* Vol. 81, #2, August 1953.

Mayovox, Vol. 2, #24, October 13, 1951.

McCoy, The Rev. John J., P.R. *History of the Catholic Church in the Diocese of Springfield.* Boston: The Hurd & Everts Co., 1900.

Meagher, Timothy J. *The Lord Is Not Dead: Cultural and Social Change Among the Irish in Worcester, Mass.* Dissertation, Brown University, June 1982.

Meagher, Timothy J. *To Preserve the Flame.* Worcester, Mass.: Mercantile Printing Company, 1984.

"Medical City: The Healthcare Center of the Future." Brochure, St. Vincent Hospital, 1992.

Morrison, Dr. James M. "Treatment of Chronic Alcoholism." *Diseases of the Nervous System,* Vol. 24, #7, July 1963.

Morrison, Dr. James M. "The Chronic Alcoholic in the General Hospital." Brochure, St. Vincent Hospital.

Morse, Dr. Leonard J., and Schonbeck, Laima E. "Hand Lotions — A Potential Nosocomial Hazard." *New England Journal of Medicine,* February 15, 1968.

Morse, Dr. Leonard J., et al. "Septicemia Due To *Klebsiella Pneumoniae* Originating From a Hand-Cream Dispenser." *New England Journal of Medicine,* August 31, 1967.

Morse, Dr. Leonard J., and Rubenstein, Dr. A. Daniel. "A Food-Borne Institutional Outbreak of Enteritis Due to *Salmonella blockley.*" *JAMA,* Vol. 202, #10, December 4, 1967.

Morse, Dr. Leonard J., et al. "The Holy Cross College Football Team Hepatitis Outbreak." *JAMA,* Vol. 219, #6, February 7, 1972.

Morse, Dr. Leonard J., et al. "Vaccine-Acquired Paralytic Poliomyelitis In An Unvaccinated Mother." *JAMA,* Vol. 197, #12, September 19, 1966.

"Most Reverend Bishop Wright." *The Catholic Mirror,* March 1950.

Mother Mary of Providence. *History of Kingston Community.* Manuscript, Sisters of Providence.

Mother Mary of Providence. *History of Sisters of Providence of Holyoke.* Manuscript, Sisters of Providence.

National Catholic Reporter, August 4, 1972.

Nespoli, John J., speech presented to Fallon medical staff, December 17, 1991.

"The New St. Vincent's Hospital." *Sacred Heart Review,* October 23, 1898.

News and Trends in Health Care, Vol. III, #10, Massachusetts Blue Cross, Inc., June–August 1970.

Nutt, Charles A.B. *History of Worcester and Its People.* Vol. II. New York: Lewis Historical Publishing Company, 1919.

O'Grady, Desmond. "An American With a Roman Connection." *National Catholic Reporter,* August 4, 1972.

O'Leary, Bishop Thomas M. "Tercentenary of Massachusetts, Centenary of Catholicity in Western Massachusetts." *The Catholic Mirror.*

"Our Hospital." Brochure, St. Vincent Hospital, 1954.

Outlook, various issues, St. Vincent Hospital.

Religious News Service, New York, November 12, 1952, November 16, 1953.

Rice, Franklin P. *The Worcester of Eighteen Hundred and Ninety Eight: Fifty Years A City.* Worcester, Mass.: F. S. Blanchard & Co. Publishers, 1899.

Rosenberg, Charles E. *The Care of Strangers.* New York: Basic Books, Inc., 1987.

"St. Vincent Hospital Pioneers New Techniques." *Ohio Chemical Items & Topics,* Vol. XII, #2, May 1966.

"Saint V's: The First 100 Years of St. Vincent Hospital." *The Catholic Free Press,* special section, 1993.

St. Vincent Hospital annual reports, various years, 1893–present.

"St. Vincent Hospital: A Brief Outline of Its Formation and Progress To Date," September 8, 1893–October 8, 1898.

"St. Vincent Hospital: 75th Anniversary, 1893–1968." St. Vincent Hospital, 1968.

"Sisters of Providence Centennial Eucharistic Celebration, 1892–1992." Program, Sisters of Providence, 1992.

Springfield Union, various articles.

Stapleton, Dr. John F. "Medical Education in the Community Hospital." *Harvard Medical Alumni Bulletin,* April 1956.

Starr, Paul S. *The Social Transformation of American Medicine.* New York: Basic Books, Inc., 1982.

Stevens, Rosemary. *In Sickness and In Wealth.* New York: Basic Books, Inc., 1989.

"A Student For Life." *Convergence,* St. Elizabeth Hospital Medical Center, Vol. 12, #1, 1991.

Sunday Telegram, various articles.

Swick, Thomas. "A Unique Guide To Medical Information," *Observer,* Vol. 5, #2, American College of Physicians, February 1985.

Telegram & Gazette, various articles.

Tracings, various articles.

Tymeson, Mildred McCleary. *Worcester Centennial, Historical Sketches of the Town and the City, 1848–1948.* Worcester Centennial, Inc., 1948.

"UMass Medical Center, An Introduction." Brochure, University of Massachusetts Medical Center.

Wall, A.E.P. "Four Americans Will Take Part in Synod; Cdl. Wright Outlines Issues, Tensions." *The Catholic Review,* October 3, 1969.

"Well-Known Nun Dies in Holyoke." *Springfield Daily News,* January 26, 1943.

The Worcester Spy, February 4, 1902.

Worcester Medical News, April 1968, May–June 1979.

Worcester Telegram, various issues.

"Worcester's New Hospital." *The Boston Globe,* September 26, 1894.

Wright, Cardinal John J., *Columbia,* January 1970.

Zikos, Joanna. "At Fallon, Physician Direction and Employee Involvement Produce Patient Satisfaction." *Business Digest,* April 1991.

Index

Sacred Heart parish, Worcester,
Mass., 2
St. Anne's Church, Worcester,
Mass., xv
St. Bernard's Church, Worcester,
Mass., 279
St. Camillus Home, Worcester,
Mass., 74, 75, 86, 87, 194
St. Charles College, Catonsville,
Md., 1
St. Elizabeth's Home, Worcester,
Mass., 3
St. Elizabeth's Hospital, Worcester,
Mass., xiv, xv, 122
St. Francis Home, Worcester, Mass.,
46
St. Francis Hospital, Rochester,
Minn., 95
St. Jerome's School for Boys,
Holyoke, Mass., 11, 16
St. John's High School, Worcester,
Mass., 2, 104
St. John's parish, Worcester, Mass.,
1, 3, 4, 6, 7, 32, 44
St. John's School, Worcester, Mass.,
3, 26
St. Joseph's Abbey, Spencer, Mass.,
189
St. Joseph's Hall, St. Vincent
Hospital, 194
St. Joseph's Hospital (St. Joseph's
Institute), Millbury, Mass., 70
St. Luke's Hall, St. Vincent Hospital,
218, 219, 273
St. Luke's Home, Springfield, Mass.,
16
St. Luke's Hospital, New Bedford,
Mass., 85
St. Luke's Hospital, Pittsfield, Mass.,
18, 110
St. Mary's Hall, St. Vincent
Hospital, 152
St. Mary's Hospital, Rochester,
N.Y., 191
St. Mary's Seminary, Baltimore,
Md., 1

St. Paul's Cathedral, Worcester,
Mass., 68
St. Stephen's parish, Worcester,
Mass., 2, 4, 137
St. Vincent Development
Foundation, 295, 312
St. Vincent Healthcare System, Inc.
See Fallon/St. Vincent
Healthcare System.
St. Vincent Home, Worcester, Mass.,
52
St. Vincent Hospital Aid
Association, 31, 33, 48, 134
St. Vincent Hospital School of
Nursing, 39, 40, 65, 66, 73–75,
85, 87, 89–91, 94, 104, 115, 134,
153, 159, 193, 212, 222, 296
St. Vincent Management
Corporation, 277
St. Vincent Physician Alliance, 285
St. Vincent Registry of Medical
Technologies, 192
St. Vincent Research Foundation,
194, 219, 236, 295
St. Vincent School of Inhalation
Therapy, 193
St. Vincent School of Medical
Technology, 193
Salerno Club, 106
Salisbury, Stephen, III, 6, 21, 22, 25,
248
Sanders, Dr. John I., 182
Sargent, Francis W., 260, 261
Scanlon, Dr. Joseph C., Sr., 155
Scanlon, Rita, 155
Scannell, Rev. Denis, 21
Schedin, Robert S., 286
Schwartz, Dr. Howard S., 241
Second Vatican Council, 205, 211
Seder, Saul, 129
Sheddan, Dr. Frank, 156
Sheraton Continuing Care Center
(later Providence House),
Worcester, Mass., 225, 226
Sheridan, Mr. Philip, 137
Shuster, Dr. Allen, 192

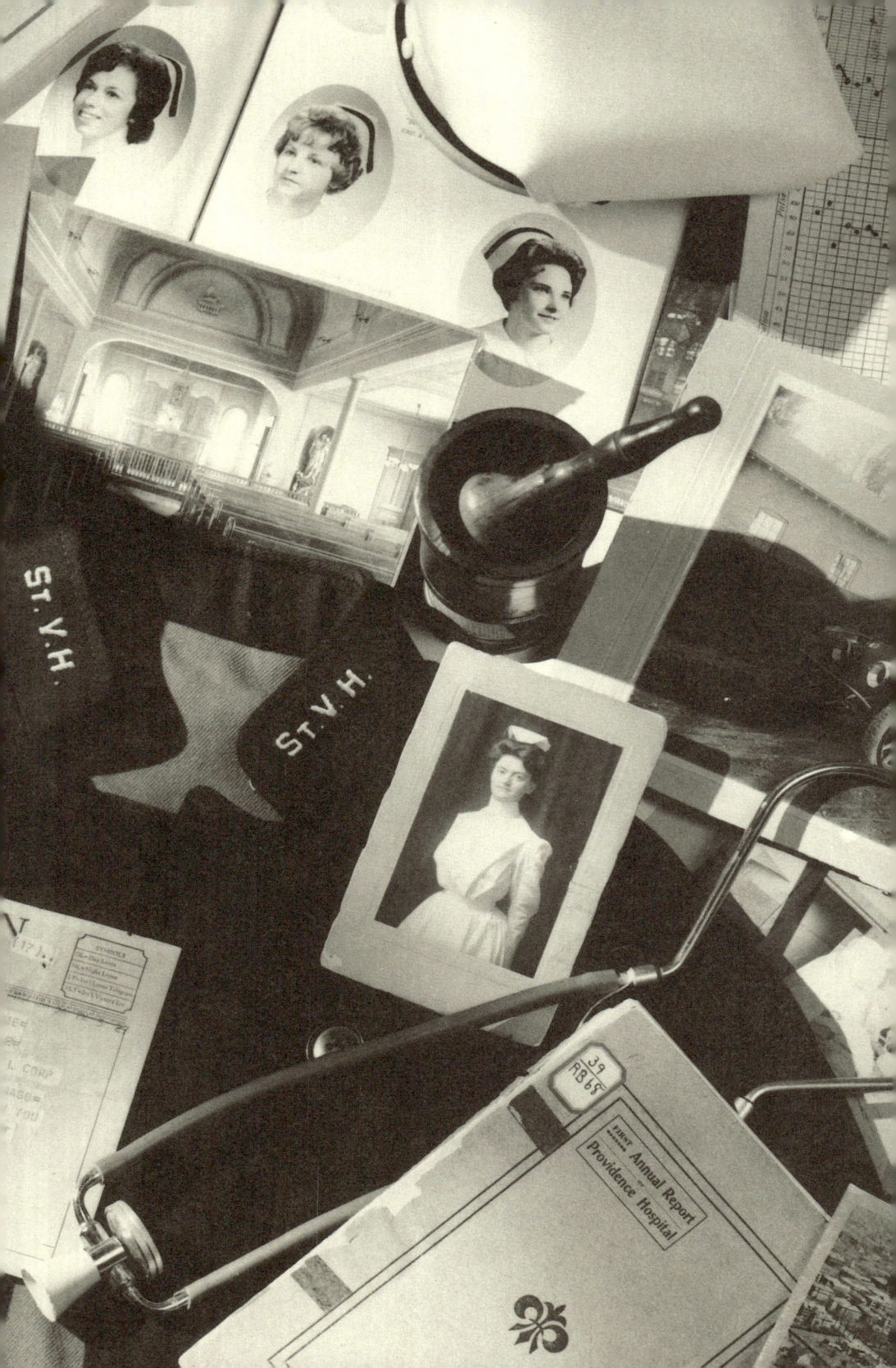